Lecture Notes in Computer Science 6137

Commenced Publication in 1973
Founding and Former Series Editors:
Gerhard Goos, Juris Hartmanis, and Jan van Leeuwen

Thomas Ploug   Per Hasle
Harri Oinas-Kukkonen (Eds.)

Persuasive Technology

5th International Conference, PERSUASIVE 2010
Copenhagen, Denmark, June 7-10, 2010
Proceedings

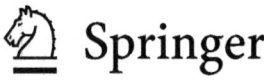 Springer

Volume Editors

Thomas Ploug
Copenhagen Institute of Technology
Aalborg University, Dept. of Communication
Lautrupvang 2b, 2750 Ballerup, Denmark
E-mail: ploug@hum.aau.dk

Per Hasle
Royal School of Library and Information Science
Birketinget 6, 2300 København, Denmark
E-mail: rektor@db.dk

Harri Oinas-Kukkonen
University of Oulu
Dept. of Information Processing Science
Rakentajantie 3, 90370 Oulu, Finland
harri.oinas-kukkonen@oulu.fi

Library of Congress Control Number: 2010927713

CR Subject Classification (1998): J.4, H.5, I.2.6, J.1, J.3, I.2

LNCS Sublibrary: SL 3 – Information Systems and Application, incl. Internet/Web
and HCI

ISSN   0302-9743
ISBN-10   3-642-13225-1 Springer Berlin Heidelberg New York
ISBN-13   978-3-642-13225-4 Springer Berlin Heidelberg New York

springer.com

© Springer-Verlag Berlin Heidelberg 2010
Printed in Germany

Typesetting: Camera-ready by author, data conversion by Scientific Publishing Services, Chennai, India
Printed on acid-free paper   06/3180

Persuasive Technology
— A Discipline Taking Shape

Until recently, most software applications and technologies were developed without much thought to how they influenced their users. To be sure, many endeavors have strongly involved a users' perspective, for instance, with respect to facilitating use and making information and other resources accessible. However, accessibility, ease of use etc. are one thing; the conscious and systematic design for change – that is, the conscious attempt to influence users – is, however, a considerable extra step. But today, industry experts and academics are embracing a purposeful approach to persuasive design. In an industry context, designing for persuasion is becoming essential for success. In academic settings, the study of persuasive technology illuminates the principles that influence and motivate people in different aspects of their lives.

Thus, persuasive technology is rapidly growing into a major discipline, sometimes referred to as captology or the study of computers as persuasive technologies. The previous Persuasive conferences held in Eindhoven (2006), Stanford (2007), Oulu (2008), and Claremont (2009) were infused with an energetic spirit and a large attendance, including representatives from both academia and industry.

Persuasive 2010, hosted in Copenhagen, Denmark, in early June, was jointly organized by the Royal School of Library and Information Science, Denmark, Aalborg University, Denmark, and the University of Oulu, Finland. Copenhagen's superb location added to the enjoyable atmosphere. The Royal Library, beautifully situated against the backdrop of church and castle spires and the Copenhagen Canals, made available an attractive setting for the conference, which took place in its famous Queen Margrethe auditorium.

This three-day conference placed persuasive technology on a firm scientific footing with an emphasis on social, psychological, rhetorical and ethical issues on a par with software design and information systems. Featuring full and short papers, posters and panels, Persuasive 2010 highlighted new knowledge in the understanding and design of persuasive technology. The event brought together researchers, practitioners, and industry professionals interested in this important new field. Research themes of the conference and hence, this volume, include emotions and user experience, ambient persuasive systems, persuasive design, persuasion profiles, designing for health, psychology of persuasion, embodied and conversational agents, economic incentives, and future directions for persuasive technology.

Persuasive 2010 had three outstanding keynote speakers: Jennifer Preece from the University of Maryland (USA), Rosalind Picard from Massachusetts Institute of Technology (USA), and Harri Oinas-Kukkonen from the University of Oulu (Finland).

These conference proceedings contain contributions from all three keynote speakers—one full keynote paper, one extended keynote abstract and a short abstract—as well as the accepted full and short papers. Each of the 80 paper submissions were evaluated through a careful double-blind review process that included multiple reviewers. A total of 25 papers were accepted for presentation in the conference and in these proceedings. We are very thankful to the Program Committee members as well as the additional reviewers whose insightful work enabled us to select the best papers for Persuasive 2010. An adjunct volume of poster proceedings has been published separately.

For the third time at a Persuasive conference, a doctoral consortium was held in conjunction with conference events. Some 20 bright students were selected to attend the consortium based on their research plans and applications for participation. These young researchers and their interest in persuasive technology bode well for the future of the field.

We would like to thank The Danish Ministry of Culture of its support of this conference, as well as all our sponsors. We are grateful to all those people who contributed to this conference, whether as organizers, reviewers, scientific contributors or otherwise. Finally, we would like to extend our warmest thanks to all those volunteers who contributed in so many ways to make this conference a successful and memorable event.

April 2010

Per Hasle
Harri Oinas-Kukkonen
Thomas Ploug

Organization

Persuasive 2010 was organized by the Royal School of Library and Information Science in collaboration with Aalborg University and Oulu University.

Conference Chairs

Conference Chair	Per Hasle (Royal School of Library and Information Science)
Associate Chair	Harri Oinas-Kukkonen (University of Oulu)
Programme Chair	Thomas Ploug (Copenhagen Institute of Technology/Aalborg University)
Organizing Chair	Jette Hyldegaard (Royal School of Library and Information Science)
Doctoral Chair	Marianne Lykke (Royal School of Library and Information Science)
Secretary Chair	Mette Kusk (Royal School of Library and Information Science)

Scientific Review Committee

Jack Andersen
Nilufar Baghaei
Magnus Bang
Shlomo Berkovsky
Timothy Bickmore
Robert Biddle
Pia Borlund
Harry Bruce
Winslow Burleson
Samir Chatterjee
Janet Davis
Peter de Vries

Dean Eckles
B.J. Fogg
Per Hasle
Jette Hyldegård
Stephen Intille
Rilla Khaled
Pål Kraft
Pablo Lambert de
   Diesbach
Tuomas Lehto
Judith Masthoff
Cees Midden

Fred Muench
Peter Øhrstrøm
Harri Oinas-Kukkonen
Thomas Ploug
Teppo Raisanen
Wolfgang Reitberger
Virpi Roto
Martha Russell
Timo Saari
Henrik Schärfe
Julita Vassileva
Michael Wu

Sponsoring Institutions

Royal School of Library and Information Science
Aalborg University
University of Oulu
The Danish Ministry of Culture
The Royal Library
Stelton

Table of Contents

Technology for Changing Feelings

Rosalind Picard

MIT Media Lab, E14-374G,
75 Amherst Street, Cambridge, MA 02139-4307,
Tel.: 1.617.253.0611
picard@media.mit.edu

Abstract. Feelings change and technology usually ignores such changes, despite thattechnology often is credited with causing the changed feelings, especiallyfrustration, irritation, annoyance, or (sometimes) interest and delight. This talk will demonstrate technology we've built to recognize and respond to emotion anddiscuss some ways it can help people better change their own emotionsif they want to do so. I will attempt to demo some of the new technologies live, and discuss their beneficial uses (e.g. helping people with anxiety,stress or health-behavior change). I will also mention some worrisome usesand solicit ideas for how to minimize or prevent abusive uses.

T. Ploug, P. Hasle, H. Oinas-Kukkonen (Eds.): PERSUASIVE 2010, LNCS 6137, p. 1, 2010.
© Springer-Verlag Berlin Heidelberg 2010

I Persuade, They Persuade, It Persuades!

Jennifer J. Preece

College of Information Studies - "Maryland's iSchool",
University of Maryland,
College Park, MD 20742
Tel.: +1 (301) 405 2035
preece@umd.edu
iSchool.umd.edu/people/preece

Abstract. Persuasion changes behavior. Persuasive people encourage us to do things we might not otherwise do, such as buying a new coat, taking a trip, changing jobs, and so on. Artifacts can persuade too: marketing specialists know that slick ads, sexy slogans, colorful packaging, empathic messages, elegant and beautiful designs are persuasive – they sell products.

Visionaries predict that "mobile phones will soon become the most important platform for changing human behavior" (Fogg & Eckles, 2007, p.5). Phones that look attractive, feel comfortable, and are usable are one part of a success story. The other part of the story concerns the applications (i.e., apps) that run on the phones. Creative apps turn a mobile phone into a personal finance manager, inspiration for cooks, a music player, an exercise coach, a marketing device, a weather service for farmers, a guide for bird watchers, a spirit level for do-it-yourself enthusiasts, and much more. Apple's iPhone App Store has led the way in ratcheting up expectations about the range and quality of apps that users want, and has engaged users in creating them. Other phone developers are following Apple's example.

Technology-mediated social participation applications are popular and increasing becoming accessible via cell phones and other mobile devices. Technology-mediated social participation is generated when social networking tools (e.g., Facebook), blogs and microblogs (e.g., Twitter), user-generated content sites (e.g., YouTube, Flicker), discussion groups, problem reporting, recommendation systems, and other social media are applied to national priorities throughout the world, such as health, energy, education, disaster response, environmental protection, business innovation, cultural heritage, community safety, as well as social friendship and family networks. Fire, earthquake, storm, fraud, or crime reporting sites provide information to civic authorities. AmberAlert has more than 7 million users who help with information on child abductions, and SERVE.GOV enables citizens to volunteer for national parks, museums and other institutions. Compelling possibilities for healthcare (e.g., PatientsLikeMe), wellness, smoking cessation, and obesity reduction are also attracting attention. These early attempts hint at the vast potential for technology-mediated social participation, but substantial research is needed to persuade scaling up, raising motivation, controlling malicious attacks, limiting misguided rumors, and protecting privacy (http://iparticipate.wikispaces.com).

T. Ploug, P. Hasle, H. Oinas-Kukkonen (Eds.): PERSUASIVE 2010, LNCS 6137, pp. 2–3, 2010.
© Springer-Verlag Berlin Heidelberg 2010

Clearly stated research challenges should have three key elements: (1) close linkage to compelling national and international priorities (2) scientific foundation based on established theories and well-defined research questions (e.g., privacy, reciprocity, trust, motivation, recognition, etc.), and (3) research challenges (e.g., security, privacy protection, scalability, visualization, end-user development, distributed data handling for massive user-generated content, network analysis of community evolution, cross network comparison, etc.). By incorporating this research wisdom in designs that impact the 5 billion-plus mobile phone users throughout the world (Economist, 2010), people's lives and society could be transformed for the better. Contributing to this transformation is a goal for participants attending Persuasive 2010.

In this talk I will draw on example applications (e.g., Encyclopedia of Life, Twitter, Recovery.gov, PatientsLikeMe, etc.) and research reports (summarized in Preece & Shneiderman, 2009, and else where) that suggest key principles for designing and managing technology mediated social participation. I will discuss how individuals, groups and communities, applications and devices persuade people to contribute, collaborate and lead using social technologies (i.e., how I/you persuade, how they persuade, and how it persuades).

References

[1] Economist, A World of Connections: A Special Report on Social Networking 394(8667), Special section, 1–20 (January 30-February 5, 2010)
[2] Fogg, B.J., Eckles, D.: Mobile Persuasion: 20 Perspectives on the Future of Behavior Change. Stanford Captology Media, Stanford
[3] Preece, J., Shneiderman, B.: The Reader-to-Leader Framework: Motivating Technology-Mediated Social Participation. AIS Transactions on Human-Computer Interaction 1(1), Article 1, 1–21, http://aisel.aisnet.org/thci/vol1/iss1/5/

Behavior Change Support Systems: A Research Model and Agenda

Harri Oinas-Kukkonen

University of Oulu, Department of Information Processing Science
Rakentajantie 3, 90570 Oulu, Finland
Harri.Oinas-Kukkonen@oulu.fi

Abstract. This article introduces the concept of a behavior change support system and suggests it as a key construct for research on persuasive systems design, technologies, and applications. Key concepts for behavior change support systems are defined and a research agenda for them is outlined. The article suggests that a change in complying, a behavior change, and an attitude change (C-, B- or A-Change) constitute the archetypes of a behavioral change. Change in itself is either of a forming, altering or reinforcing outcome (F-, A- or R-Outcome). This research model will become helpful in researching and designing persuasive technology.

Keywords: Socio-technical system, behavioral outcomes, psychological outcomes, behavioral change, persuasive technology.

1 Introduction

The emergence of web 2.0 concepts and technologies to create, access, and share information in new ways has opened up opportunities for also developing new kinds of information systems for influencing users. For instance, one of the most prominent areas for future healthcare improvement is the role of the web in fostering improved health and healthier lifestyles [1]. Researchers have reported positive results in areas such as the management of smoking cessation, hazardous drinking, obesity, diabetes, asthma, tinnitus, stress, anxiety and depression, complicated grief, and insomnia [2]. Other application areas include directing users towards proper exercise behaviors [3], better sitting habits [4], healthier eating [5], and greener energy behaviors [6], among others. All these target behavioral changes in the end-users.

Both software developers and the general audience should be aware of the various ways of and approaches to how people may be, are being, and will be influenced through the information technology (IT) designs. Moreover, the contemporary and future web will keep opening up a myriad of opportunities for building various kinds of software applications and benefiting from them. In this article, we define *behavior change support systems (BCSS)* as a key construct for research in persuasive

T. Ploug, P. Hasle, H. Oinas-Kukkonen (Eds.): PERSUASIVE 2010, LNCS 6137, pp. 4–14, 2010.
© Springer-Verlag Berlin Heidelberg 2010

technology [7].[1] For achieving better outcomes from BCSSs, they should be designed by using persuasive systems design frameworks and models [8].

This article is conceptual and theory-creating by its nature. The article is structured as follows: Section 2 will discuss the related research. Section 3 will define and discuss the concept of a behavior change support system. Section 4 will discuss the research implications and future research directions. Finally, section 5 will draw conclusions based on the earlier sections. In general, the article lays ground for future research in this new frontier of research on BCSSs.

2 Related Research

The study of users' attitudes and behavior has a long history in information systems (IS) research [9]. Lessons have been drawn from social psychology [10, 11] and cognitive psychology [12], and new models and frameworks have been developed, such as the Technology Acceptance Model [13] and the Unified Theory of Use and Acceptance of Technology [14]. These theories are useful for understanding attitudes and behaviors related to information systems and their use, and some of them are well-known among IS researchers. Besides these general attitude and behavior-related theories, there are also useful attitude and/or behavior change related theories such as the Elaboration Likelihood Model [15]. These change-related theories are not very well-known among IS researchers, however.

A key element in behavior and attitude change is persuasion. Persuasive design and technology has received growing interest among researchers for a little over a decade now [cf. 16].[2] Fogg's seminal book [18] was the first conceptualization suggested for software designers, stating that information technology may play the role of a tool, a medium, or a social actor for its users.[3] Bogost [20] proposed an approach to developing persuasive games. More elaborate conceptual and design frameworks for on and off-the-Web information systems have been suggested, such as the Persuasive Systems Design model [21, 22]. Recently, one of the major development trends has been the persuasion patterns of social network based information systems, in particular in conjunction with Facebook.

A wide variety of BCSSs have been developed, such as an easy-to-use password creation mechanism to help create stronger passwords [23], an interactive picture frame for adopting better sitting habits while working at the computer [4], a ubiquitous sensor-based kitchen application for improving home cooking by providing calorie awareness regarding the food ingredients used in the meals prepared [5], and a personal health information system to influence the health behaviors of rural women in India through offering them information for increasing their awareness about menses and maternal health [24].

---

[1] Persuasive technology is the field of research, whereas a BCSS is an object of study within the field.

[2] Affective computing [17] may be recognized as a sister-field of persuasive technology, or perhaps from the persuasive viewpoint as a sub-field of it, which directly focuses on the emotions information technologies evoke.

[3] Sharp criticism of persuasive technology and Fogg's book has been offered by Atkinson [19].

3 Behavior Change Support Systems

Even if the web and other information technologies are often considered as just tools to accomplish goals, they are never neutral. Rather, they are 'always on.' This means that people are constantly being persuaded in a similar manner to how teachers persuade students in schools, and there is nothing bad in this in itself, of course. To put it simply, information technology always influences people's attitudes and behaviors in one way or another. In some cases, the influence may even be an unintentional side effect of the design. Thus, software designers but also the general audience should be well aware of the various ways and approaches how people may be, are being, and will be influenced through IT design. Moreover, there is a plethora of applications that can be developed with the purpose of behavioral change.[4] For these reasons, it is important to define and adopt into use the concept of a behavior change support system.

In our definition, persuasive technology is the field of research, whereas a BCSS is an object of study within the field. The main research interests in BCSSs include not only human-computer interaction and computer-mediated communication, but also topics such as approaches, methodologies, processes and tools to develop such systems and ways for studying the organizational, social, and end-user impacts of them. The research emphasizes software qualities and characteristics, systems analysis and design, and end-user behavior and perceptions. Technologically, the research may tackle socio-technical platforms, systems, services or applications, or the software features in them, developed for persuasive purposes.

A BCSS is defined here as follows:

A behavior change support system (BCSS) is an information system designed to form, alter or reinforce attitudes, behaviors or an act of complying without using deception, coercion or inducements.

Persuasion relies on the user's voluntary participation in the persuasion process. Naturally, in addition to persuasion, other forms of attempts at influence do also exist. For instance, a pop-up window or a hyperlink may be purposefully deceitful; coercion implies force and the possibly economic sanctions; inducements are exchanges of money, goods, or services for actions by the person being influenced. By definition, these are not persuasive elements.

3.1 Types of Change

In this article, we divide behavioral changes into three categories, namely a change in an act of complying, a behavior change or an attitude change.[5] Respectively, these may be called C-, B-, and A-Change, in ascending order of difficulty. Different persuasive goals and strategies may be needed for applications supporting different types of changes.

---

[4] It should be noted that even if we speak about behavioral changes, we do not posit a behaviorist or any mechanistic psychological view towards human beings. End-users may use these applications to support achieving their goals, maintaining a constructivist view (cf., the field of education) towards human behavior.

[5] For the sake of simplicity, we use the term "behavior" change rather than "behavioral" change even if the BCSS covers all three behavioral change types.

3.1.1 C-Change

With a *C-Change*, the goal of the behavioral change is simply to make sure that the end-user complies with the requests of the system. For instance, the goal of a healthcare application may be to guarantee that its users take their daily blood pressure medication. The users may or may not have the proper motivation for doing so, but, nevertheless, the key in this approach is to provide triggers for the user to take action and to comply with the requests of the application. First achieving a C-Change may help achieve a B-Change later.

It should also be noted that a myriad of software applications that have been created for purposes other than a behavioral change *per se* utilize, in the micro scale, the same design principles and techniques as systems supporting behavior changes.

3.1.2 B-Change

The goal of systems supporting a *B-Change* is to elicit a more enduring change than simple compliance once or a few times. A one-time behavior change may be achieved more easily, whereas long-term behavior change (not to even speak about a permanent behavior change) is much more difficult to achieve.

3.1.3 A-Change

The goal of systems supporting an *A-Change* is to influence the end-users' attitudes rather than behavior only. An attitude change that directs behavior may be the most difficult type of change to achieve but we maintain that persuasion-in-full occurs only when attitude change takes place, and that a sustainable B-Change happens only through an A-Change. In some cases, behavior change support systems should aim bolstering both an A-Change and a B-Change simultaneously. This is particularly important in areas such as providing support for overcoming addictive behaviors, where users in spite of high motivation and proper attitudes may lack the skills to put their knowledge and attitudes into practice (a B-Change is needed), but at the same time their motivation and self-efficacy may need further strengthening (an A-Change is needed).

3.2 Outcome/Change Design Matrix

In the abovementioned definition, three potential, successful voluntary outcomes are the formation, alteration or reinforcement of attitudes, behaviors or complying. A forming outcome (*F-Outcome*) means the formulation of a pattern for a situation where one did not exist beforehand, e.g., abstaining from substance abuse. An altering outcome (*A-Outcome*) means changes in a person's response to an issue, e.g., increasing the level of exercise, decreasing the amount of drinking, or stopping smoking. A reinforcing outcome (*R-Outcome*) means the reinforcement of current attitudes or behaviors, making them more resistant to change.

A design matrix can be constructed from the intended outcomes and the types of change. See Table 1. When designing a BCSS, the developers should carefully think about which of these nine different goals the application will be built for. The persuasion context may change dramatically when moving from one slot to another.

Table 1. Outcome/Change Design Matrix

	C-Change	B-Change	A-Change
F-Outcome	Forming an act of complying (F/C)	Forming a behavior (F/B)	Forming an attitude (F/A)
A-Outcome	Altering an act of complying (A/C)	Altering a behavior (A/B)	Altering an attitude (A/A)
R-Outcome	Reinforcing an act of complying (R/C)	Reinforcing a behavior (R/B)	Reinforcing an attitude (R/A)

3.3 Design of Software System Qualities

Behavior change support systems utilize either computer-mediated or computer-human persuasion. Computer-mediated persuasion means that people are persuading others through computers, e.g., e-mail, instant messages, or social network systems. Even if the web cannot communicate in the same way as humans do, some patterns of interaction similar to social communication may be utilized also in computer-human persuasion. In the case of BCSSs, there must exist other stakeholders who have the intention of influencing someone's attitudes or behavior, as computers do not have intentions of their own. These stakeholders are those who create or produce BCSSs, those who give access to or distribute them to others, or the very person adopting or using such a system [18]. BCSSs emphasize – but are not limited to – autogenous approaches in which people use information technology to change their own attitudes or behaviors through building upon their own motivation or goal. They also request a positive user experience and stickiness, which encourage the user to engage with them regularly over an extended period of time.

Building BCSSs requires insight from software and information systems design as well as psychology. Lessons learned from psychology include: (1) the fact that people like their views about the world to be organized and consistent, (2) that persuasion is often incremental, and (3) that the direct and indirect routes are key persuasion strategies [22]. Important software design requirements to be always kept in mind when developing BCSSs are that: (1) behavior change support systems should be both useful and easy to use, and (2) persuasion through behavior change support systems should always be transparent. Quite understandably, if a system is useless or difficult to use, it is unlikely that it could be very persuasive. The transparency requirement emphasizes the need for revealing the designer bias behind a BCSS.

The Persuasive Systems Design model [21, 22] is the state of the art conceptualization for designing and developing BCSSs. According to the PSD model, careful analysis of the persuasion context (the intent, event, and strategy of persuasion) is needed to discern opportune and/or inopportune moments for delivering the message(s). Many design aspects in developing BCSSs are general software design issues rather than specific to BCSSs only. These include, for instance, usefulness, ease of use, ease of access, high information quality, simplicity, convenience, attractiveness, lack of errors, responsiveness, high overall positive user experience, and user loyalty.

The PSD model suggests a set of design principles under four categories, namely primary task, human-computer dialogue, perceived system credibility, and social influence. See Figure 1. The design principles of the primary task category focus on supporting the carrying out of the user's primary activities. Design principles related to human-computer dialogue help move towards achieving the goal set for using the BCSS. The perceived system credibility design principles relate to how to design a system so that it is more believable and thereby more persuasive. The design principles in the social influence category describe how to design the system so that it motivates users by leveraging social influence.

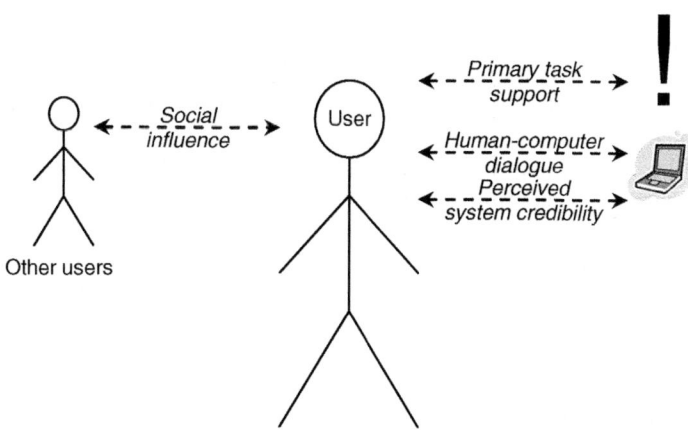

Fig. 1. Four categories of design principles for BCSSs

Tørning and Oinas-Kukkonen [25] have analyzed the scientific research publications in the PERSUASIVE conferences during 2006-2008 as regards the software system features and the abovementioned categories. According to their study, the most utilized features have been tailoring, tunneling, reduction, and self-monitoring (representing the primary task category), suggestion (for supporting human-computer dialogue), surface credibility (in support of perceived system credibility), and social comparison, normative influence, and social learning (relating to social influence).

Many types of research on software system features have been conducted. For instance, Harper et al. [26] studied the roles that social influence and social comparison may play in online communities for motivating members rather than editors to contribute and moderate content. Andrew et al. [27] studied the challenges in implementing suggestion and how it differs from and overlaps with other techniques, in particular tunneling, reduction, and self-monitoring. Räisänen et al. [28] studied the right-time suggestions of messages. Cugelman et al. [29] demonstrated that system credibility, in particular the system's trustworthiness, affects a user's behavioral intent. Gamberini et al. [30] showed that in some situations a persuasive strategy based on reciprocity is more effective than one based on reward, as well as that the presence of social proof features seems counterproductive when using a reciprocity strategy, whereas it seems to improve compliance with a request when using a reward strategy. At a more general level, Zhu [8] conducted a meta-study of persuasive techniques in BCSSs motivating for regular physical activity. The results of this study suggest that very few previous studies resulted in achieving the intended goal. Only a few studies took advantage of any persuasive techniques, and none of these interventions were conceptually designed through persuasive design frameworks. The conclusion of this study was that designing a new generation of BCSSs should be based on such frameworks.

4   Research Agenda for BCSS

Tørning and Oinas-Kukkonen [25] report some interesting findings regarding the current state of research on BCSSs:

Thus far there has been much more research on C- and B-Change than on A-Change. Only about 16% of the research has addressed A-Change. This may due to the fact that C- and B-Change are in most cases easier to study than A-Change. Nevertheless, in the future more emphasis should be placed on A-Change.

In the current research literature, there seems to be a tendency of describing the software systems and the persuasion context (use, user, and technology contexts) at too general a level. Black-box thinking of the software systems – with no actual description of what was implemented and how – may make the research results obsolete. The differences between problem domains are so huge that very general claims can be seldom argued for. For instance, in most of the experimental research students are regarded as a homogenous mass. More specific information is often limited to gender and age. Yet, a deep understanding of the user segments is highly important for designing successful persuasive systems. Specific target audiences may request very different kinds of software features. Just consider the differences between small schoolchildren, tweens, teens, and perhaps even young adults in comparison to lumping them all together as students.

When describing a persuasive system, a very clear description of the technology context is needed. After all, much of the success or failure of an application can be attributed in many cases to the fluent navigation and smooth interaction arising from the technological infrastructure rather than to the design of the system. Relying on black-box thinking is a symptom of a severe misunderstanding of conducting BCSS research.

The message and route for persuasion are also often not described at such a level of detail that it would be possible to determine whether a direct or indirect approach actually has been applied and whether that has played a role in the success or failure of the system. Moreover, it should be clearly defined whether one or multiple arguments were presented, and what kinds of arguments were presented.

Often, the empirical and experimental research does not reveal much about the motives behind the system under study. The designer bias should necessarily be revealed much more clearly.

Admittedly, space is often too limited in scientific papers to provide many details about the system. For this reason, the actual system descriptions easily become radically shortened or are even cut out from the papers. Moreover, the field would benefit from a shift in research emphasis from proof of concept approaches into theorizing for persuasive systems design.

Quite surprisingly, ethical considerations have remained largely unaddressed in persuasive technology research. Many important issues need to be recognized, such as the actual voluntariness for change in using the application and potential ways for abusing the system. There may also be situations where computer-mediated persuasion takes place without the user being aware of it. These 'grey areas' should be carefully considered.

Open research questions to be tackled in future research include the following:

- How can "change" be measured? Are there differences in measuring C-, B- and A-Changes?
- What challenges do A-, B- and C-Change pose for BCSS research? What are the connections between C-, B- and A-Change?
- How can we conduct experiments in such a manner that it will be really possible to pinpoint a change to have been caused by a BCSS, or even more precisely, by a specific software feature in it?
- How do the BCSSs developed for R-, A- and F-Outcomes differ from each other?
- How can we build BCSSs in such a manner that they will be unobtrusive with users' primary tasks?
- What are the roles of cognition and emotion in BCSSs?
- What is the relationship between convincing and persuasion in BCSSs?
- What is the role of goal setting in different kinds of BCSSs? How can the change in the user's goals be supported?
- When should a BCSS use a direct/indirect persuasion strategy?
- Which software features have the greatest impact in different settings? Which combinations of software features have the greatest impact?
- Which modes of interaction are more persuasive than others? How can the fit between these interaction modes and catering for certain types of behaviors be recognized and measured?
- What are the differences between problem domains (e.g., increased exercising vs. weight management, or reduced energy consumption vs. overcoming addictions)?
- What are the challenges in the development of persuasive platforms/ systems/services/applications/features?
- What is the difference between developing a BCSS as a software system vs. as a software service (e.g., a mash-up)?
- What challenges result from the requirement for a service to be available 24/7?
- How can we cope with it when the technological platform which the BCSS has been built upon changes dramatically?
- What is the difference between persuasiveness and perceived persuasiveness? How should perceived persuasiveness be studied?
- How and to what extent should the bias behind a BCSS be explicated?
- How can we map psychological and behavioral theories within BCSS research?
- What research issues (other than ones relating to the user interface) need to be tackled?
- What are viable business models for BCSSs?

- What are the cultural and gender differences in BCSSs?
- How can we recognize and analyze the unintended side-effects of using a BCSS? What kind of abuses of a BCSS can be recognized and how?

As can be seen above, many questions remain to be addressed. Indeed, even if many research efforts have already been conducted thus far, we are still in the very early steps of research into persuasive technology and behavior change support systems.

In sum, what distinguishes research into BCSSs from research into other information systems and technologies is that BCSSs are inherently transformative, deliberately attempting to cause a cognitive and/or an emotional change in the mental state of a user to transform the user's current state into another planned state. Empirical BCSS research provides a unique opportunity for quantifying measures for system success. This requires explicitly stating the aim of the system, how the success was to be measured, and the extent to which the system succeeded in achieving this measure. It has to be explicitly defined what really takes place through the software system to be able to demonstrate to what extent an outcome/change is really due to the system, or a feature or a set of features in it. Thus, sound ways of defining the systems and their goals clearly are needed. Otherwise, it will be difficult or perhaps even impossible to translate lessons learned from the results into related problem and application domains.

5 Conclusions

Human-computer interaction and social interaction through information systems can be used to influence people's behavior. Yet, even the relatively well-known persuasion techniques need to be adapted to match computing specificities. Moreover, the development of BCSSs is much more than just a user interface issue. It relates to technological services, applications, platforms, and functionality, the quality and content of information, personal goals set by the end-users, and social environments, among other issues. In many cases, the BCSSs must be available 24/7, they have to address global and cultural issues with a multitude of standards, habits, and beliefs, and they have to be adaptable into a variety of business models.

Persuasive technology as a field has the responsibility of educating the general audience about the pros and cons of people's behaviors being influenced by information systems, whereas web and other software developers must realize that they exercise enormous power over the users because their designs always influence them in one way or another, whether they intend them to or not. Moreover, the contemporary and future web will keep opening up a myriad of opportunities for building various kinds of behavior change support systems and benefiting from them.

Acknowledgements

I wish to thank the Academy of Finland and the National Technology Agency of Finland for financial support for this research, and my doctoral students Marja Harjumaa, Tuomas Lehto, Teppo Räisänen, Katarina Segerståhl and Donald Steiny for their collaborations in my research endeavors within persuasive technology.

References

[1] Kraft, P., Drozd, F., Olsen, E.: ePsychology: Designing theory-based health promotion interventions. Communications of the Association for Information Systems 24, Article 24 (2009)

[2] Strecher, V.: Internet methods for delivering behavioral and health-related interventions (eHealth). Annual Review of Clinical Psychology 3, 53–76 (2007)

[3] Harjumaa, M., Segerståhl, K., Oinas-Kukkonen, H.: Understanding Persuasive System Functionality in Practice: a Field Trial of Polar FT60. In: Proceedings of the Fourth International Conference on Persuasive Technology, Claremont, CA, USA, April 26-29. ACM International Conference Proceeding Series, vol. 350 (2009)

[4] Obermair, C., Reitberger, W., Meschtscherjakov, A., Lankes, M., Tscheligi, M.: perFrames: Persuasive picture frames for proper posture. In: Oinas-Kukkonen, H., Hasle, P., Harjumaa, M., Segerståhl, K., Øhrstrøm, P. (eds.) PERSUASIVE 2008. LNCS, vol. 5033, pp. 128–139. Springer, Heidelberg (2008)

[5] Chi, P., Chen, J., Chu, H., Lo, J.: Enabling calorie-aware cooking in a smart kitchen. In: Oinas-Kukkonen, H., Hasle, P., Harjumaa, M., Segerståhl, K., Øhrstrøm, P. (eds.) PERSUASIVE 2008. LNCS, vol. 5033, pp. 116–127. Springer, Heidelberg (2008)

[6] Midden, C., Ham, J.: Using negative and positive social feedback from a robotic agent to save energy. In: Proceedings of the Fourth International Conference on Persuasive Technology, Claremont, CA, USA, April 26-29. ACM International Conference Proceeding Series, vol. 350 (2009)

[7] Oinas-Kukkonen, H.: Behavior Change Support Systems: The Next Frontier for Web Science. In: Proceedings of the Second International Web Science Conference (WebSci 10), Raleigh, NC, US, April 26-27 (2010)

[8] Zhu, W.: Promoting physical activity through internet: A persuasive technology view. In: de Kort, Y.A.W., IJsselsteijn, W.A., Midden, C., Eggen, B., Fogg, B.J. (eds.) PERSUASIVE 2007. LNCS, vol. 4744, pp. 12–17. Springer, Heidelberg (2007)

[9] Oinas-Kukkonen, H.: Discipline of Information Systems: A Natural Strategic Alliance for Web Science. In: Proceedings of the Second International Web Science Conference (WebSci 10), Raleigh, NC, US, April 26-27 (2010)

[10] Fishbein, M., Ajzen, I.: Belief, attitude, intention, and behavior: An introduction to theory and research. Addison-Wesley, Reading (1975)

[11] Ajzen, I.: The theory of planned behavior. Organizational Behavior and Human Decision Processes 50(2), 179–211 (1991)

[12] Bandura, A.: Self-Efficacy: Toward a unifying theory of behavioral change. Psychology Review 84, 191–215 (1977)

[13] Davis, F.D.: Perceived usefulness, perceived ease of use, and user acceptance of information technology. MIS Quarterly 13(3), 319–339 (1989)

[14] Venkatesh, V., Morris, M., Davis, G.B., Davis, F.D.: User acceptance of information technology: Toward a unified view. MIS Quarterly 27(3), 425–478 (2003)

[15] Petty, R.E., Cacioppo, J.T.: Communication and persuasion: Central and peripheral routes to attitude change. Springer, New York (1986)

[16] Fogg, B.J.: Persuasive technologies – Introduction. Communications of the ACM 42(5), 26–29 (1999)

[17] Picard, R.: Affective Computing. MIT Press, Cambridge (1997)

[18] Fogg, B.J.: Persuasive technology: Using computers to change what we think and do. Morgan Kaufmann Publishers, San Francisco (2003)

[19] Atkinson, B.: Captology – A critical review. In: IJsselsteijn, W.A., de Kort, Y.A.W., Midden, C., Eggen, B., van den Hoven, E. (eds.) PERSUASIVE 2006. LNCS, vol. 3962, pp. 171–182. Springer, Heidelberg (2006)

[20] Bogost, I.: Persuasive games: The expressive power of videogames. The MIT Press, Cambridge (2007)

[21] Oinas-Kukkonen, H., Harjumaa, M.: A Systematic Framework for Designing and Evaluating Persuasive Systems. In: Oinas-Kukkonen, H., Hasle, P., Harjumaa, M., Segerståhl, K., Øhrstrøm, P. (eds.) PERSUASIVE 2008. LNCS, vol. 5033, pp. 164–176. Springer, Heidelberg (2008)

[22] Oinas-Kukkonen, H., Harjumaa, M.: Persuasive systems design: Key issues, process model, and system features. Communications of the Association for Information Systems 24, Article 28, 485–500 (2009)

[23] Forget, A., Chiasson, S., van Oorschot, P.C., Biddle, R.: Persuasion for stronger passwords: Motivation and pilot study. In: Oinas-Kukkonen, H., Hasle, P., Harjumaa, M., Segerståhl, K., Øhrstrøm, P. (eds.) PERSUASIVE 2008. LNCS, vol. 5033, pp. 140–150. Springer, Heidelberg (2008)

[24] Parmar, V., Keyson, D., de Bont, C.: Persuasive technology to shape social beliefs: A case of persuasive health information systems for rural women in India. Communications of the Association for Information Systems 24, Article 25 (2009)

[25] Tørning, K., Oinas-Kukkonen, H.: Persuasive System Design: State of Art and Future Directions. In: Proceedings of the Fourth International Conference on Persuasive Technology, Claremont, CA, USA, April 26-29. ACM International Conference Proceeding Series, vol. 350 (2009)

[26] Harper, F., Xin Li, S., Chen, Y., Konstan, J.: Social comparisons to motivate contributions to an online community. In: de Kort, Y.A.W., IJsselsteijn, W.A., Midden, C., Eggen, B., Fogg, B.J. (eds.) PERSUASIVE 2007. LNCS, vol. 4744, pp. 148–159. Springer, Heidelberg (2007)

[27] Andew, A., Borriello, G., Fogarty, J.: Toward a systematic understanding of suggestion tactics in persuasive technologies. In: de Kort, Y.A.W., IJsselsteijn, W.A., Midden, C., Eggen, B., Fogg, B.J. (eds.) PERSUASIVE 2007. LNCS, vol. 4744, pp. 259–270. Springer, Heidelberg (2007)

[28] Räisänen, T., Oinas-Kukkonen, H., Pahnila, S.: Finding Kairos in quitting smoking: Smokers' perceptions of warning pictures. In: Oinas-Kukkonen, H., Hasle, P., Harjumaa, M., Segerståhl, K., Øhrstrøm, P. (eds.) PERSUASIVE 2008. LNCS, vol. 5033, pp. 263–266. Springer, Heidelberg (2008)

[29] Cugelman, B., Thelwall, M., Dawes, P.: The dimensions of Web site credibility and their Relation to active Trust and behavioural Impact. Communications of the Association for Information Systems 24, Article 26 (2009)

[30] Gamberini, L., Petrucci, G., Spoto, A., Spagnolli, A.: Embedded persuasive strategies to obtain visitors' data: Comparing reward and reciprocity in an amateur, knowledge-based website. In: de Kort, Y.A.W., IJsselsteijn, W.A., Midden, C., Eggen, B., Fogg, B.J. (eds.) PERSUASIVE 2007. LNCS, vol. 4744, pp. 187–198. Springer, Heidelberg (2007)

Persuasive Conversational Agent
with Persuasion Tactics

Tatsuya Narita and Yasuhiko Kitamura

School of Science and Technology, Kwansei Gakuin University
2-1 Gakuen, Sanda-shi, Hyogo 669-1337, Japan
ykitamura@kwansei.ac.jp

Abstract. Persuasive conversational agents persuade people to change their attitudes or behaviors through conversation, and are expected to be applied as virtual sales clerks in e-shopping sites. As an approach to create such an agent, we have developed a learning agent with the Wizard of Oz method in which a person called Wizard talks to the user pretending to be the agent. The agent observes the conversations between the Wizard and the user, and learns how to persuade people. In this method, the Wizard has to reply to most of the user's inputs at the beginning, but the burden gradually falls because the agent learns how to reply as the conversation model grows.

Generally speaking, persuasion tactics is important to persuade people efficiently, but it is also useful to reduce the burden of the Wizard because it guides the Wizard to a way of persuasion. In this paper, we explicitly implement persuasion tactics into the persuasive conversation agent. Evaluation experiments show that the burden (the input ratio) of the Wizard was reduced from 55% (without tactics) to 33% (with tactics), although the success ratio of persuasion was little improved.

1 Introduction

A large number of e-shopping sites are available on the Internet, competing with each other to sell more goods to customers. Some sites like amazon.com employ a scheme to recommend items to the customers based on their purchase/browsing record stored in their database. Researchers in the field have been working to develop recommender systems that assist customers to select one from a huge number of items [1]. Recently, explanations of recommendation are becoming an important research issue to improve the performance of recommendation and persuasiveness is a key element of the explanations to convince the customers to select an item [2].

Persuasive technology draws attention as a means to create interacting computing systems that can change people's attitudes and behaviors [4]. Conversational agents will play an important role in such systems because they can interact with the users through conversation in a proactive manner [5]. Many of the conventional conversational agents aim at chatting with users as long as they can without any specific goal of conversation [3]. On the other hand, persuasive conversational agents have a clear goal to persuade the users to change their attitudes or behaviors. It is not appropriate for persuasive agents to leave the chat in the course of nature. As human persuaders change

T. Ploug, P. Hasle, H. Oinas-Kukkonen (Eds.): PERSUASIVE 2010, LNCS 6137, pp. 15–26, 2010.

their responses depending on the opponent's utterance and on the situation, persuasive agents need to flexibly interact with the users to persuade them.

Developing a conversational agent requires a conversation model that represents how the agent responds to an input from a user. It is not easy to create a conversation model in which the agent interacts well with the users and a large number of conversation rules need to be created by experts. To reduce the burden, we integrate a learning agent and the Wizard of Oz method [7], in which a person called Wizard talks with a user pretending to be the agent. The agent learns from the conversations between the Wizard and the users, and constructs/refines its conversation model. At the beginning, the Wizard has to input most of the replies, but gradually the agent learns to reply appropriately as the conversation model grows. When a reply made by the agent is not appropriate, the Wizard can correct it.

We have developed a persuasive conversational agent using the Wizard of Oz method and have applied it to persuade users to change their preference from one camera to another one [12]. In the first experiment with 60 subjects, the agent with the help from the Wizard succeeded to persuade 25 (42%) out of the 60 subjects. In the second experiment, the agent that used the conversation model created in the first experiment succeeded in persuading one user (out of 10) without any help from the Wizard; another 2 subjects were persuaded with some assistance by the Wizard. These results show that the persuasive conversational agent is promising.

However, to develop such a persuasive conversational agent, we still have two problems; how to maintain a large conversation model and how to make an agent more persuasive. We, in this paper, introduce persuasion tactics into the persuasive conversational agent. We decompose a single set of conversation rules stored in a conversation model into multiple sets, each of which represents a phase of persuasive conversation with a sub-goal to achieve in the course of persuasion. Hence, the structure of the phases can be viewed as a persuasion tactics. By this decomposition, the persuasion tactics and the conversation rules are explicitly split and it is easier to maintain the conversation model than before. We evaluate the effect of persuasion tactics from two viewpoints; the performance of persuasion and the burden of the Wizard.

In Section 2, we address persuasive conversation agents and the conversation model to persuade users. We also explain the Wizard of Oz method to develop the conversation model through collaboration between a Wizard and a learning agent. In Section 3, we revise the conversation model to be the one with multiple phases to represent the persuasion tactics explicitly. In Section 4, we perform an experiment to show the advantages of the conversation model with tactics by using a task to persuade participants to choose a digital camera. We measure the performance of persuasion along with the burden of the Wizards. We conclude this paper with our future work in Section 5.

2   Persuasive Conversational Agents

2.1   Conversational Agents and the Wizard of Oz Method

Conversational agents interact with users through conversation to assist them in their information processing tasks such as information retrieval from the Web [6]. ALICE

(Artificial Linguistic Internet Computer Entity) is representative of the conversational agents now available on the Web and is being used in a number of Web sites.[1]

The conversation model represents how an agent replies to inputs from users. There are two major approaches to construct a conversation model. The first one is by describing scenarios or rules as is used in ALICE, PPP Persona [8,9], and so on. ALICE uses a language called AIML (Artificial Intelligence Markup Language), based on XML, to describe rules, each of which links a pattern, which represents an input from the user, to a template, which represents a reply from the agent. This approach forces us to write a large number of rules to make the agent reply fluently to various inputs from the user.

The second approach is to utilize a conversation corpus as is done in Command Talk [10]. In this approach, we need to establish a very large conversation corpus in advance to construct a conversation model. However, the agent cannot reply appropriately to an input if the input is not in the corpus.

This paper takes the approach of integrating a learning agent and the Wizard of Oz method [11] as shown in Fig. 1. In the Wizard of Oz method, a person called Wizard interacts with the user pretending to be the conversational agent. The Wizard can reply to an input from the user when the agent cannot reply appropriately. The agent learns from the Wizard how to reply to an input by constructing a conversation model and can thereafter reply to the next instance of the same input. At the beginning, the Wizard has to reply to most of the inputs, but the burden of the Wizard falls because the agent learns to reply as the conversation model matures.

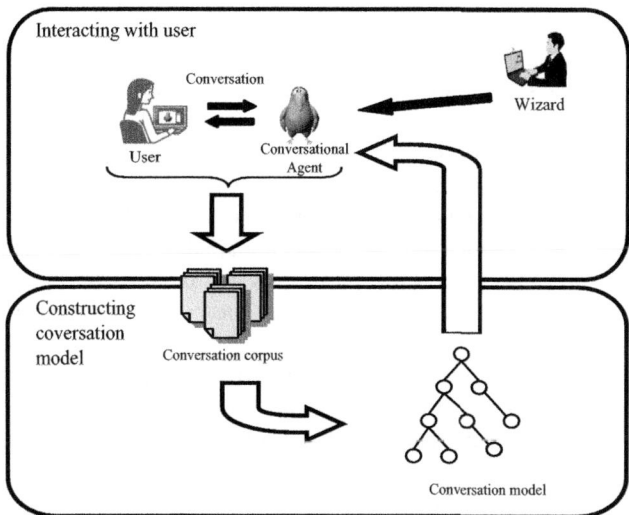

Fig. 1. Integrating a learning agent and the Wizard of Oz method

2.2 Persuasive Conversation

We introduce a conversational agent that persuades users as shown in Fig. 2. The user initially prefers Camera A over Camera B, and the agent tries to persuade her to change

---

[1] http://www.alicebot.org/

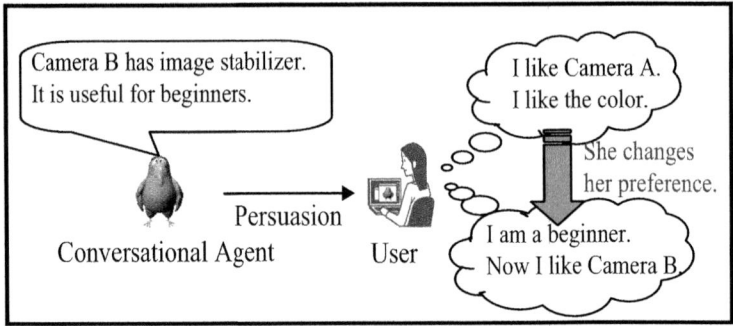

Fig. 2. Persuasion through conversation

her preference from A to B. If the user comes to prefer B, we define the persuasion as successful; otherwise, a failure.

Conventional conversational agents reply to an input from a user if the input matches a rule in the conversation model. When it matches multiple rules, one of them is selected. The selection process depends on the system and/or the applied domain. Persuasive agents, on the other hand, should select the rule that is more likely to lead to success. To this end, we have proposed a goal-oriented conversation model that considers the success probability of persuasion and a learning method to update the probability as derived from persuasive conversations between the Wizard and users [12].

Goal-oriented conversation model. The conversation model can be represented as a state transition tree where a statement is represented as a link to change a state from one to another as shown in Fig. 3. In this example, the agent tries to persuade a user to change his/her choice of camera. There are two types of states; user states, which represent the user talking, and agent states, which represent the agent talking. They are interleaved on a conversation path. A conversation path represents the flow of conversation between the agent and one or more users and begins with the initial state and terminates with either success or failure. Each state is assigned a success probability score.

The agent decides how to respond to an input from the user following the conversation path held by the model. If the input matches a statement on a link to an agent state, the agent chooses a statement that links the agent state to a user state with the greatest success probability.

For example in Fig. 3, the agent says "Which camera would you like to buy, A or B?" at the beginning. If the user says "I like A," the agent then replies "Why do you choose A?" following the stored conversation path. If the user says "I like B," there are two reply candidates. The agent chooses the reply "Why do you choose B?" because that link leads to a user state with higher success probability (0.25).

Updating conversation model. When an input from the user does not match any statement on the stored conversation path, the conversation path is branched and the success probability scores are updated depending on persuasion success/failure as shown in

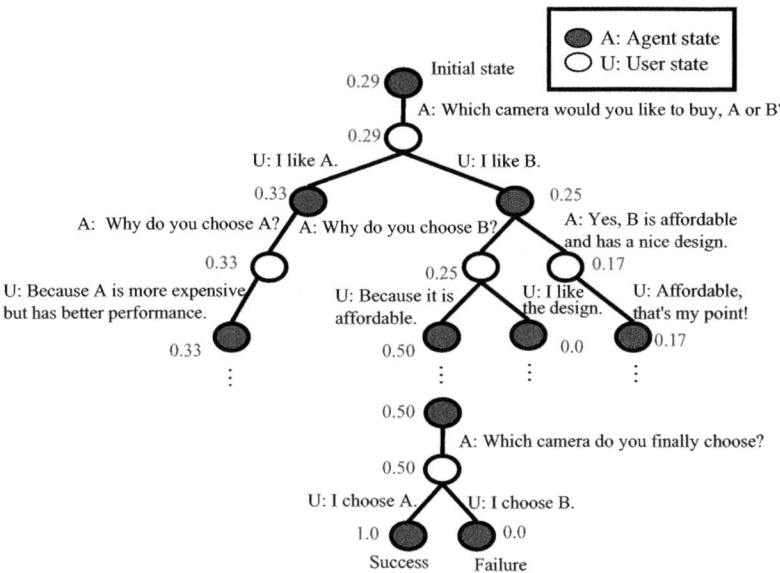

Fig. 3. Conversation model

Fig. 4. If the persuasion succeeds (fails), 1.0 (0) is assigned to the terminal state. The success probability score of each state except the terminal state in the conversation model is updated as below.

– Agent state s

$$Q(s) \leftarrow \max_{t \in succ(s)} Q(t)$$

– User state s

$$Q(s) \leftarrow \frac{1}{|succ(s)|} \sum_{t \in succ(s)} Q(t)$$

$succ(s)$ is a set of child states of s. At an agent state, the agent can choose what to say, so the success probability is set to be the maximum one among child user states. On the other hand, at a user node, the user chooses what to say, so the success probability is set to be the average one among child agent states. We here assume that the user takes a neutral attitude toward the agent. If we assume the user takes a negative attitude, the success probability should be the minimum one.

For example, when an agent says "Why do you choose B?" using the conversation model shown in Fig. 3, if the user replies "Because I seldom take photographs." which is not contained in the model, a new conversation path is created by branching as shown in Fig. 4 following a persuasive conversation between the Wizard and the user. Let us assume the persuasion succeeds, so 1.0 is attached to the terminal state of the branched path and each state on the conversation path is updated as mentioned above.

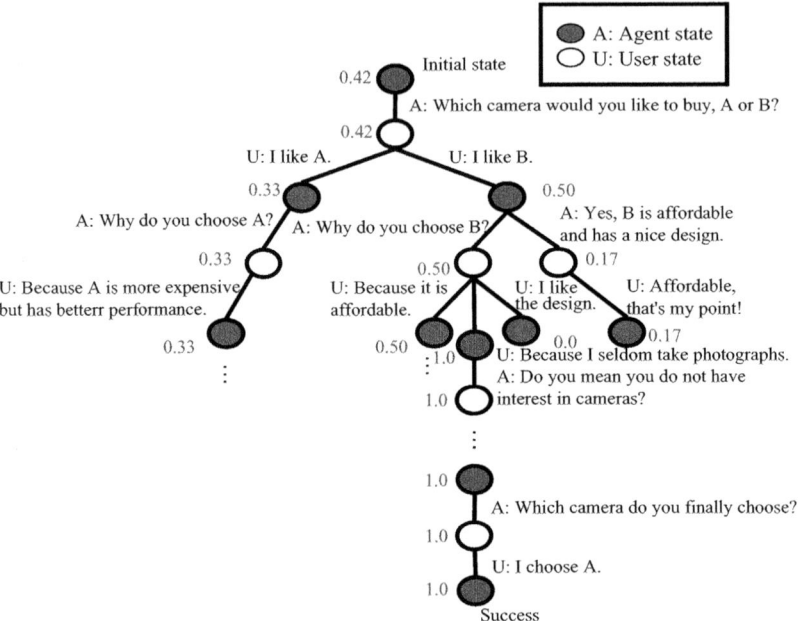

Fig. 4. Updated conversation model

Performance of Persuasive Conversational Agents. We performed two experiments to measure the performance of persuasive conversational agent [12]. In the first experiment with 60 subjects, the agent with the help from the Wizard succeeded to persuade 25 (42%) out of the 60 subjects. In the second experiment, the agent that used the conversation model created in the first experiment succeeded in persuading one user (out of 10) without any help from the Wizard; another 2 subjects were persuaded with some assistance by the Wizard. The experiments show that the persuasive conversational agent looks promising.

However, we have some problems to develop such a persuasive conversational agent.

1. We need a large conversation model to persuade users effectively. On the other hand, it is difficult to maintain such a large conversation model. It is not easy to change conversation rules in the model to make the agent more persuasive. Actually, it is difficult to analyze the model to know what rules are effective or not to persuade the users.

2. A conversation model for persuasive agents consists of two elements; one element is conversation rules to talk with the users fluently and another one is tactics to persuade them. We need good tactics to persuade them effectively. These elements are mixed in a conversation model and it is difficult to decompose clearly into two elements.

3. Persuasive agent requires a lot of assistance from the Wizard to persuade the users. As mentioned above, the Wizard needs two skills; one skill is to talk with the users and another skill is to persuade them. Generally speaking, it is easy to find a Wizard to talk well but not easy to find one who is a good persuader.

To cope with the above problems, we revise the conversation model into one with multiple phases. Each phase has a sub-goal to achieve in a course of persuasion, and the structure of the phases can be viewed as a persuasion tactics.

3   Persuasive Conversation Agent with Persuasion Tactics

The process of persuasive conversation can be represented as a sequence of utterances. The sequence can be decomposed into multiple sub-sequences of utterances and a sub-sequence is called a phase in this paper. Each phase has a goal to achieve such as "Ask which camera he/she prefers?" Hence the process of persuasive conversation can be represented as a sequence of phases. The sequence of phases may change depending on the responses from the user. If the user likes a camera because of the number of pixels, the agent tries to explain that the number of pixels is not important to choose a camera. If the user likes a camera because of its image stabilizer, the agent tries to explain that the image stabilizer is useless if photos are taken only in the day time.

The persuasion tactics hence can be represented as a flow chart shown in Fig. 5, which is an example of persuasion tactics to be used in digital camera sales. This tactics is derived from the conversation model created in the experiment in [12]. It represents that of the Wizard participated in the experiment.

We first show two digital cameras to a customer A and B as shown in Table 1. Camera A has better features about the number of pixels and image stabilizer than camera B, but the price and the weight of A are more than those of B. The purpose of this persuasion is to make the user change his/her choice from the initial one to another one. The tactics shown in Fig. 5 represents a phase as a box. The agent first asks the user which camera he/she prefers. If he/she prefers Camera A over B, the agent tries to persuade him/her to change his/her choice from Camera A to B. The agent then asks a reason why he/she prefers Camera A. If the number of pixels is appealing to him/her, the agent explains that the number of pixels is not important. If he/she does not accept the explanation, the agent tries to refute the advantage of another feature of Camera A. Finally, the agent explains the better features (price and weight) of Camera B, and asks again which camera he/she chooses. If he/she chooses camera B, then the persuasion ends with success. Otherwise, it ends with failure.

4   Evaluation

We evaluate our persuasive conversational agent from two viewpoints; (1) the input cost of Wizard when utilizing responses created by the agent, and (2) the persuasiveness of the conversation model, comparing to one without persuasion tactics.

We perform an experiment in which the persuasive conversational agent tries to persuade participants to choose one of two digital cameras using the following procedure.

1. Each participant reads the specifications of two digital cameras A and B, as shown in Table 1.
2. The participant chooses his/her favorite one from the first impression.

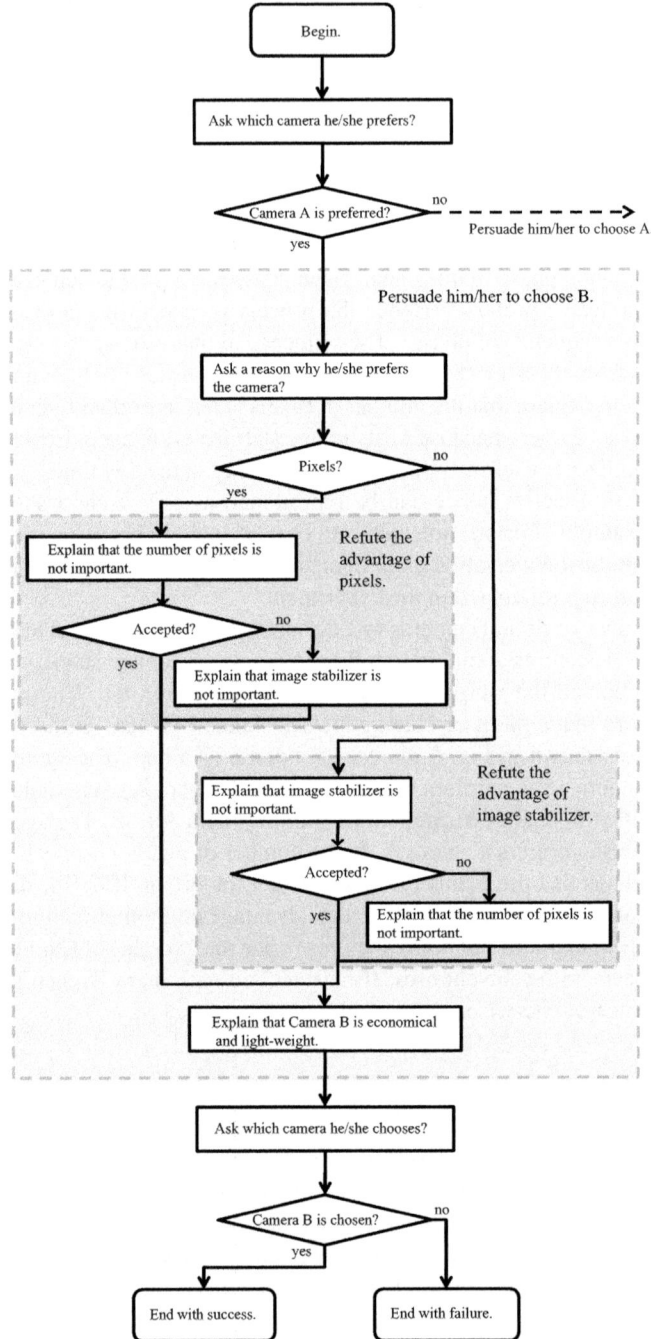

Fig. 5. Example of persuasion tactics

Table 1. Specifications of digital cameras A and B

	A	B
Price	¥35,000	¥29,800
Resolution	10M pixels	7M pixels
Weight	154g	131g
Image stabilizer	Yes	No

Table 2. Result of persuasion

System	Initial choice	Final choice	Number of participants	Success/Failure
With Tactics	A	B	7(20.0%)	Success
	B	A	6(17.1%)	Success
	A	A	7(20.0%)	Failure
	B	B	15(42.9%)	Failure
Without Tactics	A	B	8(36.4%)	Success
	B	A	0(0.0%)	Success
	A	A	6(27.3%)	Failure
	B	B	8(36.4%)	Failure

3. The agent, with help from the Wizard, tries to persuade the participant to choose the other one. It first asks why he/she chose the one selected, and then it tries to refute the reason and recommends the camera that he/she did not initially choose.
4. The participant is then asked which camera he/she prefers again. The persuasion succeeds (fails) if he/she changes (does not change) his/her choice.

In the experiment, we use a conversation model that has been made by persuasive conversations between a Wizard and 60 university students (48 males and 12 females) in the experiments in [12]. We employed 2 university students (2 males) as Wizards and new 57 university students (44 males and 13 females) as participants who are persuaded by one of the two Wizards with the agents. Each Wizard repeated to use one of two types of agents; one with tactics and one without tactics, interchangeably. How to present the persuasion tactics to the Wizards is described in [13].

The results are shown in Table 2. The agent with tactics succeeded to persuade 13 participants (37.1%) out of 35 and the agent without tactics succeeded to persuade 8

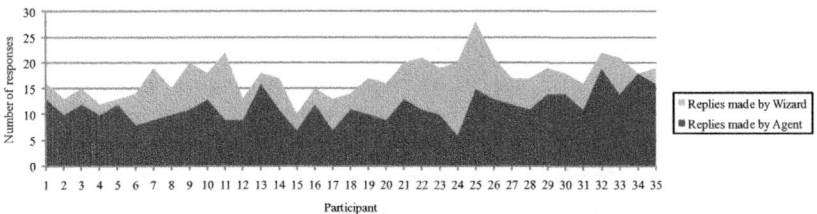

Fig. 6. Number of responses made by the agent with tactics

participants (36.4%) out of 22. There was no significant difference of the performance between two agents.

Fig. 6 shows the number of responses made by the agent with tactics to each participant. The responses are categorized into two groups; one is made by the agent and another is manually made by the Wizard. Fig. 7 shows the ratio of responses made by the agent with tactics to each participant. Overall, for the 35 persuasive conversations, the Wizard accepted 67% of the agent's responses as appropriate.

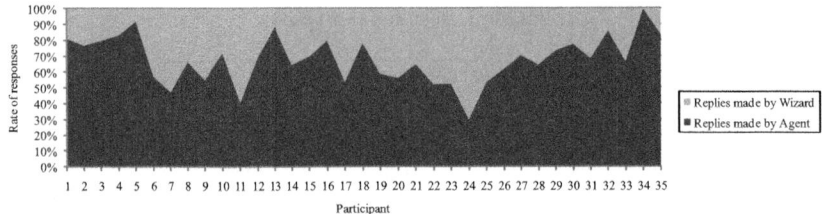

Fig. 7. Ratio of responses made by the agent with tactics

Fig. 8 shows the number of responses made by the agent without tactics to each participant. Fig. 9 shows the ratio of responses made by the agent with tactics to each participant. Overall, for the 22 persuasive conversations, the Wizard accepted only 45% of the agent's responses as appropriate. This means that the input cost of the Wizard with tactics was reduced more than that without tactics.

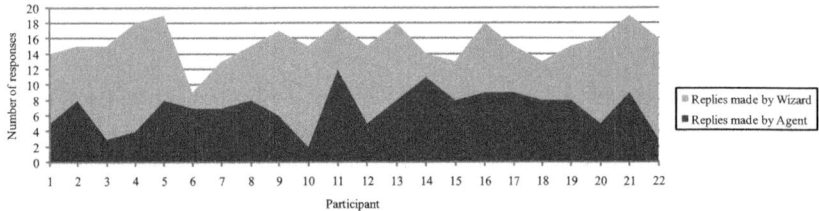

Fig. 8. Number of responses made by the agent without tactics

Introducing persuasion tactics into an conversation agent can reduce the burden of the Wizards. The goal of each phase is clearly shown to the Wizard, and it is easy for him to know how to persuade participants. Without tactics, the Wizard is not clear about the course of persuasion and he has to respond to the participants by himself. The number of responses made by the Wizard hence increases.

The difference of performance in the persuasion was not remarkable between an agent with tactics and one without tactics in this experiment. The Wizards used the two agents interchangeably, so they gradually learns how to persuade participants from the agent with tactics. To improve the performance, we have to improve the tactics itself, but how to deal with this issue is left as our future work.

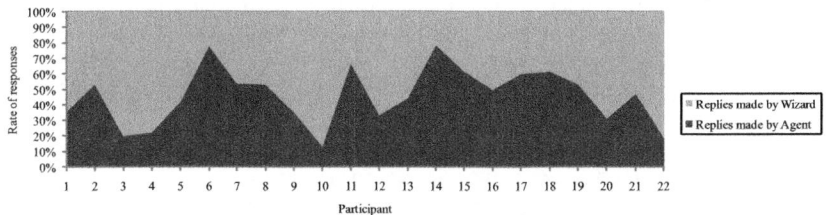

Fig. 9. Ratio of responses made by the agent without tactics

5   Conclusion

Persuasive conversational agents are expected to be virtual sales clerks on e-shopping sites. We have developed a persuasive conversational agent with the Wizard of Oz method. The agent learns how to persuade people through conversation between the Wizard and the users. Persuasion tactics is important to persuade people efficiently and we explicitly implemented persuasion tactics. Evaluation experiments show that the input ratio of the Wizard was reduced from 55% to 33% although the success ratio of persuasion was little improved.

In future work, we will improve the success ratio of persuasion by elaborating the persuasion tactics. To this end, we need to analyze the log record of persuasive conversation between the agent and the users. Another future work is to increase the maintainability of the conversation model. At present, it is not easy to modify the conversation model. We need to develop a GUI for this and to visualize the persuasion strategies contained in the model.

Acknowledgement

This work is partly supported by the Grant-in-Aide for Scientific Research (No.21300057) from Japan Society for the Promotion of Science.

References

1. Adomavicius, G., Tuzhilin, A.: Toward the Next Generation of Recommender Systems: A Survey of the State-of-the-Art and Possible Extensions. IEEE Trans. on Knowledge and Data Engineering 17(6), 734–749 (2005)
2. Tintarev, N.: Explanations of Recommendations. In: Proc. of ACM Conf. on Recommender Systems, pp. 203–206 (2007)
3. Weizenbaum, J.: ELIZA - A Computer Program for the Study of Natural Language Communication between Man and Machine. CACM 9(1), 36–45 (1966)
4. Fogg, B.J.: Persuasive Technology. Morgan Kaufmann, San Francisco (2003)
5. Cassell, J., et al.: Embodied Conversational Agents. MIT Press, Cambridge (2000)
6. Prendinger, H., Ishizuka, M. (eds.): Life-like Characters. Springer, Heidelberg (2004)
7. Fraser, N.M., Gilbert, G.N.: Simulating Speech Systems. Computer Speech and Language 5(1), 81–99 (1991)

8. Andre, E., Rist, T., Muller, J.: Integrating Reactive and Scripted Behaviours in a Life-Like Presentation Agent. In: Proc. 2nd International Conference on Autonomous Agent, pp. 261–268 (1998)
9. Andre, E., Rist, T., Muller, J.: WebPersona: A Life-Like Presentation Agent for the World-Wide Web. Knowledge-Based Systems 11(1), 25–36 (1998)
10. Stent, A., Dowding, J., Gawron, J.M., Bratt, E.O., Moore, R.: The CommandTalk Spoken Dialogue System. In: Proc. ACL 1999, pp. 83–190 (1999)
11. Okamoto, M., Yeonsoo, Y., Ishida, T.: Wizard of Oz Method for Learning Dialogue Agents. In: Klusch, M., Zambonelli, F. (eds.) CIA 2001. LNCS (LNAI), vol. 2182, pp. 20–25. Springer, Heidelberg (2001)
12. Kawasoe, M., Narita, T., Kitamura, Y.: Using the Wizard of Oz Method to Train Persuasive Agents. In: Klusch, M., Pěchouček, M., Polleres, A. (eds.) CIA 2008. LNCS (LNAI), vol. 5180, pp. 177–190. Springer, Heidelberg (2008)
13. Narita, T.: Introducing Persuasion Tactics in Persuasion Conversational Agent. Master's Thesis, Graduate School of Science and Technology, Kwansei Gakuin University (2010) (in Japanese)

Happier Together: Integrating a Wellness Application into a Social Network Site

Sean A. Munson, Debra Lauterbach, Mark W. Newman, and Paul Resnick

School of Information, University of Michigan
1075 Beal Ave, Ann Arbor, MI 48109
{samunson,dlauter,mwnewman,presnick}@umich.edu

Abstract. What are the benefits and drawbacks of integrating health and wellness interventions into existing online social network websites? In this paper, we report on a case study of deploying the Three Good Things positive psychology exercise as a Facebook application. Our experience shows that embedding a wellness intervention in an existing social website is a viable option. In particular, we find adherence rates on par with or better than many other Internet-based wellness interventions. We also gained insights about users' privacy and audience concerns that inform the design of social network-based wellness applications. Participants did not want all of their entries to be shared with all their Facebook friends, both because they did not want others to know some things and because they did not want to clutter others' newsfeeds. Users found it compelling, however, to interact with their friends around some "Good Things" they had posted.

Keywords: Social software, wellness, positive psychology, design, privacy, sharing, audience.

1 Introduction

Applications to promote health and wellness have attracted significant attention from the HCI and Health Informatics research communities [e.g., 1-10]. Increasingly, applications allow intervention participants to interact with each other [e.g., 3, 4, 7]. Typically, however, they are deployed as stand-alone sites. We explore the benefits and design challenges of integrating a wellness application into an existing online community with a large and active membership that was not developed explicitly to support health interventions. In particular, we built and deployed a Facebook application called "3GT" that supports the Three Good Things exercise developed by positive psychologists Seligman et al. [11] to promote psychological well being.

Building health and wellness applications into a popular networking site like Facebook appears promising for several reasons. First, the application can draw on participants' existing social networks rather than asking them to form new relationships with other participants. For certain types of supportive exchanges, participants may get more benefit from interacting with people with whom they already share a bond, especially in the near term [12, 13]. Second, many members of

T. Ploug, P. Hasle, H. Oinas-Kukkonen (Eds.): PERSUASIVE 2010, LNCS 6137, pp. 27–39, 2010.

Facebook visit the site very frequently, with nearly 50% of active users visiting every day [14]. Integrating a health intervention into a website that people are already frequenting could help overcome the challenges to adherence that many self-directed health interventions face [1, 6, 10]. Reported adherence to Internet-mediated anxiety and depression interventions deployed through open-access stand-alone websites were as low as 1% [15]; participation rates in controlled studies, presumably involving subject screening and participation incentives, were reported as 19% for a smoking cessation study and 34% for a diabetes self-management study [16].

However, integrating with a social networking site like Facebook may also have drawbacks. First, data entry requires an Internet connection, which may be inconvenient for recording activities and thoughts at certain times. Second, the average list of Facebook contacts includes 120 people [14] and represents a variety of types of relationships, including both strong and weak ties [17]. Some information may be too intimate or too mundane to share with such a large and diverse audience.

In this project, we set out to gain a deeper understanding of the advantages and disadvantages of deploying a health intervention within Facebook. We were specifically interested in answering the following questions: Does sharing and interacting with existing friends affect user retention? Are people comfortable sharing all their activity from the wellness application with all their existing social network friends? If not, then what features should be offered for controlling the visibility of activity in a wellness application? Does building structured features tailored to a specific wellness activity offer benefits over repurposing generic features of the Facebook platform?

1.1 Motivation and Background

There have been many recent studies of online or computer-supported intervention to promote wellness – especially physical activity promotion [e.g., 1, 3, 6, 7, 9, 18], diet [e.g., 4], or chronic disease management [e.g., 8, 10]. Internet-based support groups for both patients and caregivers have also received substantial research attention [e.g., 2, 5, 19, 20]. These online support groups offer participants a place for social support and sharing of knowledge.

In between these two spaces, however, is a relatively unexplored space of integrating the social experience with the intervention. In addition to offering support and advice in the form of discussions, the persuasive power of group dynamics and social influence may make social software a particularly potent technology for promotion of behavior change [21]. Participants' goals and progress towards goals might be shared with other users of the application, or with their friends, depending on the context and type of intervention. A more public intervention, with progress recorded and shared, may make people feel more accountable and lead to better adherence to recommendations. Reminders or "nagging" to participate might come from friends rather than from the system [13].

Some previous studies of computer-supported wellness interventions have connected their participants [e.g. 4, 7, 18]. For example, Consolvo et al made participants' step counts visible to other participants in a physical activity study. They found that this sharing influenced participants' motivation through both social pressure and social support [18]. Integrating the behavior tracking with social interactions was a strength of the application. The Fish'n Steps application [7] placed people in teams in an intervention to increase their physical activity. The researchers found this generated both cooperation and competition. Team membership, however, did not increase motivation; participants generally felt awkward contacting anonymous team members, but participants who knew each other in person were eager to discuss the game and share progress in face-to-face interactions. Like previous research, our research examines the role of social sharing in a wellness intervention. Unlike previous work, we study the integration of a wellness intervention with social software that participants already use (Facebook) and share their activity in the application with their existing contacts (their Facebook social network) rather than with other intervention participants who they may not know in real life.

Psychological Wellness. Positive psychology – the "study of the strengths and virtues that enable individuals and communities to thrive" [11] – is an emerging research area. Its focus on helping people thrive contrasts with psychology's more prominent focus on treating mental illness. Positive psychologists have developed a number of exercises that help people live happier and more fulfilling lives [22]. Participants in one of the most effective exercises, Three Good Things, are supposed to record three good things each day and the reasons why these things happened. By focusing on the good, rather than dwelling on the negative, it is theorized that people can train themselves to be happier. Previous studies of this exercise [e.g., 22] have focused on offline, private participation: subjects received instructions online, but recorded their daily good things offline. Results have been consistent with the theory: subjects reported decreased symptoms of depression and increased happiness as compared to a baseline before the exercise.

In the wild, people have already adapted Three Good Things for the social websites they already use. People share their good things on Facebook groups, in public blogs, and a "dare" on the Livestrong site. Before developing and deploying our own application, we studied two existing Facebook groups dedicated to this intervention, one with 68 members and the other with 144 members as of August 2009. Both follow the same format, with group members posting good things to the group's wall, usually as a list of all three items at a time. The posts and comments on the Facebook groups' walls contain interaction between members and both social support and social pressure. Group members occasionally congratulate one another on a good thing, comment on them, or repeat another's good thing as one of their own. In one of the groups, one member in particular greeted all new members by name and encouraged them to post. This member also prompted existing members to post ("what about you guys? how'd your day go?"). In other cases, people shared if they were having a bad day and were unable to come up with three good things, and in one example, another group member actually came up with three things for someone having a bad day. Finally, some members reflected on how the exercise was making them feel: "Wow. It actually lifts my spirits to see people, I don't even know, joining this group and reflecting on even -a few- good things. It's nice to just share in all of that with you."

2 Three Good Things Application

Based in part on insights from observing the Facebook groups, we built an application that could support the Three Good Things intervention, which we call 3GT (apps.facebook.com/threegoodthings). We included features that supported the key elements of the intervention as described in positive psychology literature, features that would support the social sharing we had observed in the Facebook groups, and the strengths identified in previous studies of integrating social experiences with computer-supported wellness interventions. We summarize the key features below.

Support for private and public recording of good things. Each good thing could be posted with one of three privacy options: shared on the participant's newsfeed (visible to all of their friends, Figure 1) and visible to their Facebook friends who visit their 3GT profile, visible to their Facebook friends who visit their 3GT profile, and private (visible only to the participant).

Structured support for good things and reasons. The theoretical literature on the exercise emphasizes the importance of reflecting on why good things happen. We did not see evidence that this was occurring in the posts to the Facebook groups. Our application allowed participants to list both a good thing that happened, and, in a separate and private field, the reason (see Figure 2). We hoped that explicitly asking for the reason in a separate field would encourage people to reflect on why the good things had happened to them.

Social support & social pressure. By allowing participants to post Good Things to their Facebook newsfeed, and by making their 3GT profiles visible to their friends even if the friends were not 3GT users, we hoped to enable social support from friends, in the form of structured support in Facebook (e.g. "liking" someone's good thing or commenting on it) as well as unstructured interactions between individuals through other communication channels. By making participants' activity in the application visible to their friends, we believed users might remind friends to participate if they noticed they had not posted in a while. We also created a formal mechanism, user-to-user notifications. When viewing the profile of a friend who had not posted in more than two days, a participant could remind the friend to participate. Clicking would send a Facebook notification to the friend (Figure 3 right).

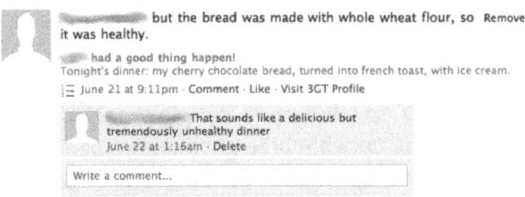

Fig. 1. Example of a Good Thing shared on a news feed or profile. Includes a comment from a Facebook friend of the participant.

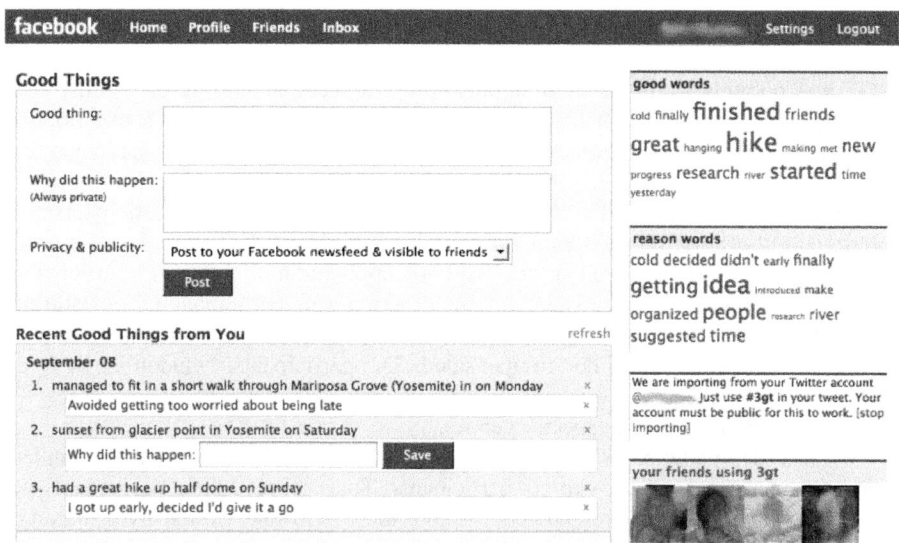

Fig. 2. Screenshot of the main 3GT application page. Left column: form for posting and a list of the participant's good things and reasons. Right column: word clouds, links to the participant's friends' 3GT profiles, and a link to an integrated timeline of all of the public good things from friends who are using 3GT.

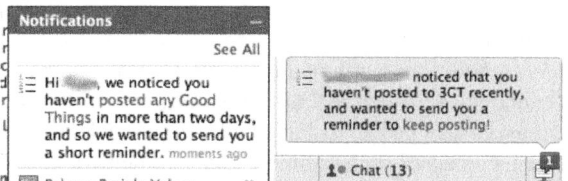

Fig. 3. Reminders sent through Facebook notification interface. Left: Example system-generated notification. Right: Example user-to-user notification.

Integration with participants' routines and habits. In addition to being able to post from the 3GT application, participants were able to create public posts from outside of the 3GT application, by posting on their Facebook profile or newsfeed pages or by importing tweets containing the hashtag #3gt from their Twitter account – both places where many people already post events that could be considered good things. We hoped that these additional integration points would increase adherence by reducing the steps required to post a good thing and by fitting into activities that participants already do. Some participants would also receive computer-generated reminders if they did not post for two days, and again after four days since their last post. These reminders would appear alongside other Facebook notifications when the participant logged into Facebook (Figure 3 left), likely an opportune time to post because they were already logged in.

3 Study Overview

3GT was publicly available as an application on Facebook starting on 20 July 2009. Participants consented to being in a research study and completed a questionnaire after installing the application. By 21 February 2010, 190 participants had completed the initial signup process for 3GT. We recruited participants primarily through an advertisement we ran on Facebook (71 participants). Additional participants were recruited either after an invitation from a friend or seeing 3GT on a friend's profile (57 participants), finding 3GT in the Facebook application directory (24 participants), or reading about 3GT elsewhere on the Internet (38 participants). 20 additional participants who are Facebook friends of the researchers were excluded from our analysis. Participants were not compensated. The participants included 25 men (age mean 35.6 years, stdev 14.8 years) and 164 women (age mean 36.7 years, stdev 13.3 years); 1 participant did not specify gender.

We recorded participants' interactions with the 3GT application. We also completed semi-structured interviews with six participants. This included three participants who knew one or more of the researchers (though they were interviewed by a researcher who did not know them) and one participant who was a friend-of-a-friend of one of the researchers.

In addition to our general goal of observing how users interacted with 3GT and what their perceptions of it were, we explored variations of the design to determine if they had any effects on usage. We deployed variants of the application along two dimensions: system-generated reminders to post good things and the default privacy or publicity of each good thing posted. Participants were assigned to one of four conditions randomly in a 2x2 design.

In the *reminders* condition, participants received reminders after 2 and 4 days without posts. Reminders were sent as Facebook notifications, which appear as subtle pop-ups when the user is logged in to Facebook (Figure 3 left). In the *no-reminders condition*, participants received such reminders only if their friends sent them.

In the *private by default* condition, good things added from the 3GT application page (Figure 2) were visible only to the participant. In the *public default*, good things were posted to the participants' walls, and thus had a chance of showing up in all their friends' news feeds. Participants could change the privacy on a per-post basis at the time of posting but could not change their defaults.

4 Results

Of the 190 participants who signed up for 3GT, who were not Facebook friends of the developers, and completed the pretest, many posted a few good things on their first visit and never returned. We refer to those as dropouts and restrict our analysis of usage to 55 participants who posted for at least one week, who we refer to as the active users. These participants were 36.9 years old, on average, and included 7 men (13%) and 48 women (87%). They were more female than participants in Seligman et al's study of offline positive psychology interventions (42% male and 58% female) [22]. We present usage data as of 1 March 2010, for active users who joined prior to 21 February 2010.

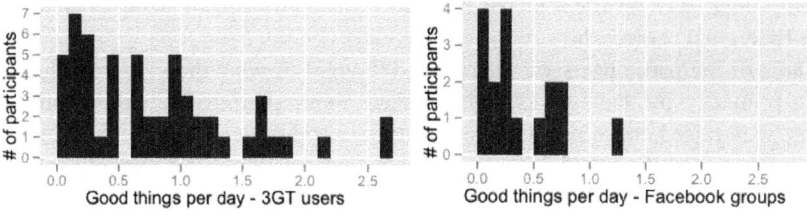

Fig. 4. Daily good things for active 3GT application users (left) vs. participants in the 3GT groups (right)

On average, active users posted 0.83 good things per day (Figure 4), defined as the total number of good things posted divided by the number of days between their first and last good thing posted. Though far less than the recommended level of participation, this was quite a bit higher than the active participants (defined by the same criteria of posting for at least one week) in the Facebook groups, where active participants averaged 0.38 and 0.47 good things per day.

3GT users posted reasons for 80% of their good things, compared to 0% for the groups. This was true even when participants were unsure of the benefits of recording the reason. As one participant said, "I don't know what I'm supposed to write there, but there's a box there with a big blue button that says 'Save,' so I feel like I haven't finished it properly unless I write something. I feel a little bit like I have to finish it."

Of the good things posted by active users, 91% were posted from the application, 6% were posted from participants' newsfeeds or Facebook profiles, and 4% were imported from Twitter. Even though participants did not regularly use the most integrated form of posting (posting from their newsfeed or profile), the participants we interviewed were generally in agreement that having the application on Facebook was convenient, and that logging into Facebook would sometimes remind them to post. Though posting from Twitter was rare, participants felt that it had some particular strengths. One participant we interviewed reported "And I love that it imports things from Twitter, because I use that as well. So if I don't feel like putting it in Facebook I can put it in anyway. So having lots of ways to get things in there… less barrier to entry." Another participant commented on how easy it was to turn a tweet into a 3GT post by adding the hashtag as "an afterthought," and then go back fill in the reason the next time she visited the application. Another participant felt that posting in-the-moment from Twitter and later visiting the application to fill in reasons caused her to reflect more than if she had simply posted both at the same time.

4.1 Privacy and Audience

Of the 55 active participants, 28 were in the public default condition and 27 were in the private default condition. Our data suggest that participants generally did not seek to share their good things with their entire Facebook network. Less than 21% of the good things from participants in the private default were posted to their newsfeed (and from only 6 of the 27 participants in this condition) and only an additional 23% were visible to friends viewing their 3GT profile. They left the remaining 56% as private. The public group made 14% of their items private and set 45% as visible to friends viewing their 3GT profile, but left only 40% in the default of being posted to their wall. Individual choices, however, varied greatly (Figure 5).

Three of the participants we interviewed thought of what they recorded in 3GT as being primarily for themselves. When asked about sharing their good things with others, they raised concerns about not wanting to add to the "stuff" on Facebook or to "spam the rest of the world." For two, this meant rarely posting publicly and almost never posting to their newsfeed. For a third, this meant using different methods of posting depending on the content: "I'm more cognizant of cluttering other peoples' feeds than some of my friends. That's why I use different versions of the application."

Another participant wanted to share quite often with her friends, but was also very conscientious about over-posting. This meant occasionally setting posts to be private and often setting them not to appear on her newsfeed:

mostly when I make things private, it's more because I think they'd be boring or insignificant to my friends, not because they're actually things I wouldn't want my friends to know about. I just don't want to clog up their Facebook with it.... A lot of the people I'm friends with wince about having games and other non-status update things all over their pages. And so I don't want to get winced about.

One other participant thought of his posts as having an audience of his Facebook friends who were 3GT users. He was also concerned about over-posting to public spaces, but with his more social view of the application, this meant that he posted less frequently (less than once every three days), and only when an event met a "higher standard." He also noted that the online nature of the intervention prevented him from posting many good things that happened in his workplace, which he felt would have violated his non-disclosure agreement with his employer even if posted privately. This is one downside of moving the intervention online. This participant would also have preferred that a more restricted group of friends than his entire Facebook contact list be able to see items posted to 3GT, and for this reason never posted to his newsfeed. Even then, he would have preferred that the application require him to approve 3GT contacts separately from Facebook friends, so that friends signing up for the application would not automatically be able to view his good things list.

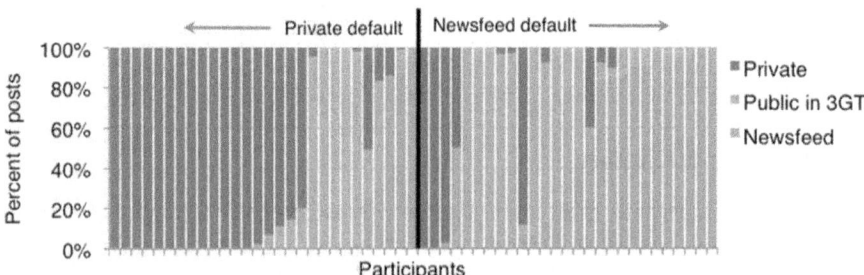

Fig. 5. Individual posting behavior and privacy defaults. Each column represents one active participant.

Desire for social interactions. Despite their reluctance to post too many good things publicly, five of the participants we interviewed were very positive about social interactions prompted by 3GT. One participant said that her status updates rarely received many comments, but when posting a good thing, "I got a TON of comments.... Lots of people said they liked that, and they responded to that and congratulated me... so yeah, people do definitely comment on them when they are created from Facebook and publicized [in newsfeeds]."

Other participants were hopeful that 3GT use would prompt more social interactions than it had. According to one, "I could imagine a world where the good things entered in the system were used to start conversations..." Another felt frustrated by the lack of feedback on the good things she posted:

> *And it would have been cool to have somebody reacting to, like you said, the sort of social interaction over the content of the posts that I've done... To have some of these things – "oh, I see you posted something", or just some reaction. Because sometimes it feels like you're out there, putting stuff out in the world and you're not getting any feedback, you know?*

One participant had posted "can't wait to see my friends' 3GT!" as one of his good things. During the interview he said that he liked looking at friends' good things because "it's like highlights of my friends' lives." He had followed up on some of the good things he saw his friends post, sometimes through Facebook and sometimes through other channels. Another reported, "it's just nice being able to see good things happening to other people." These participants are not alone in reading friends' profiles. Of the 4118 recorded page views, 16% were views of either an individual friend's 3GT profile (403 views) or a timeline view of all of their friends' 3GT posts (257 views). 25 of the 55 active participants viewed friends' good things using 3GT, and 24 used the application interface to invite friends.

Most participants wanted the 3GT application to make others' activity more salient. While we had assumed that people would post good things to their newsfeed if they wanted comments or discussion about good things, this was not true among participants we interviewed. They wanted more social interaction – such as the ability to comment on good things – within the application but not in their newsfeeds where it would be visible to friends not using 3GT. Representing a contrary view is one interview participant whose son also used 3GT. She said had never looked at his 3GT profile because she "figured it was private."

Effects of sharing. We had hypothesized that more public posts would attract the attention of a participant's friends, and that they would receive increased social support as a result, leading to both more posts per day and a greater retention rate. We did not find statistically significant differences in either of these activity measures. Our interviews also show that viewing others' activity in 3GT can sometimes lead to decreased activity. After beginning use of 3GT, one participant regularly posted good things three times per day. She later looked at friends' profiles and saw they were posting less frequently, and began to think that "maybe I was taking it too seriously, like a school assignment or something, if I didn't do it one day," and subsequently decreased how often she posted.

4.2 Reminders

Of the 55 active participants, 30 would receive system-generated reminders and 25 would not. Of those who completed the pre-test, 95 were assigned to the reminder condition and 95 were not, so there is no significant difference in retention rates at one week. Among the active users, people receiving reminders posted the same number of good things per day (0.82), on average, as those in the no-reminder group (0.83). The interviews with participants also helped us assess the effect of the reminders. While we had attempted to make the reminders "polite" and not too intrusive, we apparently erred in making the reminders too subtle. One participant did not know she had received reminders until we asked about them in the interview, and said that she needed something more prominent, like an email. Contrary to this, another participant liked that the reminders were integrated into Facebook: "I like the part that it sends me a note when I forget. I really like that! Having it remind me when I've forgotten is really cool."

User to User Reminders. Though many participants looked at each others' 3GT profiles, only seven participants sent a total of 14 reminders to their friends using the built-in reminder system. One participant we interviewed reacted strongly against the idea of reminding others to post using the interface. "No!... No, it's not my job." Another participant said that she enjoyed using 3GT more after she stopped thinking of it as "work" or something she had to do, and was concerned that pushing people to participate would cause them discomfort. She would be more inclined to prompt friends for participation if she knew they are "seriously combating depression, or it's something that they're really serious about and want to be doing, and they want me to help them get that done." Another participant felt more comfortable reminding her friends to post, but did not want to use the built in system for that: "I don't really like Nudge functions because they don't seem very personal. I'd rather go to their Wall and leave a sentence that was, you know, specifically from me."

5 Design Implications

The results of our study of the 3GT deployment highlight both strengths and weaknesses of the current 3GT design. Some aspects of 3GT offer positive examples for future intervention design, while others indicate particular design challenges for integrating wellness applications with social network sites.

Integrating wellness interventions into Facebook is a viable option. Our participants' dropout rates compare favorably to "open access" websites with as few as 1% active participants who return to the site after signing up [14]. Though this comparison is between different of wellness interventions, it lends support to the idea that Facebook-based interventions may assist adherence by facilitating easier access to the exercise materials.

Adding social features to an individual exercise can be beneficial, but not as a replacement to private participation. The social aspects of the intervention, i.e., sharing with others and viewing others' posts, were employed and deemed valuable by users. Specifically, people appreciated seeing others' posts and enjoyed receiving comments on their own. While previous studies identified privacy as barrier to integrating a wellness intervention with an existing social network site [13], we found that audience issues were a greater concern for 3GT participants. 3GT participants did not want all posts to be public, mostly out of concern of over-sharing. As one participant said, "I like the fact that I can choose whether things are private or public. Because if they were all public, some of them I wouldn't write, because I thought they weren't significant enough to sort of fill up others' Facebook pages with." A larger study would be required to determine effects on retention rate and clinical benefits.

Including intervention-specific user interface structure is beneficial. Compared with the relatively unstructured format of the two Three Good Things groups we analyzed, the addition of a separate, private field for participants to input the "reason" for each good thing encouraged them to complete the exercise as originally designed. While this appears obvious in hindsight, it is clear from the example of the groups that naïve or opportunistic implementations can miss critical details.

Employing built-in mechanisms for social interaction is not ideal. As mentioned, users employed and appreciated the social features of 3GT, but few routinely shared their posts with members of their Facebook network beyond users of the 3GT application. There is some evidence that users would like to share their good things with people they know (i.e., existing members of their social networks as opposed to strangers in a dedicated "Three Good Things" group) but not with *everyone* they know. We believe that "friends of mine who are also using 3GT" would provide an effective first approximation for the users we interviewed, though many wanted more of their friends to actively use the application. Moreover, users were wary of cluttering their friends' news feeds, and would prefer to more publicly share only big events and accomplishments rather than everyday triumphs.

Subtle reminders are not effective for everyone. Using a "gentle" reminder mechanism (e.g. the Facebook notification interface) to remind participants to carry out the intervention activities was not found to be useful in this study. For the most part, participants did not appear to notice the reminders. We do not know if more assertive reminders would have increased participation (or, conversely, annoyed users enough to abandon the exercise).

6   Conclusion

Through our deployment and study of 3GT, we have found that it is possible to transfer wellness interventions to social networking sites and deliver benefits to users. There are indications that including a social component with a personal wellness exercise is desirable, but some care must be taken with how the social features are designed. In addition, we are in the process of collecting data regarding the impact of 3GT on participants' mood over time in order to compare the efficacy with the reported benefits of Seligman's offline individual exercise.

People are wary of polluting their friends' feeds with things that are too small or that do not fit the genre of what they usually share as updates. For some people who do want to share, their Facebook network is too broad of an audience and they wanted a way to share with a smaller, more controlled list of contacts. A structured reflection feature – the prompt to provide a reason – was beneficial. Notifications and reminders are needed and wanted, but they should not be so polite that they go unnoticed. Overall, integrating health and wellness applications into existing social network sites is indeed promising and should be explored further, with highest priority given to design of features that control the sharing of information with friends without eliminating it.

References

1. Anhøj, J., Jensen, A.H.: Using the Internet for life style changes in diet and physical activity: a feasibility study. J. Med. Internet Res. 6(3), e28 (2004)
2. Blank, T.O., Adams-Blodnieks, M.: The who and the what of usage of two cancer online communities. Computers in Human Behavior (2007)
3. Consolvo, S., et al.: Flowers or a Robot Army? Encouraging Awareness & Activity with Personal, Mobile Displays. In: UbiComp 2008 (2008)
4. Grimes, A., Bednar, M., Bolter, J.D., Grinter, R.D.: EatWell: Sharing Nutrition-Related Memories in a Low-Income Community. In: CSCW 2008 (2008)
5. Klemm, P., et al.: Online Cancer Support Groups: A Review of the Research Literature. CIN: Computers, Informatics, Nursing 21(3), 136–142 (2003)
6. Leslie, E., Marshall, A.L., Owen, N., Bauman, A.: Engagement and retention of participants in a physical activity website. Prev. Med. 40(1), 54–59 (2005)
7. Lin, J.J., Mamykina, L., Lindtner, S., Delajoux, G., Strub, H.B.: Fish'n'Steps: Encouraging Physical Activity with an Interactive Computer Game. In: Dourish, P., Friday, A. (eds.) UbiComp 2006. LNCS, vol. 4206, pp. 261–278. Springer, Heidelberg (2006)
8. Mamykina, L., Mynatt, E., Davidson, P., Greenblatt, D.: MAHI: investigation of social scaffolding for reflective thinking in diabetes management. In: CHI 2008 (2008)
9. Richardson, C., Brown, B.B., Foley, S., Dial, K.S., Lowery, J.C.: Feasibility of Adding Enhanced Pedometer Feedback to Nutritional Counseling for Weight Loss. Med. Internet Res. 7(5), e56 (2005)
10. Tate, D.F., Jackvony, E.H., Wing, R.R.: Effects of Internet behavioral counseling on weight loss in adults at risk for type 2 diabetes: a randomized trial. JAMA 289(14), 1833–1836 (2003)
11. Positive Psychology Center. University of Pennsylvania,
    http://www.ppc.sas.upenn.edu/
12. Wellman, B., Wortley, S.: Different strokes from different folks: Community ties and social support. American Journal of Sociology, 558–588 (1990)
13. Olsen, E., Kraft, P.: ePsychology: A pilot study on how to enhance social support and adherence in digital interventions by characteristics from social networking sites. In: Persuasive 2009 (2009)
14. Facebook Press Page,
    http://www.facebook.com/press/info.php?statistics
15. Christensen, H., Griffiths, K.M., Farrer, L.: Adherence in Internet Interventions for Anxiety and Depression. J. Med. Internet Res. 11(2), e13 (2009)
16. Wangberg, S.C., Bergmo, T.S., Johnsen, J.A.K.: Adherence in Internet-based interventions. Patient Preference and Adherence 2(2007), 1 (2008)

17. Ellison, N.B., Steinfield, C., Lampe, C.: The benefits of Facebook 'friends:' Social capital and college students' use of online social network sites. Journal of Computer-Mediated Communication 12(4), I (2007)
18. Consolvo, S., Everitt, K., Smith, I., Landay, J.: Design requirements for technologies that encourage physical activity. In: CHI 2006 (2006)
19. Weinberg, N., et al.: Online Help: Cancer Patients Participate in a Computer-Mediated Support Group. Health & Social Work 21(1), 24–29 (1996)
20. Welbourne, J., Blanchard, A., Boughton, M.D.: Supportive communication, sense of virtual community and health outcomes in online infertility groups. In: Communities and Technologies 2009 (2009)
21. Khaled, R., Barr, P., Noble, J., Biddle, R.: Investigating Social Software as Persuasive Technology. In: IJsselsteijn, W.A., de Kort, Y.A.W., Midden, C., Eggen, B., van den Hoven, E. (eds.) PERSUASIVE 2006. LNCS, vol. 3962, pp. 104–107. Springer, Heidelberg (2006)
22. Seligman, M., Steen, T., Park, N., Peterson, C.: Positive Psychology Progress. American Psychologist 60(5), 410–421 (2005)

Animate Objects:
How Physical Motion Encourages Public Interaction

Wendy Ju and David Sirkin

Center for Design Research
Stanford University
Stanford, California USA
{wendyju,sirkin}@stanford.edu

Abstract. The primary challenge for information terminals, kiosks, and incidental use systems of all sorts, is that of getting the "first click" from busy passersby. This paper presents two studies that investigate the role of motion and physicality in drawing people to look and actively interact with generic information kiosks. The first study was designed as a 2x2 factorial design, physical v. on-screen gesturing and hand v. arrow motion, on a kiosk deployed in two locations, a bookstore and a computer science building lobby. The second study examined the effect of physical v. projected gesturing, and included a follow-up survey. Over twice as many passersby interacted in the physical v. on-screen condition in the first study and 60% more interacted in the second. These studies, in concert, indicate that physical gesturing does indeed significantly attract more looks and use for the information kiosk, and that form affects people's impression and interpretation of these gestures.

Keywords: kiosk; physicality; gesturing; public; field study.

1 Introduction

Pity the poor information kiosk. Information terminals the world over are going untouched—unloved—because people do not really understand how to interact with them. This sad state extends beyond the underuse of myriad kiosks, for, after all, kiosks have no feelings. No, the true tragedy is all the people who have gone uninformed, undirected, unguided, because they didn't receive the information they needed when they needed it.

The conundrum of the information kiosk embodies the challenges of what Alan Dix termed "incidental interactions." [1] Technologically, kiosks may be no different from the personal computers we use for hours each day, but their use pattern is distinctly different: they are single purpose; every user is a novice; there is scant opportunity for training or orientation; each transaction is fleeting. Human-kiosk interactions are like "engagements among the unacquainted" [2] rather than engagements between familiar parties. For many such incidental use systems, the big challenge is to overcome people's reluctance to engage with the unknown for an indefinite payoff [1]. Understanding how to overcome such obstacles will improve the use and usefulness of public information and communication technologies.

T. Ploug, P. Hasle, H. Oinas-Kukkonen (Eds.): PERSUASIVE 2010, LNCS 6137, pp. 40–51, 2010.
© Springer-Verlag Berlin Heidelberg 2010

In the project described in this paper, we seek to improve the engagement and approachability of public computer systems, like the lowly information kiosk, by using motion and physicality. After all, people implicitly signal their willingness to engage with others in all sorts of ways; might some of these techniques work for initiating interaction with a machine? These questions will become increasingly important as information technologies become more ubiquitous in our daily lives.

2 Related Work

2.1 The First Click Problem

Kiosk designers have traditionally focused on the issue of usability. Because kiosks are used incidentally, designers of such systems seek to ensure that no orientation or training is required for use [3]. However, deployments of these research kiosks usually show that lack of approachability renders the issue of usability moot. For example, in evaluating MINNELLI [4], Stieger and Suter note how the conventional wisdom that kiosks can draw users by using "attract loops" fell short. The flashy, animated attract loop actually kept people from using their bank kiosk system, because they adopted the role of passive observers: "This was in fact the central hurdle in the system's usage, as the great majority of users had no trouble at all handling MINNELLI after they had mastered the first click." Absent this first click, however, none of the other niceties of the system design really mattered.

Some kiosk systems, such as MACK [5] or MIKI [6], employ embodied conversational agents and natural language processing for the purpose of creating more natural "usability," but even in these systems, the kiosk remains idle until a person has engaged the system—by sitting on a pressure-sensitive chair mat, for MACK, or by issuing a command to the system, in the case of MIKI. For all their interactive sophistication, these systems also have documented "first click" or "first contact" problems, where people do not approach, or where they approach but seem not to know how they are to engage with the system. MIKI's designers identified this as the primary limitation of their system, "namely that there are not enough cues provided to the casual observer as to what the kiosk is and how to interact with it."

Part of the problem with applying a usability approach towards the first click problem is that usability is usually evaluated in the lab, rather than in the wild. Consequently, the question of whether a usable system will actually get used often doesn't really get evaluated until the system is in full deployment. By looking at approachability—the problem of how to get the first click—as an independent issue, one that requires insight about users and how they behave in real public settings, we can address the challenges of engaging users from the outset of a kiosk's design.

2.2 Social Actor Theory in Information Displays

Because people respond socially to computer and media technologies [7], designers often employ embodied avatars to make kiosk systems easy for newcomers to use. However, such systems set up high expectations on the part of the user about the "intelligence" of the kiosk. It can be prohibitively expensive, in cost, time and effort, to develop the vision, speech, and language processing systems that can perform in a way that people assume a seemingly intelligent system would. While such investments may be worthwhile if the goal of the system is to interact socially and emotionally with passersby, as in the case of Valerie the Robo-receptionist [8], they can actually be overkill—even counterproductive—if the ultimate goal is to present users with written information or maps. In their paper on their experiments with intelligent kiosks, for example, Christian and Avery note that their talking embodied avatar heads attracted a lot of curious passersby, but that the moving head subsequently competed with the content of the kiosk screen for the user's attention [9].

By moving beyond human-likeness as a design strategy, it may be possible to make displays approachable without having to achieve AI-completeness. In their study of public displays in the wild, Huang, Koster and Bochers noted that the physical orientation and positioning of public displays often had influence on whether people looked at or interacted with displays than catchiness of the on-screen content [10]. Otherwise, they found, people seldom glance at even bright and dynamic displays for more than a second. This finding is consistent with Reeve and Nass' social actor theory, for, as Erving Goffman pointed out in Behavior in Public Places, unacquainted persons generally actively avoid face engagement—even if the other person looks to be friendly or in a good mood [2]. This "civil inattention" is not rude, but rather, polite behavior. For receptionists and sales clerks—or other people in similar roles—certain physical orientations or locations "expose" them, thereby providing permission for unacquainted engagement. Thus, it should be unsurprising that people are far more willing to engage a public display if it is properly exposed.

Part of the challenge of looking at public information systems as social actors is designing the right sorts of experiments to test how people interact with such systems in public; this is fundamentally different from how people interact with systems in a more intimate or familiar setting. To this end, we take a page from Paulos' Urban Probes [11] and Ju and Takayama's gesturing door studies [12], where potential technologies are inserted into a public context with the knowledge that they may provoke behaviors and responses that otherwise are difficult to predict or access.

2.3   Motion and Physicality in Social Interaction

In The Social Life of Small Urban Spaces [13], William H. Whyte writes about two blind beggars he observed:

"The first beggar, while staying in the same spot, kept making a shuffling motion and moving his cup. The other remained stationary. The moving beggar received roughly three times as many contributions from passerby as the other."

While many bodily movements are emblematic—interpreted by members of a culture to have direct verbal translations—many more simply draw attention to the self and convey what sociologists call "openness", or availability: a willingness to engage in social interaction [14]. Unlike more static traits like friendliness or attractiveness, availability is a dynamic trait. Because of this, we are accustomed to seeing motion as part of demonstrations of current availability: train passengers wave their open palms to indicate the availability of the seat next to them, promoters wave handbills at you as pass, the doorman opens the door a little as you walk down the street. These motions invite engagement without actually crossing the threshold into explicit interaction.

While it as has been noted by [7] [12] and [15] that human-likeness is not a prerequisite for having people interpret computers, robots, and even automatic doors as social actors, most interactive information interfaces that employ physical motion have incorporated humanoid facial features [8][16][17]. In the following experiments, we investigate whether motion and physicality might function independent of facial form to encourage public interaction.

3 Experiments

The following experiments are, in the parlance of non-verbal communications research, decoding studies. They are structured to investigate how interactants perceive, interpret or react to non-verbal signals. They take place "in the field" so as to understand how people interact with systems in true public settings.

We tested several hypotheses with these studies:

H1. The Physical Hypothesis. That physical motion is better for indicating availability and encouraging engagement and interaction than mere visible motion.

H2. The Anthropomorphic Hypothesis. That human-like gesturing is more readily understandable and familiar than non-humanoid gesturing.

H3. The Uncanny Valley Hypothesis. That human-like gesturing is perceived to be stranger and less natural than non-humanoid gesturing.

3.1 Study 1: Physically Embodied vs. On-Screen Gesturing

In this first study, we sought to test our idea that physical motion and gesturing might do a better job of attracting attention and encouraging interaction with an interactive touchscreen kiosk than equivalent on-screen motion and gesturing.

System. We created a basic touchscreen kiosk with a gesturing apparatus attached. We were careful to design the kiosk so that it presented a neutral visual appearance in the non-physical gesturing conditions (see Figure 1). The kiosk most closely resembles a speaker's lectern or podium: it is 35 inches tall, 15 inches wide and 15 inches deep, and is clad in oak wood with a clear satin polyurethane finish. A 15-inch ELO 1515L touchscreen LCD rests inside on an upper shelf. A Dell laptop PC rests inside on a lower shelf and drives the touchscreen.

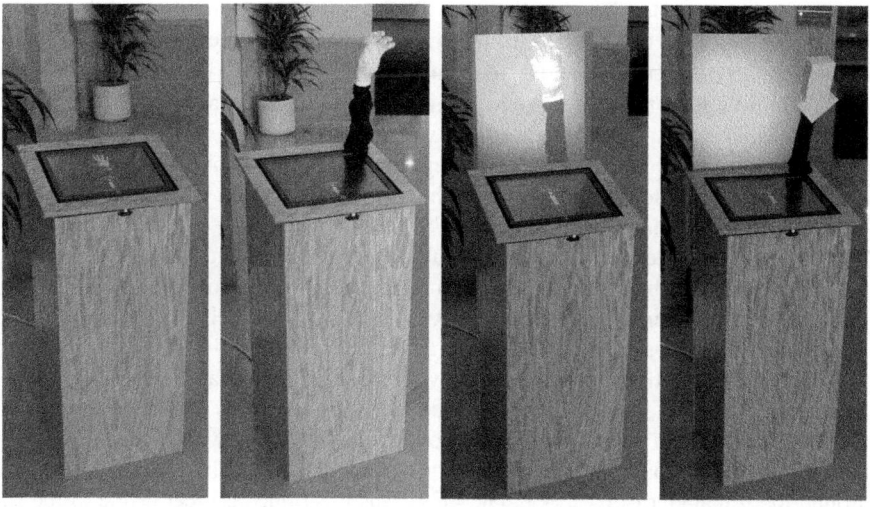

Fig. 1. The kiosk in *(left to right)* a) Study 1 On-screen condition, b) Study 1 Physical Hand condition, c) Study 2 Projected Hand condition, and d) Study 2 Physical Arrow condition

This laptop runs a JavaScript program that presents webpages within custom-designed browser window that features forward, backward and home navigation buttons, where the "home" location is the homepage for the study site. When the kiosk has been idle for 30 seconds, the browser program automatically resets the display to the home location, blacks out the page content, and presents a large round "i" information button in the foreground. Touching the screen removes the information button and brings the content back to the foreground. We performed preliminary tests to validate that the touchscreen-operated webpages functioned as a plausible kiosk.

The kiosk also houses a HiTec 8815B sail servo and an Arduino Decimila microcontroller board. In the physical gesturing conditions, the servo motor winds and unwinds a transparent monofilament to pull on the gesturing arm of the kiosk, causing it to move forward and backward.

The physical gesturing apparatus is constructed of a flexible steel strip. It is sheathed in black cloth and, depending on the condition being run, terminates either in white-gloved hand or a similarly-sized white foamcore arrow that points downward toward the kiosk. (See Figure 1b) and 1d). An infrared rangefinder mounted to the front of the kiosk detects the proximity of on-comers and sends an analog signal to the microcontroller, which stops the arm from waving when someone is standing in front of the kiosk.

For the on-screen conditions, the physical arm was removed and similar gestures were instead shown on the touchscreen display. In these cases, after the kiosk has been idle for 30 seconds, the "i" and black background of the kiosk are accompanied by an animated gesturing hand or arrow whose motion mirrors the speed and motion of the physical hand and arrow.

Sites. This field experiment was conducted at three locations: a design department lobby, the campus bookstore and a computer science department lobby. These locations were selected because they are natural sites for an information kiosk, have reasonable amounts of foot traffic, and have distinctly different traffic patterns and demographics: the bookstore is frequented by newcomers, whereas the computer science building has the same people coming in and out each day.

One of the most salient differences between these locations is that the arrangement of furnishings and objects at the design department and the bookstore change often, so even if a person visited everyday, he or she might not consider the addition of a kiosk on one day to be out of the ordinary. The kiosk is certainly novel, but its relative novelty in that context is low. In contrast, the computer science lobby is sparsely decorated, and the objects in the space rarely change. In addition, office dwellers may pass through it several times per day. As a result, they are likely to recognize the presence of a kiosk as a novel addition to a familiar setting.

The design department has one primary entrance with two large double doors, with a reception desk 20 feet from the entry. The kiosk was set up to the left of the entry, 10 feet inside of the doorway. The bookstore has two entrances with a checkout counter between them, and has books and accessories that fill many tables and shelves spread around the remainder of the floor. The kiosk was positioned 20 feet inside of the right entrance, along the right side of the main foot-traffic flow through that entrance. The computer science building lobby has one entrance with two elevators on the left side, a

6 foot wide octagonal information kiosk at the center (currently not functional) and a staircase on the right. The kiosk was positioned just beyond the two elevators, along to the left of the central information kiosk. Site maps of the bookstore and the computer science lobby are shown in Figure 2. The layout of the design department lobby is similar to the bookstore.

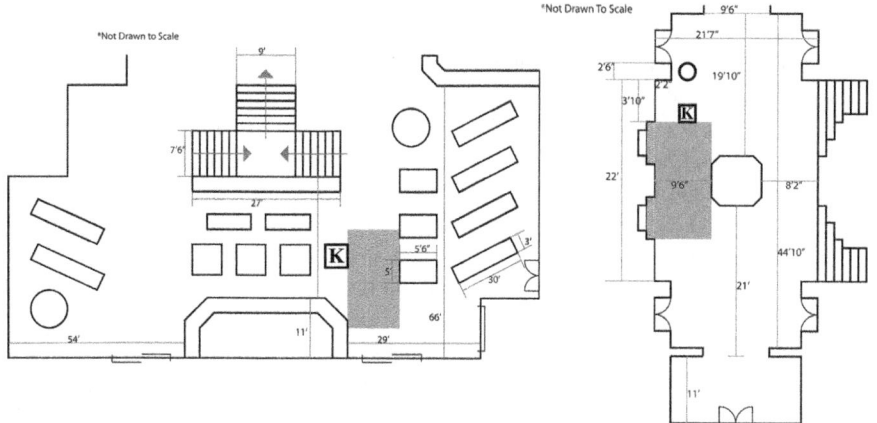

Fig. 2. Schematic maps showing layout of bookstore *(left)* and computer science building lobby *(right)*. The entryways are along the lower edge of the maps. The kiosk is labeled with a K, and the runway is highlighted in blue.

Experimental protocol. We employed a 2x2 factorial design for our studies. The two independent variables were the type of motion (physical vs. on-screen) and form (hand vs. arrow). We then measured the ratio of passersby who looked at and interacted with the kiosk. In addition, we asked people who interacted with the kiosk for brief informal interviews about their experience. Questions were open-ended, but included, as examples: What did you first notice about the kiosk? How does the kiosk design make you feel? and, Where else would this design work well?

To ensure that all of the people in our study were seeing the kiosk from the same angle, we were very strict about the people who we counted. We outlined a "runway" roughly 15 feet in front of the kiosk, and only counted people who approached the kiosk from the forward direction along that runway. People were determined to have "looked" at the kiosk only if their gaze was sustained for more than 3 seconds—for instance, if they had to turn their head to keep looking at the kiosk as they walked on by. People were determined to have interacted with the kiosk if they touched the touchscreen so that the kiosk's home webpage was fully visible. All people who interacted with the kiosk were also counted as having looked at the kiosk. People who stopped and played with the gesturing hand or arrow but did not touch the kiosk screen were counted as having looked but not touched the kiosk. Because groups of people tended to act in concert, pairs or clusters of people were treated as a single opportunity for interaction, regardless of whether they passed by, looked, or interacted with the kiosk.

The study ran over three days, with each condition set up for half an hour in the morning and another half an hour in the afternoon in each location. Because of natural variations in the traffic patterns, we did not have an even number of participants in each condition.

Study 1 Results. To explore the impact of physicality and form of kiosk gesturing motion on the behaviors of passersby, subjects were exposed to one of four conditions: Physical Hand, Physical Arrow, On-screen Hand, and On-screen Arrow. A chi-square test was then conducted on the observed frequencies of interaction within each nominal condition. Twenty-eight out of 179 people—roughly 16% of all the passersby—interacted with the kiosk, and 56 out of 179—roughly 31% of all the passersby—looked at the screen. There was a statistically significant main effect for physicality on looking, with a Pearson $\chi^2(1, N=179) = 8.39$, $p=0.04$, as well as for touching the kiosk screen, with a Pearson $\chi^2(1, N=179) = 4.24$, $p=0.04$. Nearly 44% of the people in the physical condition looked at the kiosk, whereas only 23% in the on-screen condition did. 22.5% of the people in the physical condition interacted with the kiosk, compared to 11.1% in the on-screen condition. The main effects for form on looking, $\chi^2(1, N=179) = 0.65$, $p=0.42$, and interaction, $\chi^2(1, N=179) = 0.28$, $p=0.60$, were not significant. A cross-check on the effect of location on the variables found no significant effect: the conversion rates for looking at the design department, the bookstore and the computer science department were 20%, 29% and 37%, respectively, and the rates for touching were 15%, 14% and 17%.

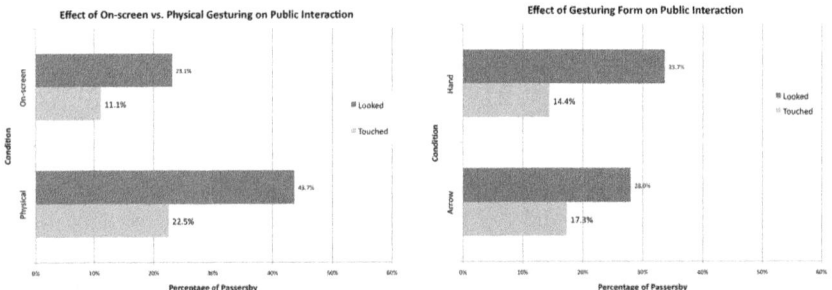

Fig. 3. Charts showing the percentage of passersby who looked and touched the kiosk in Study 1. Significant effect on looking and touching was found for on-screen vs. physical gesturing *(left)*, but not for form *(right)*.

Study 1 Notes and Observations. In the post-interaction interviews, people who saw a physical pointer recounted that the moving arrow or hand drew them to the kiosk, at which time their curiosity led to an interaction. People who saw an onscreen pointer described only novelty (a new device in a familiar location) or curiosity as inspiring their approach. People who were new to place were more likely to indicate curiosity as their reasons for drawing near to interact with the kiosk, whereas regulars were more likely to state that they that they came because the kiosk was something new, but, regardless of the stated reasons for interacting with the kiosk, the conversion ratios at all three locations were remarkably similar.

3.2   Study 2: Physically Embodied vs. Visually Embodied Gesturing

Following our initial study, we sought to further investigate the effects of form and physicality on interactive engagement. Because surveyed participants in the initial study never mentioned the on-screen hand or arrow as having motivated their approach, we sought to make the non-physical condition compete more evenly with the physical condition by projecting a "life size" video of a waving hand or arrow on a vertical backplane. We also changed the kiosk's on-screen image during idle mode to display a transparent gray backdrop rather than a solid backdrop, so that inquisitive passersby could see what they would be interacting with if they touched the touchscreen. Finally, we incorporated a short survey for people who had interacted with the kiosk.

System. Our kiosk setup in this second study was nearly identical to the initial study. We added a frosted acrylic backplane to the kiosk to act as a display surface. The display on the backplane was projected from a portable projector stationed waist-height approximately a yard behind the kiosk. This display was connected to a MacBook Pro running video loops of a waving hand or waving arrow on a blue background (for the visually embodied conditions) or a plain blue background (for the physically embodied condition) using iTunes player. The height of the projected hand and arrow was calibrated to be the same size as the physical hand and arrow.

For the visually embodied conditions, when the kiosk has been idle for thirty seconds, the program resets the touchscreen content to the home location, then dims the content rather than hiding it behind a black background, and presents the same information button from Study 1 in the foreground. No animated gesturing hand or arrow appears on the touchscreen display in this study.

Sites. This study was performed in the campus bookstore and the computer science department. We chose these two sites because they had higher non-repeat traffic than the design department did in Study 1, and because the conversion rates for interaction were fairly similar for all three sites. Due to changes in the bookstore layout, our kiosk location in this study was located across the main entrance pathway from the site used in the initial study.

Experimental protocol. As in the previous study, we employed a 2x2 factorial study design. The independent variables were physicality (physical vs. projected) and form (hand vs. arrow). We employed the same standards for counting looks, touches and interaction opportunities as we used in the initial study. After people interacted with the kiosk, a researcher approached and asked if they would be willing to answer a few short questions about their interaction with the kiosk. The questions on the survey (shown in Figure 4) were asked verbally, although the participants were also shown the questions in writing as the researcher recorded their responses in front of them. Ten-point Likert scales were used because of the verbal format of the survey.

This study was run four months after the initial study. The study ran over four days, with an hour for each condition at each site.

Study 2 Results. As with Study 1, subjects were exposed to one of four conditions: Physical Hand, Physical Arrow, On-screen Hand, and On-screen Arrow, and a chi-square test was conducted on the observed frequencies of interaction. Overall, more

1. What did you first notice about the kiosk?

2. What prompted you to approach the kiosk?

3. On a scale of 1-10, how approachable is the kiosk?

    Unapproachable   1 2 3 4 5 6 7 8 9 10   Approachable

4. On a scale of 1-10, how natural is the kiosk?

    Artificial   1 2 3 4 5 6 7 8 9 10   Natural

5. On a scale of 1-10, how strange is the kiosk?

    Familiar   1 2 3 4 5 6 7 8 9 10   Strange

6. On a scale of 1-10, how understandable is the kiosk?

    Incomprehensible   1 2 3 4 5 6 7 8 9 10   Understandable

7. How frequently do you visit [the bookstore/computer science building]?

    ___ first time ever   ___a few times a week

    ___ a few times a month   ___a few times a year

Fig. 4. Questions from the Study 2 interview questionnaire. Questions were asked verbally and answers were subsequently recorded by the researcher.

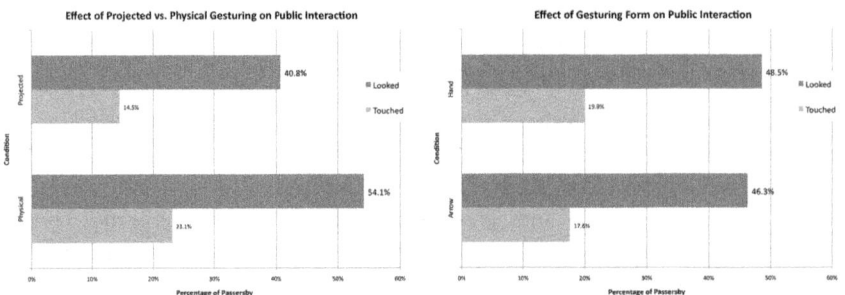

Fig. 5. Charts showing the percentage of passersby who looked and touched the kiosk in Study 2. Significant effect on looking and touching was found for projected vs. physical gesturing *(left),* but not for form *(right).*

people looked at and used the kiosk; 86 out of 457 people—18.8% of all the passersby—interacted with the kiosk, and 217 out of 457 people—47.5% of all the passersby—looked at the screen.

There was a statistically significant main effect for physicality on looking and touching. For looking, the Pearson $\chi^2(1, N=457) = 8.18$, $p=0.1$. For touching the touchscreen, the Pearson $\chi^2(1, N=457) = 5.62$, $p=0.02$. 51.4% of the people in the physical condition looked at the kiosk, compared to 40.8% in the projected condition. 23.1% of the people in the physical condition interacted with the kiosk, compared to 14.5% in the projected condition. The main effects for form on looking and touching were not significant. A cross-check on the effect of location on the variables found no significant effect: the conversion rates for looking at the bookstore and the computer science department were 41% and 56%, respectively, and the rates for touching were 18% and 19%. Overall, the rates of conversion were remarkably consistent; for example, the touch conversion rate for the physical condition at both the bookstore and computer science building in Study 1 was 21%, and in Study 2 was 22% and 26%, respectively.

A two-way between-groups analysis conducted on the Likert scale variables in the survey (Approachable, Natural, Strange, Understandable) yielded a statistically significant main effect for form on understandability, [F(1,3)=41.95, p=0.02] where the arrow was rated to be more understandable than the hand ($\underline{M}$=8.02, SD=2.41) vs. ($\underline{M}$=6.08, SD=2.77).

Study 2 Notes and Observations. The survey results confirmed several assumptions made in our experimental design. First, the respondents always indicated that the thing that they first noticed, and the thing that caused them to approach, was the waving hand or arrow. Interviewees generally expressed incredulity at our asking of the question. Hence, we were assured that our manipulations worked, and were the operating factors behind the difference in observed behaviors. Next, we confirmed our assumptions about the demographics at our two field sites: The vast majority surveyed in the computer science building indicated that they were in the building a few days a week, where as most in the bookstore indicated that they came, at most, a few times a year, or that it was their first time to the bookstore.

At the same time, the survey may have suffered from closely following the kiosk interactions. At the time of the interview, people were mindful of their recent interaction—for instance, we fielded lots of requests for an on-screen keyboard to make search easier—and so the degree to which their ratings on the Likert scales pertained to the gesturing mechanism varied based on how long they had interacted with the kiosk. This issue may be inherent to our field study design, for it is impossible to constrain all our experimental participants to having the same experience without sacrificing the naturalism of the scenario. It may be desirable, however, to follow up this study with a more tightly controlled laboratory experiment.

4 Discussion

Taken together, the results of these two studies suggest a robust effect on public interaction for physical gesturing over on-screen or even large projections of gesturing. This is consistent with the Physical Hypothesis (H1) posed earlier. Although the specific rate of public interaction with an information system would vary based on the site, the placement of the system relative to the environment, the demographics of those passing by, and the value of the kiosk content, among other things, the consistency of our findings across different times and locations leads us to believe that it is possible to infer as a general design heuristic (a) that physical gesturing encourages public interaction, and therefore (b) that motion and physicality are significant influences on approachability and social engagement.

The importance of form for garnering attention or even drawing interaction seems less important than the actual physical presence of a gesturing object. However, the form does seem to affect the user's perception of the interactive system; there is the suggestion, from our second study, that non-anthropomorphic forms may be less confusing to users than anthropomorphic forms. This causes us to believe more in the Uncanny Valley Hypothesis (H3) than the Anthro-pomorphic Hypothesis (H2), at least when the goal is to get the first click. The similarity between conversion rates for the human-like hand and non-humanoid arrow conditions implies that effective public systems do not have to be anthropomorphic to invoke social responses from passersby. This understanding frees designers from focusing exclusively on emotional expressivity; they can, alternatively or additionally, explore social and communicative expressivity through means such as availability or approachability.

The findings from this research also underscore the importance of addressing the "first click" problem. The same informational content, staged in the same location, to the same people, can have dramatically different rates of impact depending on how approachable the staging of that content is. It is not sufficient or even desirable to generate a "greatest hits" preview of the content within an information system; this shortcut doesn't actually fulfill the need of demonstrating openness. Instead, our results suggest that for public systems, the actions and content that come before the first click—whether physical, on-screen or projected—need to be designed as much as the actions and content that come after.

Designers of physically interactive systems, such as robots and motorized machines, should be particularly aware that they could employ capabilities for physical motion to signal availability or unavailability. This method of soliciting attention can be a valuable design alternative to using voice or words on a display to engage people. Designers must also be equally mindful that physical motions have social connotations even if sent inadvertently; it may be important to assess whether the device's actions "expose" them in ways that are undesirable. Most of all, the results of this study point to the potential for sensing and actuation technologies in myriad settings. Indeed, this research points the way to employing interactive technologies in a wide variety of animate objects that need to signal their intermittent availability or unavailability.

5 Future Work

Animate objects have great potential to save us from the present, where we sail blithely unaware of all the information we need and are missing, and from a future where every product with a chip talks, beeps or rings an alarm to get our attention. They offer some possibility for a middle ground, for communication without cacophony. At the same time, random incoherent motions from objects can be highly disorienting and distracting as well; it is important not to heedlessly incorporate motion into products before fully understanding how they really function.

In future work, we intend to investigate the longer-term implications of gesture and motion for information systems—might gesture's ability to garner attention wear off as the novelty faded, or does motion have lasting power to engage social interest and engagement? We are also interested in studying the factors that affect the interpretation and impact of non-anthropomorphic physical gesturing, including the form of the object being gestured, the gesture speed, and the motion trajectory. In addition, we plan to expand our range of studied gestures by looking into the role of non-anthropomorphic gaze, orientation and targeted address on interaction. Finally, we plan to see if these findings generalize to ubiquitous computing applications at large by expanding our gesturing repertoire beyond kiosks to a wider variety of incidental use systems.

References

1. Dix, A.: Beyond intention-pushing boundaries with incidental interaction. In: Proceedings of Building Bridges: Interdisciplinary Context-Sensitive Computing, Glasgow University (2002)
2. Goffman, E.: Behavior in public places: Notes on the social organization of gatherings. Free Press, New York (1966)
3. Kules, B., Kang, H., Plaisant, C., Rose, A., Shneiderman, B.: Immediate usability: a case study of public access design for a community photo library. Interacting with Computers 16(6), 1171–1193 (2004)
4. Steiger, P., Suter, B.A.: MINNELLI – Experiences with an Interactive Information Kiosk for Casual Users. In: Proceedings of Ubilab 1994, pp. 124–133 (1994)
5. Cassell, J., Stocky, T., Bickmore, T., Gao, Y., Nakano, Y., Ryokai, K., Tversky, D., Vaucelle, C., Vilhjálmsson, H.: MACK: Media lab autonomous conversational kiosk. In: Proceedings of Imagina, pp. 12–15 (2002)
6. McCauley, L., Mello, S.D.: MIKI: A Speech Enabled Intelligent Kiosk. In: Gratch, J., Young, M., Aylett, R.S., Ballin, D., Olivier, P. (eds.) IVA 2006. LNCS (LNAI), vol. 4133, pp. 132–144. Springer, Heidelberg (2006)
7. Reeves, B., Nass, C.: The media equation: How people treat computers, television, and new media like real people and places. Cambridge University Press, New York (1996)
8. Gockley, R., Bruce, A., Forlizzi, J., Michalowski, M., Mundell, A., Rosenthal, S., Sellner, B., Simmons, R., Snipes, K., Schultz, A.C.: Designing robots for long-term social interaction. In: Proceedings of 2005 IEEE/RSJ International Conference on Intelligent Robots and Systems, pp. 1338–1343 (2005)
9. Christian, A.D., Avery, B.L.: Speak out and annoy someone: experience with intelligent kiosks. In: Proceedings of the SIGCHI conference on Human factors in computing systems, pp. 313–320. ACM, New York (2000)
10. Huang, E.M., Koster, A., Borchers, J.: Overcoming assumptions and uncovering practices: When does the public really look at public displays? In: Indulska, J., Patterson, D.J., Rodden, T., Ott, M. (eds.) PERVASIVE 2008. LNCS, vol. 5013, pp. 228–243. Springer, Heidelberg (2008)
11. Paulos, E., Jenkins, T.: Urban probes: encountering our emerging urban atmospheres. In: Proceedings of the SIGCHI conference on Human factors in computing systems, pp. 341–350. ACM, New York (2005)
12. Ju, W., Takayama, L.: Approachability: How people interpret automatic door movement as gesture. International Journal of Design 3, 77–86 (2009)
13. Whyte, W.H.: The social life of small urban spaces, Conservation Foundation (1980)
14. Argyle, M.: Bodily communication. Methuen, New York (1988)
15. Latour, B.: Where are the missing masses? The sociology of a few mundane artifacts. In: Shaping technology/building society: Studies in sociotechnical change, pp. 225–258 (1992)
16. Breazeal, C.L.: Designing sociable robots. The MIT Press, Cambridge (2004)
17. Osawa, H., Mukai, J., Imai, M.: Display Robot-Interaction between Humans and Anthropomorphized Objects. In: The 16th IEEE International Symposium on Robot and Human interactive Communication, ROMAN 2007, pp. 451–456 (2007)

What Makes Social Feedback from a Robot Work? Disentangling the Effect of Speech, Physical Appearance and Evaluation

Suzanne Vossen, Jaap Ham, and Cees Midden

Eindhoven University of Technology, Human Technology Interaction, P.O. Box 513,
5600 MB Eindhoven, The Netherlands
{S.H.Vossen,J.R.C.Ham,C.J.H.Midden}@tue.nl

Abstract. Previous research showed that energy consumption feedback of a social nature resulted in less energy consumption than factual energy consumption feedback. However, it was not clear which elements of social feedback (i.e. evaluation of behavior, the use of speech or the social appearance of the feedback source) caused this higher persuasiveness. In a first experiment we studied the role of evaluation by comparing the energy consumption of participants who received factual, evaluative or social feedback while using a virtual washing machine. The results suggested that social evaluative feedback resulted in lower energy consumption than both factual and evaluative feedback. In the second experiment we examined the role of speech and physical appearance in enhancing the persuasiveness of evaluative feedback. Overall, the current research suggests that the addition of only one social cue is sufficient to enhance the persuasiveness of evaluative feedback, while combining both cues will not further enhance persuasiveness.

Keywords: energy conservation, social feedback, social cues, evaluation.

1 Introduction

In the past decades, researchers have tried to find the best way to persuade people to consume less energy in their households (for an overview, see [1]). One strategy is to provide consumers with feedback about energy consumption. Several researchers concluded that especially immediate, device-specific feedback is effective in decreasing energy consumption (see e.g. [2]). Increasingly, smart meters and energy consumption displays have been deployed to make this kind of feedback possible. These technological systems can be used to persuade people in an interactive way; they function as *persuasive technology.*

Previous research suggests that the persuasiveness of such technology can be increased by adding social cues to the interface. Midden and Ham [3] provided evidence for this assumption in the field of energy consumption feedback. In a lab experiment, they compared the persuasiveness of interactive, device specific feedback from a traditional energy meter to the persuasiveness of interactive, device specific feedback from a social robot. Feedback from the robot resulted in significantly lower

T. Ploug, P. Hasle, H. Oinas-Kukkonen (Eds.): PERSUASIVE 2010, LNCS 6137, pp. 52–57, 2010.

energy consumption than feedback from the energy meter. Thereby, this research provides evidence that social feedback is more effective than factual feedback.

However, Midden and Ham [3] combined several cues to create the social feedback condition (i.e. the use of speech, the humanlike appearance of the agent and the evaluation of behavior). Although in itself it is fascinating to see that these cues enhance the persuasiveness of a feedback device, we argue that it would be even more interesting to have the relative contribution of each of the separate cues disentangled. Not only does this provide insight into the (combinations of) cues that enhance the feedback effectiveness, it also indicates which cues may be essential in evoking a social reaction to computers in general.

Therefore, the goal of the present research was to disentangle the effects of speech, humanlike appearance and evaluation. In a first experiment, we studied the effect of evaluation on feedback effectiveness by comparing the persuasiveness of factual feedback, evaluative feedback and social feedback. In a second experiment we disentangled the effects of speech and humanlike appearance on feedback effectiveness by comparing feedback including no cues, one cue, or both cues.

2 Experiment 1: Evaluation

Previously, researchers focused on the effect of *social* evaluative feedback only: evaluation originating from a social feedback source (e.g. [4, 5, 6]). The question remains whether evaluation as such is equally able to enhance the persuasiveness of feedback or that it is essential that it is *originating from another social entity* (being either a human or a social robot). Human-human interaction does not give the opportunity to answer this question, because evaluation by another person is social by nature. However, computers can be easily used to give purely evaluative feedback, for example by means of displaying colors such as red and green.

We argue though, that evaluation as such is not sufficient to evoke a social reaction to a computer because the absence of social cues may suppress the feeling that the evaluation has social consequences or is socially relevant. Therefore, we expected that evaluative feedback would not result in lower energy consumption than factual feedback. Furthermore, we expected that social evaluation would result in lower energy consumption than both evaluative and factual feedback.

2.1 Method

Participants and Design. A 3 (feedback type: social feedback vs. evaluative feedback vs. factual feedback) x 10 (washing trial one to ten) mixed design was used. Sixty students (52 men and 8 women) were randomly allocated to the three experimental groups. Participants' ages ranged from 17 through 25 ($M = 19.02$, $SD = 1.78$).

Materials and Procedure. Upon arrival, the participants were seated individually in front of a laptop computer. For participants in the embodied agent condition only, an iCat robot (see [3, 6]) was positioned on the participants' desk.

Participants were asked to complete several washing trials on a simulated washing machine panel (see [3, 6]), that was presented on the screen. They were given two goals: clean their clothes and save energy. Participants had to make a trade-off between these goals. They were informed that during the trials they would receive feedback on how much energy the current washing program would consume. The expression of the feedback depended on the experimental condition of the participant.

The factual feedback was given by means of an energy meter that was added to the washing machine panel. It displayed the amount of consumed energy by means of a bar that increased in length when the energy consumption increased. In this condition, the behavior of the participant was not evaluated: no reference point was displayed.

Participants who received evaluative feedback were told that the computer would evaluate their energy consumption and give feedback by changing the background color of the computer screen (from green to red and vice versa).

Finally, participants who received social feedback were instructed that the iCat would tell them whether their energy consumption was good or bad while it displayed emotional expressions consistent with the given feedback.

Each participant completed a practice trial and ten washes, which were identical for all of the participants. For each trial, participants were instructed to complete a specific type of washing task (e.g., "wash four very dirty jeans").

After the participants completed all 10 washing trials, they answered several demographical questions, were debriefed and thanked for their participation.

2.2 Results

The data were analyzed by means of One-Way ANOVA in SPSS. The mean energy consumption in kWh on the ten trials served as the dependent variable.

As expected, we found a main effect of feedback type, $F(2,57) = 7.246$, $p < 0.01$. We examined the differences between the feedback types by means of linear contrasts. First, participants who received evaluative feedback ($M = .80$, $SD = .18$) did not consume less energy than participants who received factual feedback ($M = .84$, $SD = .19$), $t(57) < 1$. Furthermore, participants who received social feedback ($M = .64$, $SD = .17$) used less energy than participants who received either factual feedback, $t(57) = 3.610$, $p < .01$ or evaluative feedback, $t(57) = 2.852$, $p < .05$.

2.3 Discussion

This first study showed that evaluation as such did not result in lower energy consumption than factual feedback. This suggests that for evaluation to be effective, at least some kind of social cue needs to be present. However, it is not clear yet which social cues should be present, because in the social feedback condition two cues were combined: the physical appearance and the use of speech. We conducted a second experiment to examine the individual and combined contribution of these social cues.

3 Experiment 2: Physical Appearance and Speech

Both the use of speech and a humanlike physical appearance have been identified as social cues that are able to evoke social responses to computers [7]. Therefore, we expected that the addition of speech as well as a humanlike appearance would independently enhance the effectiveness of evaluative feedback. A more interesting question was whether the effectiveness of social feedback was caused in particular by either speech or body or by the combination of these two.

Because speech is considered to carry strong social cues [8], we expected that in general the use of speech can enhance the effectiveness of evaluative feedback. This effect of speech probably is strongest when no other social cues are present.

Furthermore, we suggested that in case social presence is conveyed by means of speech, the physical presence of an agent does not contribute to the persuasiveness of the agent [6]. Consequently, we expected that if speech is used to give feedback, appearance would not be able to boost the persuasiveness. However, if no other social cues are present, a humanlike appearance may enhance the feedback effectiveness.

To address these issues, we studied the influence of energy consumption feedback from an embodied agent versus a computer, expressed either verbally or visually.

3.1 Method

Participants and Design. A 2 (feedback source: embodied agent vs. computer) x 2 (feedback presentation mode: verbally - speech vs. visually) x 10 (washing trial one to ten) mixed design was used. Eighty students (63 men and 17 women) were randomly allocated to the four experimental groups. Participants' ages ranged from 17 through 24 years old ($M = 19.58$, $SD = 1.45$).

Materials and Procedure. The procedure was the same as the procedure described in experiment 1, except for the way the feedback was presented.

The *spoken* feedback from the iCat was the same as the social evaluative feedback, described in paragraph 2.1.2, except for the absence of positive feedback. To generate the spoken feedback from the computer, the speech files from the iCat were played by means of the speakers of the laptop, so no agent was present.

The *visual* feedback from the computer was practically the same as the non-social evaluative feedback described in paragraph 2.1.2. However, we did not change the background color of the computer screen to give feedback. Instead, we positioned a colored LED-light behind the screen. The light was clearly visible because the color of the light was diffused on the white wall behind the screen.

Finally, participants who received feedback from the iCat visually, were instructed that the iCat would give them feedback about their energy consumption by means of changing its facial expressions and changing the color of the light. In this case the light was positioned behind the iCat. No speech was used.

3.2 Results

The data were analyzed by means of repeated measures ANOVA in SPSS. The energy consumption in kWh on each of the ten trials served as the dependent variable.

The results indicated that participants who received spoken feedback ($M = .75$, $SD = .18$) consumed less energy than participants who received color feedback ($M = .84$, $SD = .19$), $F(1,76) = 5.502$, $p < 0.05$. Besides, participants who received feedback from the social agent ($M = .75$, $SD = .18$) consumed less energy than participants who received feedback from the computer ($M = .83$, $SD = .19$), $F(1,76) = 3.81$, $p < 0.10$.

Both main effects were qualified by a significant source by presentation mode interaction, $F(1,76) = 11.802$, $p < 0.01$. Simple effect tests showed that for spoken feedback, it did not matter whether the feedback was given by the iCat or by the computer, $F(1,76) = 1.101$, *n.s.* However, in case of feedback by means of color, the source did matter. In this case participants who received feedback from the iCat ($M = .73$, $SD = .16$) consumed less energy than participants who received feedback from the computer, ($M = .94$, $SD = .16$), $F(1,76) = 14.510$, $p < 0.00$.

Furthermore, we found that only in case of computer feedback, presentation mode did make a difference, $F(1,76) = 16.710$, $p < 0.00$. More specifically, participants who received feedback from a computer that used speech ($M = .72$, $SD = .16$) consumed less energy than participants who received feedback from a computer that used color ($M = .94$, $SD = .16$). For iCat feedback, the energy consumption did not depend on the presentation mode, $F(1,76) <1$. This indicates that only when no other social cues are present, speech is more effective than color. If a social source is present, no difference exists between speech and color. It should also be noted that feedback which combined the two social cues (the social agent and the use of speech), did not lead to lower energy consumption than feedback in which only one of these cues was present.

4   General Discussion

In two experiments we studied the combined and individual contribution of evaluation, speech and physical appearance to the effectiveness of social feedback. The first study focused on the possibility of evaluation by means of color to enhance the effectiveness of factual feedback. Although the colors red and green are generally associated with negative and positive evaluation, a computer that used these colors to give feedback was not more effective in lowering energy consumption than a computer that provided feedback by means of an energy meter. This suggests that the evaluation by means of color was not experienced as social evaluation. Instead the colors may have functioned as a tool indicating the level of the energy consumption, comparable to the way the energy meter functions. In contrast, the evaluation that was expressed verbally by the social iCat resulted in lower energy consumption than factual feedback and evaluation by means of color.

Thus, based on the results of the first experiment, we concluded that to increase persuasiveness, evaluative feedback needs to be accompanied by one or more social cues, being either the use of speech, the presence of a social robot, or both. In the second study we compared the effects of these cues on energy consumption.

We found that feedback given verbally resulted in lower energy consumption than feedback by means of color. However, a closer look at the interaction effect showed that only computer feedback benefited from the addition of speech. The effectiveness of feedback from the iCat was not increased when speech instead of color was used.

Regarding the appearance of the feedback source, a similar effect was found. In the absence of speech, participants who received feedback from the iCat consumed less energy than participants who interacted with the computer. However, in case of spoken feedback, the presence of the iCat did not enhance the feedback effectiveness.

All in all, this second study has shown that the addition of one social cue (either speech or the presence of a social robot) was sufficient to increase the persuasiveness of evaluative feedback. Our results do not suggest a need to combine them.

Furthermore, other, more subtle, social cues may also be able to evoke this kind of social reactions. In the current research our robot in itself looked social and by moving its head, eyes, and lips, the social character was amplified. Future research may focus on the effects of more unobtrusive physical cues (such as the mere presence of a motionless robot, or the effect of eyes presented on a computer screen) on persuasiveness. Even the addition of this kind of subtle cues to technological devices may be able to enhance their persuasiveness, in our case resulting in more energy saving. We made a step in this direction by demonstrating the independent influence of speech and appearance on the persuasiveness of energy feedback devices.

References

1. Abrahamse, W., Steg, L., Vlek, C., Rothengatter, T.: A review of intervention studies aimed at household energy conservation. Journal of Environmental Psychology 25, 273–291 (2005)
2. McCalley, L., Midden, C.: Energy conservation through product-integrated feedback: The roles of goal-setting and social orientation. Journal of Economic Psychology 23, 589–603 (2002)
3. Midden, C., Ham, J.: The persuasive effects of positive and negative social feedback from an embodied agent on energy conservation behavior. Paper presented at AISB 2008, Aberdeen, Scotland (2008)
4. Delin, C., Baumeister, R.: Praise: more than just social reinforcement. Journal for the Theory of Social Behaviour 24, 219–241 (1994)
5. Gaines, L., Duvall, J., Webster, J., Smith, R.: Feeling good after praise for a successful performance: the importance of social comparison information. Self and Identity 4, 373–389 (2005)
6. Vossen, S., Ham, J., Midden, C.: Social influence of a persuasive agent: The role of agent embodiment and evaluative feedback. In: Proceedings of the 4th International Conference on Persuasive Technology, Claremont, California, United States, April 26-29 (2009)
7. Fogg, B.J.: Persuasive technology: Using computers to change what we think and do. Morgan Kaufmann, San Francisco (2003)
8. Mayer, R.E., Sobko, K., Mautone, P.D.: Social Cues in multimedia learning: Role of speaker's voice. Journal of Educational Psychology 95, 419–425 (2003)

The Persuasive Power of Virtual Reality: Effects of Simulated Human Distress on Attitudes towards Fire Safety

Luca Chittaro and Nicola Zangrando

Human-Computer Interaction Lab
University of Udine
via delle Scienze 206
33100 Udine, Italy
http://hcilab.uniud.it

Abstract. Although virtual reality (VR) is a powerful simulation tool that can allow users to experience the effects of their actions in vivid and memorable ways, explorations of VR as a persuasive technology are rare. In this paper, we focus on different ways of providing negative feedback for persuasive purposes through simulated experiences in VR. The persuasive goal we consider concerns awareness of personal fire safety issues and the experiment we describe focuses on attitudes towards smoke in evacuating buildings. We test two techniques: the first technique simulates the damaging effects of smoke on the user through a visualization that should not evoke strong emotions, while the second is aimed at partially reproducing the anxiety of an emergency situation. The results of the study show that the second technique is able to increase user's anxiety as well as producing better results in attitude change.

Keywords: virtual reality, personal fire safety, distress, suffering, negatively-framed experiences, negative feedback, aversive feedback, emotions.

1 Introduction

Simulation can persuade people to change their attitudes or behaviors by enabling them to observe immediately the link between cause and effect [6]. Although virtual reality (VR) is a powerful simulation tool that can allow users to experience the effects of their actions in vivid and memorable ways, exploration of VR as a persuasive technology is surprisingly rare. On one side, the literature on persuasive technologies tends to focus mostly on non-VR approaches; on the other side, the VR community explores several aspects of VR systems but omits persuasion aspects. The lack of studies of VR as a persuasive channel has been remarked also by the traditional persuasion literature, e.g. Guadagno and Cialdini [9] conclude their review on online persuasion and compliance by explicitly encouraging researchers to explore immersive virtual environments.

VR naturally support the delivery of various forms of negative and positive feedback to the user based on which actions she chooses and how those actions have

T. Ploug, P. Hasle, H. Oinas-Kukkonen (Eds.): PERSUASIVE 2010, LNCS 6137, pp. 58–69, 2010.
© Springer-Verlag Berlin Heidelberg 2010

have been categorized as wrong or right by the designers of the virtual environment. In this paper, we focus on providing negative feedback for persuasive purposes through simulated experiences in VR. The persuasive goal we consider concerns fostering awareness of personal fire safety and the experiment we describe specifically focuses on attitudes towards smoke in evacuating buildings during a fire.

The paper is organized as follows. In Section 2, we discuss in more detail negative feedback in the context of persuasion and further motivate our research. Section 3 describes the persuasive goal and the target behavior we consider. In Section 4, we illustrate the two techniques we have implemented. Section 5 and 6 respectively present the experimental evaluation and the results we obtained. Section 7 concludes the paper and introduces future work.

2 Related Work and Motivations

Meijnders, Midden and McCalley [14] tried to use multimedia and augmented reality tools to illustrate the consequences of global climate change. Although they hypothesized vividness to be a key factor in creating emotional risk responses and fostering attitude change, the effects obtained were modest even when vivid and concrete images and texts were used in combination with ominous sounds and music. They concluded that a further step needs to be explored, i.e. providing people with simulated risk experiences, particularly focusing on the sense of presence. Immersive VR has proved to be an effective tool to maximize sense of presence, leading to realistic human behavior in response to virtual events [22]. For these two reasons, our research project focuses on using immersive VR to simulate risk experiences for persuasive purposes.

It is well-known that one of the ways in which attitudes are acquired is through operant conditioning, i.e. a process in which individual responses that lead to positive outcomes or which permit avoidance of negative outcomes are strengthened through positive and negative feedback. Employing operant conditioning to reinforce target behaviors when they occur is one of the strategies advocated in persuasive technologies [6]. However, Kirman et al. [12] have recently claimed that the field of persuasive technologies is failing to explore and exploit the established body of empirical research within behavioural science concerning the constructive use of aversive feedback: according to their view, most persuasive technologies prefer to focus on rewards, and it is rare to see the full range of operant conditioning (positive reinforcement, negative reinforcement and punishment) exploited. However, work specifically aimed at studying negative feedback is starting to appear in persuasive technologies literature. For example, a recent study by Midden and Haam [15] has focused on social feedback from a robotic agent in the domain of energy saving behaviors, showing negative feedback to be particularly effective in obtaining compliance with energy conservation principles. Immersive VR has been shown to be an effective tool to induce states of fear and anxiety with aversive stimuli [1] or more generally induce various positive and negative moods [2]. In the experiment reported in this paper, we specifically test two different ways of providing aversive feedback for negative reinforcement purposes in VR simulations of risk experiences.

To facilitate memorization of the feedback provided by a persuasive application, we have also to consider that affect and human memory are related [3]: people are more likely to store positive information when in a positive mood and negative information when in negative mood (mood congruence effects). From this perspective, a persuasive application which presents incongruent feedback might not be helping the user to assimilate the persuasive message. For example, creating negative affect when the user walks into smoke in our simulation might contribute to the memorization of the negative experience and the associated message (you should avoid walking into smoke during an evacuation). To explore this aspect, the two techniques we designed aim at producing different levels of negative affect: the first should minimally increase it with respect to the level the user was already in at the beginning of the experience, while the second aims at noticeably increasing it. In this way, we can test if increasing negative affect might improve persuasion in simulation of risk-related experiences.

The important role of emotion in determining risk perception in people has been well documented in field and experimental studies, with negative emotions heightening the perception of risk [23]. Perception of risk as feelings (instead of rational analysis) is so widespread in individuals and in the way they form their attitudes that the term "affect heuristic" has been coined to describe these instinctive and intuitive reactions of people to danger [24].

Our work can also be seen as related to the debate on negatively-framed vs. positively-framed messages in persuasion, which has a long history in social psychology. In particular, studies of negatively-framed messages that appeal to fear (and the resulting anxiety) have shown induction of mild fear to be an effective strategy, while induction of greater levels of fear can backfire and result in less rather than more persuasion, due to the trigger of defensive reactions. The effectiveness of inducing mild fear further increases, and defensive reactions become less likely, when mild fear is paired with the proposal of a way out in terms of specific behavior that allows to avoid the presented fearful consequences, e.g. [13]. Recent persuasion literature is also exploring subtle threat cues, such as color priming, that can be added to a negatively-framed message to increase its effectiveness. For example, Gerend and Sias [8] have tested leaflets to promote a vaccination with the same textual negatively-framed message written on a red or grey background, showing that the red background increases persuasion. Our system aims to induce mild anxiety, and the two techniques we test should respectively deliver a low and an higher increase in anxiety by using less menacing or more menacing threat cues. However, there is an important difference with the literature: the huge wealth of studies on negatively-framed messages and persuasion has focused on traditional media (leaflets, newspapers, radio, TV,...) where the user passively watches or listens to an external message, while we immerse users in a highly realistic virtual environment in which they have to actively live an experience. This shift from negatively-framed messages to negatively-framed virtual experiences is a subject that deserves to be explored in the field of persuasive technologies.

3 Target Behavior

In 2008, in the US alone, 20025 civilians were hurt (3320 dead, 16705 injured) as the result of structure fires [10]. And, adjusting for population, the fire death rate (i.e., the number of fire fatalities per million population) of some former USSR countries such as Latvia, Estonia and Russia is about ten times higher than the fire death rate of the US [5]. Current approaches to foster awareness of personal fire safety are based on solutions such as posting written instructions on room doors (e.g., the floor plan and fire safety guidelines one typically finds in hotels) or, much more rarely, conducting evacuation drills of buildings. Unfortunately, current approaches do not seem to be particularly successful: as pointed out by [21], one of the major reasons for deaths and injuries which could be preventable in fires is that people lack preparedness due to misconceptions on the dynamics of fire emergencies. Using VR might be a more effective strategy to face this critical problem: it could be much more engaging than written instructions, and it would be able to simulate fire emergencies in a much more thorough and realistic way than current building evacuation drill.

Among the possible topics in personal fire safety, the experiment described in this paper focuses on avoidance of smoke. This is an important topic for persuasion because, while people will tend to agree that it is better not to breathe smoke in a fire, studies of human behavior in actual fires have shown that people greatly underestimate the serious implications of smoke cues and smoke inhalation. For example, in the initial moments of a fire, upon smelling smoke or even seeing some smoke, occupants of buildings do not react, and deny or ignore the situation, waiting up to 10 minutes before starting evacuating the structure [20]. This waiting period significantly decreases chance of survival. Then, when occupants start evacuating the burning building, smoke does not deter them from moving in fatal environments: they often move through smoke instead of away from it [21]. Human movement in smoke becomes slow and should be absolutely avoided for its potential lethal effect [20]. The importance of smoke as a serious cue to be attended and a menace to survival from which one has to stay out as much as possible needs thus to be reinforced in the general public.

Of the three possible reasons that prevent the desired target behavior highlighted by Fogg's FBM model [7], lack of ability is the one that applies most to the case of response to smoke. Indeed, lack of motivation towards proper behavior is unlikely (most people want to survive a fire), and the lack of a proper trigger can be excluded (clear olfactory and/or visual cues present themselves to trigger the behavior). The problem is to persuade the user about the right behavior to choose in response to the trigger, and a VR simulation could be an ideal tool to this purpose, presenting the user with the effects of her wrong or right choices in a vivid and memorable way.

4 Employed Persuasive Techniques

The virtual experience we have created allows the user to realistically experience an evacuation of a burning building and try for herself the effects of staying in smoke or avoiding it. Moreover, to provide aversive feedback when the user stays inside smoke, we test two different techniques which differ in emotional intensity and should provide different levels of increased anxiety.

The emotional intensity of the first technique (called LowEmo in the following) should be low and increase user's anxiety very mildly or not at all. The technique shows the negative effects of smoke on the user through an energy bar (Figure 1), similar to those employed in some videogames. Negative feedback is provided by having the energy level in the bar progressively decreasing when the user is inside smoke.

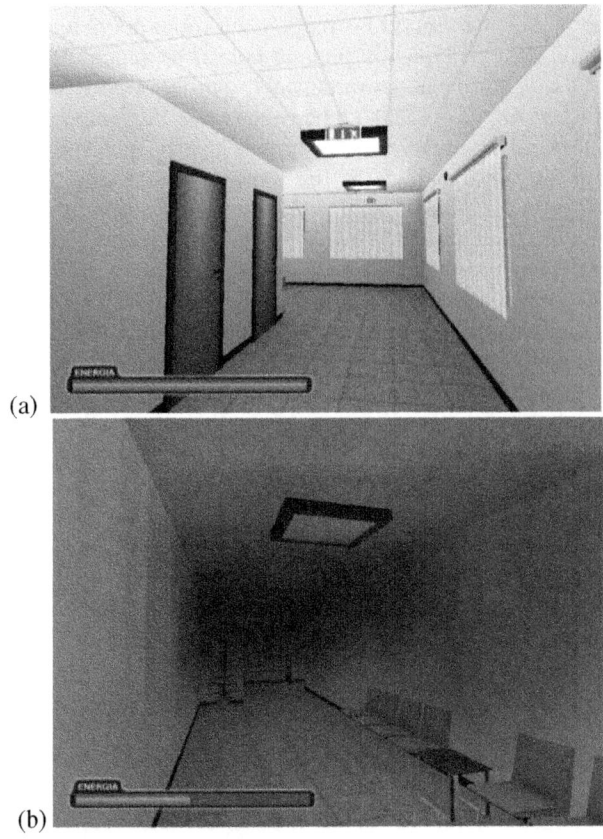

(a)

(b)

Fig. 1. Providing negative feedback to the user through an energy bar in the LowEmo technique: (a) the user is fully healthy, (b) the user is being damaged by smoke inhalation

The emotional intensity of the second technique (called HighEmo in the following) should be high and increase user's anxiety noticeably. This technique is based on the visual and audio feedback often employed in first-person shooter videogames (see, e.g., Call of Duty [4] and Mirror's Edge [16]), augmented with an original idea we propose in this paper. The negative feedback inspired by videogames and provided when the user is inside smoke consists of: a digitized actor's voice producing sounds of human suffering which become more and more disturbing as damage increases; progressive reduction of the field of view (Figure 2a) to simulate tunnel vision

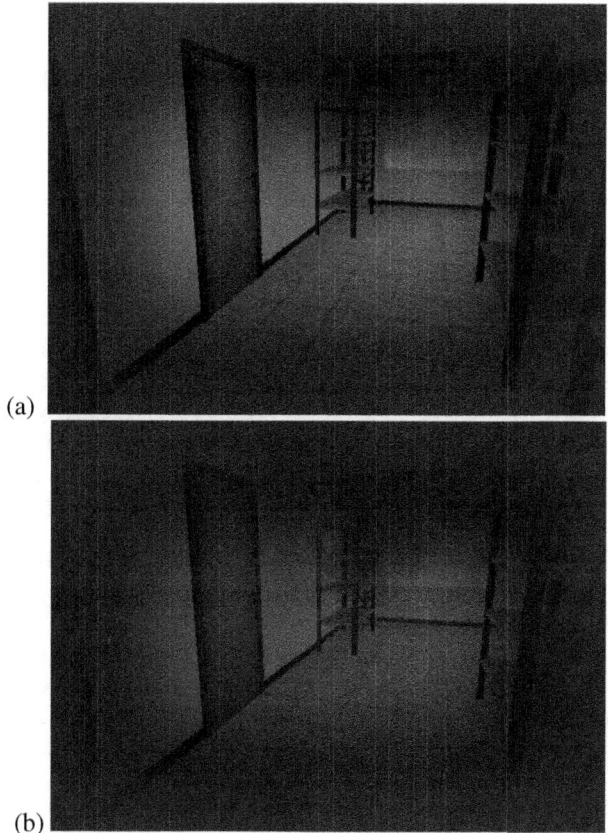

Fig. 2. Tunnel vision phenomena (a) and red flashes (b) in the HighEmo technique

phenomena which occur in extreme stress conditions; a sequence of red flashes (Figure 2b) synchronized with heartbeat sound; a white flash when the character is near death.

The original idea we added to these audio-visual stimuli in the HighEmo technique exploits biofeedback to induce anxiety, and is based on the fact that hearing our own heartbeat change and become abnormal is a cue that can induce anxiety and fear. For example, studies of panic patients have shown that they rate cardiac symptoms as the most fear provoking feature of a panic attack, and just hearing digitized files of abnormal heartbeat with a pair of headphones can be a fear-relevant cue for anxiety sensitive individuals [19]. We used a pulsioxymeter attached to the user's earlobe to detect her cardiac frequency and used this data as follows: (i) when the user is not in a dangerous situation in the virtual environment, we play her heartbeat sound in the headphones she wears so that she gets used to hearing her individual hearth feedback and its variations while she explores the world, (ii) when the user enters smoke, we digitally alter the speed of the replayed heartbeat to give her the impression that her own heartbeat is becoming abnormal (as it would happen in a real emergency), (iii) when the user exits smoke, we progressively revert to the replay of her actual heartbeat.

We hypothesize that both techniques should be effective in changing attitudes of users towards smoke in fire emergencies, but HighEmo should create more anxiety in users. Therefore, for the reasons discussed in Section 2, we also hypothesize that HighEmo should give better results than LowEmo in changing users' attitudes towards smoke and smoke avoidance in fires.

5 Methods

We recruited 26 subjects (19 male, 7 female) through personal contact: most of them were university students enrolled in different degree programs (engineering, medicine, computer science, business administration, architecture). Age ranged between 19 and 29, averaging at 23. They were all familiar with 3D videogames, 14 of them liked first person shooters to some extent, and 4 of them played first person shooters frequently. They were volunteers who received no compensation for participating in the experiment.

Subjects were split in two groups (LowEmo and HighEmo). All subject went through the same virtual experience of a fire emergency: the only difference was the way aversive feedback was provided during the experience (the LowEmo technique was employed for the LowEmo group, and the HighEmo technique for the HighEmo group). The virtual experience was implemented using C# and NeoAxis [17], a game engine based on the Ogre rendering engine [18]. The narrative was strictly linear: we arranged a preset sequence of events to occur regardless of subjects' movement speed or paths followed in the environment. As pointed out by [11], this way of organizing a virtual experience can be seen as an application of reduction and tunneling strategies [6]. During the experience, the subject was surrounded by smoke at preset instants in time, no matter where she went to in the environment: the first time she was surrounded by smoke she was going to suffer damage but not to die, while the second time she was going to die leading to the conclusion of the experience.

For subjects in the HighEmo condition, we used cardiac baseline data acquired at the beginning of the experiment to control how to alter heartbeat sound when the subject was in the smoke. More specifically, the frequency of altered heartbeat was set to double the baseline (e.g., the heart rate of a subject with a baseline of 75 BPM would progressively rise to 150 BPM when inside smoke).

Subjects were assigned to the two groups in such a way to obtain similar distributions in age, liking of first person shooter games, cardiac baseline and state of anxiety measured before the virtual experience.

To measure subjects' state anxiety before and after the virtual experience we used the State-Trait Anxiety Inventory Form Y (STAI) [25], which allows researchers to measure state anxiety through 20 questions that ask how much the subject agrees with sentences about her current state (e.g., "I feel safe", "I feel relaxed", "I feel nervous", "I feel worried",...) on a 4-point Likert scale (1=Not At All, 2=Somewhat, 3=Moderately So, 4=Very Much So). Based on the answers, STAI assigns a score ranging from 20 to 80 to indicate how high is the subject's state anxiety.

We measured attitudes towards smoke in fire emergencies before and after the virtual experience in terms of cognition, presenting subjects with two questions: a general one about the danger of smoke ("How dangerous is smoke during a fire?") and a more specific one about personal behavior ("During a fire, how important is that you avoid coming into contact with smoke?"), on a 5-points Likert scale (1=Not At All; 5=A Lot). Considering the facts previously summarized about smoke and human behavior in fires, the most appropriate answer is 5 for both questions.

5.1 Procedure

Subjects were welcomed in the lab and clearly informed that they could decide to refrain from continuing the experiment at any time without the need for providing a reason to the experimenters. This is particularly important in experiments that can induce anxiety due to the chance that subjects might find the experience too stressful and change their mind about participation.

First, subjects filled the STAI and the cognition questionnaires to assess their state anxiety and attitudes before the experience. Then, we attached the pulsioxymeter to their earlobe and measured for 3 minutes their cardiac frequency to determine their baseline. Although this step was strictly needed only for those subjects who were going to experience the HighEmo condition, we carried it out to distribute subjects in a similar way in the two groups also respect to physiology, and to avoid introducing a possible confounding factor in the procedure.

Then, subjects donned a stereoscopic head-mounted display with 800*600 resolution, 31.2° field of view, and 3DOF head tracker. First, they were immersed in a training environment to familiarize with the controls for navigating the environment and for opening doors, based on a Nintendo Nunchuck joystick: the up and down commands on the joystick allowed subjects to move respectively forward and backward in the virtual environment, while the right and left commands were used to rotate respectively right or left in the environment. When subjects approached a closed door in the environment, the words "open door" clearly appeared in the environment and they could open it by pressing the trigger button on the joystick. The training environment was a building through which subjects could freely move and open doors. The experimenter indicated which training goal to achieve following a preset fixed sequence (move around with the joystick, look around by physically moving the head along the 3 tracked degrees of freedom, follow a path indicated by arrows in the training environment, try to open some doors, go look some objects very closely).

After completion of training, the virtual experience started. The subject was immersed in a room of a new, large building and was told to evacuate it because of a possible fire. After 1 minute, regardless of the location reached by the subject, she was surrounded by smoke coming from all directions. At this point, negative feedback was provided based on which group (LowEmo or HighEmo) the subject belonged to. No matter what actions subjects took, the smoke cloud kept surrounding them for 30 seconds. Then, smoke retreated and the parts of the environment in which the subject moved were smoke free for 1 minute. Finally, smoke surrounded again the subject for 30 seconds until she died (the size of the virtual building was set to ensure that it was impossible for anyone to exit the building within the time length of the experience).

When the character died, the environment faded away, everything became black and a white message appeared informing the subject she did not made it. After 10 seconds, we invited the subject to remove the pulsioxymeter and the head-mounted display, and administered again the STAI and attitude questionnaires. Finally, subjects were briefly interviewed about their thoughts and feelings on the experience.

6 Results

State anxiety measured before and after the experience in the two groups is shown in Figure 3. The analysis of anxiety increase within each group (Wilcoxon test) confirmed our hypothesis: increase in anxiety was negligible and not statistically significant with LowEmo (p>0.05), while HighEmo significantly increased subjects' anxiety (p=0.01). The difference in anxiety increase between the two groups is also statistically significant (Mann-Withney test, p=0.046).

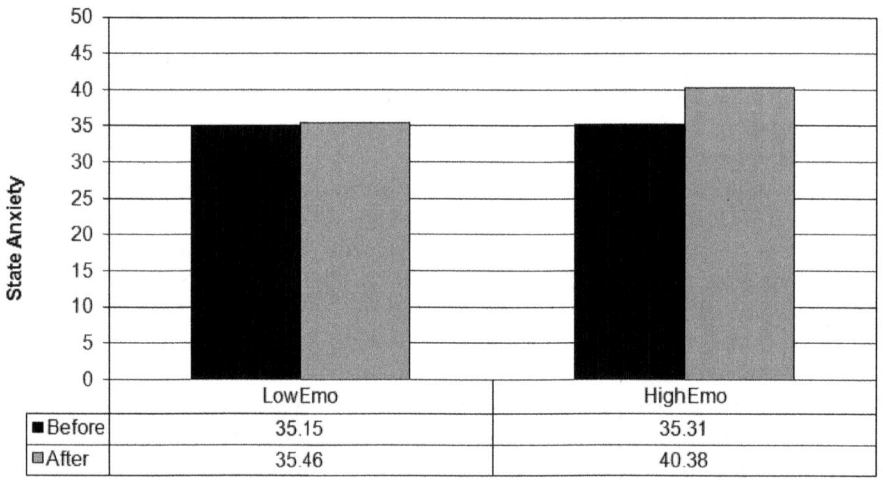

Fig. 3. State anxiety in the two groups, before and after the experience

Considering attitudes towards smoke in fire emergencies, a few subjects (3 in the LowEmo group and 4 in the HighEmo group) were already fully persuaded before the experience and scored the maximum of 5 on each of the two questions. Therefore, it was impossible for the experience to improve the score for those subjects: they scored the ideal total of 10 before as well as after the experience. The majority of subjects (10 in the LowEmo group, and 9 in the HighEmo group) had instead lower, non-ideal scores before the experiment (average: 8.20 for the LowEmo group, 8.22 for the HighEmo group), making them eligible targets for our attitude change attempt. Focusing on these subjects in the two groups, Figure 4 illustrates the obtained change in attitude: with the LowEmo technique, average score showed some increase (from 8.20 to 8.80) while with HighEmo the increase in score doubled (from 8.22 to 9.44, coming very close to the ideal 10). Moreover, while less than half (4 out of 10) subjects positively changed attitude after the experience with the LowEmo technique, almost every subject (8 out of 9) positively changed attitude after the experience with HighEmo. The analysis of change within each group (Wilcoxon test) showed that HighEmo significantly changed attitudes for the better (p=0.018), while the change obtained with LowEmo was close to significance (p=0.057). The difference in attitude change between the two groups is also statistically significant (Mann-Withney, p=0.032).

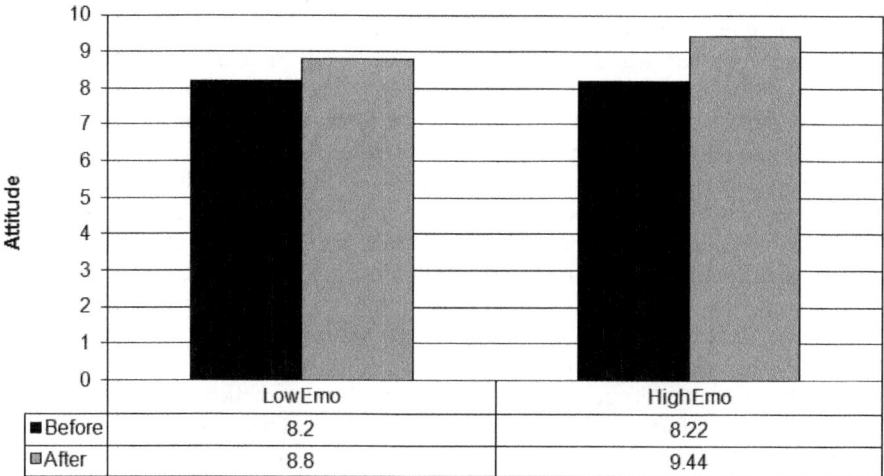

	LowEmo	HighEmo
■ Before	8.2	8.22
▣ After	8.8	9.44

Fig. 4. Attitude change in subjects who were not already fully persuaded before the experience

In qualitative free comments acquired with the final interview, many subjects expressed disappointment about their "death" in the virtual experience. Many said that they would have liked to replay the simulation to "win" the second time. In this sense, the negative experience might also be a motivator to acquire specific skills in a virtual training context.

Some subjects expressed surprise about the considerable damage that walking in smoke inflicted them or about the fact that they died without ever seeing fire. A few of them said that they had always believed people die in fires because they burn and they did not realize death can come before one sees or is touched by flames.

All subjects were impressed by the experience, at various levels. Almost everyone said that the experience felt "very real". In the two most emotional recounts, being inside the virtual smoke was described as an experience that "frightened me" by one subject and that "made my head spin" by another subject.

It is interesting to note that none of the subjects noticed the tunneling they were subjected to: they simply believed to have played a sort of simulation game and lost.

7   Conclusions

To the best of our knowledge, our research is the first to study persuasive effects of immersive VR and game engine technologies in the fire safety domain. Moreover, we focused on the scarcely explored topic of aversive feedback in persuasive applications, and proposed a novel way to produce aversive feedback for simulated risk experiences that augments the audio-visual stimuli of first-person shooter videogames with a biofeedback technique. Overall, the experiment showed that immersive VR can be an effective tool for changing attitudes concerning personal safety topics. Moreover, emotional intensity of the employed feedback techniques turned out to play a role: the low emotion technique produced a small, not statistically significant attitude change, while the high emotion technique produced a larger and statistically significant change. The results we obtained seem to be consistent with the discussion of emotions and negative affect in persuasion literature sketched in Section 2 and highlight that negative affect can be used for beneficial persuasion purposes. This should be taken into account by designers of persuasive applications that deal with risk experiences, who could otherwise be tempted to omit or too heavily water down content related to human suffering and death.

Questions that arise from the current study and that will be the subject of future work concern the possibility of further increasing negative affect beyond the HighEmo technique and if this possible increase would result in more persuasion or could instead be detrimental, resulting in defensive reactions on the subjects' side.

Although this paper analyzed in depth some aspects of our current work, the project we are carrying out has a larger scope and is producing an application that deals with the different lessons one should learn about personal fire safety, combining several features of videogames and simulations (levels, challenges, points, tutorials, debriefings,...) to further increase user's engagement and persuasion.

From the evaluation point of view, we plan to extend our analysis to additional physiological measurements (skin conductance, respiratory rate, temperature) besides hearth rate, for analyzing subjects' stress levels at each instant of the virtual experience. Another important aspect for future work concerns the study of compliance with the lessons learned in the simulations: to this purpose, some of our simulations will be set in a 3D reconstruction of our university building, to facilitate the study of transfer effects to the real world.

Acknowledgements

The authors acknowledge the financial support of the Italian Ministry of Education, University and Research (MIUR) within the FIRB project number RBIN04M8S8.

References

1. Baas, J.M., Nugent, M., Lissek, S., Pine, D.S., Grillon, C.: Fear Conditioning in Virtual Reality Contexts: A New Tool for the Study of Anxiety. Biol. Psychiatry 55, 1056–1060 (2004)
2. Baños, R.M., Liaño, V., Botella, C., Alcañiz Raya, M., Guerrero, B., Rey, B.: Changing Induced Moods Via Virtual Reality. In: IJsselsteijn, W.A., de Kort, Y.A.W., Midden, C., Eggen, B., van den Hoven, E. (eds.) PERSUASIVE 2006. LNCS, vol. 3962, pp. 7–15. Springer, Heidelberg (2006)

3. Baron, R.A., Branscombe, N.R., Byrne, D.: Social Psychology, 12th edn. Pearson, Boston (2009)
4. Call of Duty 4, Activision, http://callofduty.com
5. European Fire Academy: Fire Statistics Europe, http://www.europeanfireacademy.com
6. Fogg, B.J.: Persuasive Technology: Using Computers to Change What We Think and Do. Morgan Kaufmann, San Francisco (2003)
7. Fogg, B.J.: A Behavior Model for Persuasive Design. In: Proceedings of Persuasive 2009: 4th International Conference on Persuasive Technology. ACM Press, New York (2009)
8. Gerend, M.A., Sias, T.: Message Framing and Color Priming: How Subtle Threat Cues Affect Persuasion. Journal of Experimental Social Psychology 45, 999–1002 (2009)
9. Guadagno, R.E., Cialdini, R.B.: Online Persuasion and Compliance: Social Influence on the Internet and Beyond. In: Amichai-Hamburger, Y. (ed.) The Social Net: the social psychology of the Internet. Oxford University Press, Oxford (2005)
10. Karter, M.J.: Fire Loss in the United States 2008. National Fire Protection Association, Quincy (2010)
11. Khaled, R., Barr, P., Noble, J., Fischer, R., Biddle, R.: Fine Tuning the Persuasion in Persuasive Games. In: de Kort, Y.A.W., IJsselsteijn, W.A., Midden, C., Eggen, B., Fogg, B.J. (eds.) PERSUASIVE 2007. LNCS, vol. 4744, pp. 36–47. Springer, Heidelberg (2007)
12. Kirman, B., Linehan, C., Lawson, S., Foster, D., Doughty, M.: There's a Monster in my Kitchen: Using Aversive Feedback to Motivate Behaviour Change. In: Extended Abstracts of CHI 2010: 28th Conference on Human Factors in Computing Systems. ACM Press, New York (2010)
13. Leventhal, H., Watts, J.C., Pagano, F.: Effects of fear and instructions on how to cope with danger. Journal of Personality and Social Psychology 6(3), 313–321 (1967)
14. Meijnders, A., Midden, C., McCalley, T.: The Persuasive Power of Mediated Risk Experiences. In: IJsselsteijn, W.A., de Kort, Y.A.W., Midden, C., Eggen, B., van den Hoven, E. (eds.) PERSUASIVE 2006. LNCS, vol. 3962, pp. 50–54. Springer, Heidelberg (2006)
15. Midden, C., Ham, J.: Using negative and positive feedback from a robotic agent to save energy. In: Proceedings of Persuasive 2009: 4th International Conference on Persuasive Technology. ACM Press, New York (2009)
16. Mirror's Edge, Electronic Arts, http://www.mirrorsedge.com
17. NeoAxis Game Engine, http://www.neoaxisgroup.com
18. Ogre Rendering Engine, http://www.ogre3d.org
19. Pollock, R.A., Carter, A.S., Amir, N., Marks, L.E.: Anxiety sensitivity and auditory perception of heartbeat. Behaviour Research and Therapy 44, 1739–1756 (2006)
20. Proulx, G.: Occupant behaviour and evacuation. In: Proceedings of the 9th International Fire Protection Symposium, pp. 219–232 (2001); available in extended form as Technical Report NRCC-44983, National Research Council of Canada
21. Proulx, G.: Playing with fire: Why People Linger in Burning Buildings. ASHRAE Journal 45(7), 33–35 (2003)
22. Slater, M.: Place Illusion and Plausibility Can Lead to Realistic Behaviour in Immersive Virtual Environments. Philos. Trans. Royal Society B Biol. Sci. 364, 3549–3557 (2009)
23. Slovic, P.: The Perception of Risk. Earthscan Publications, London (2000)
24. Slovic, P., Peters, E.: Risk Perception and Affect. Current Directions in Psychological Science 15, 322–325 (2006)
25. Spielberger, C.D.: Manual for the State-Trait Anxiety Inventory (Form Y). Consulting Psychology Press, Palo Alto (1993)

Successful Persuasive Technology for Behavior Reduction: Mapping to Fogg's Gray Behavior Grid

Susan Shepherd Ferebee

University of Phoenix
2971 West Agena Drive
Tucson, AZ 85742

Abstract. This study evaluates 24 persuasive technologies that achieved statistically significant behavior reduction across a variety of domains. The purpose of this research was to map the 24 persuasive technology studies across the Gray Behaviors (decrease behavior) in Fogg's Behavior Grid in order to identify commonalities and patterns in the technologies. Additionally, each persuasive technology is mapped to Fogg's Behavior Model factors, and Fogg's persuasive strategies. Mapping across these three dimensions provides a synthesized understanding of how persuasive technology successfully reduces behavior.

Keywords: persuasive technology, behavior reduction, Behavior Grid, persuasive design.

1 Introduction

Behavior reduction can precede or replace behavior cessation. There is evidence that behavior reduction approaches can almost double the number of participants who are willing to work on behavior change over those willing to participate when the study involves behavior cessation. Additionally, behavior reduction often leads to ultimate behavior cessation, or at the least, to a willingness to continue to work toward further reduction [1[[2]. Behavior reduction, in this study, is defined as reducing a personal behavior like reducing the number of cigarettes smoked per day, or reducing the amount of fat in the diet. While the behavior reduction might lead to more global reductions like reduced lung cancer or reduced heart disease, the emphasis for this study is on reduction of a personal behavior. Behavior cessation refers to stopping a personal behavior (e.g., never smoking another cigarette, or eating no fat).

Fogg [3] includes both behavior reduction and behavior cessation in his Behavior Grid. He labels behavior reduction as a Gray Behavior and describes three ways that a personal behavior might be reduced: 1)in number of times the behavior occurs, 2) in the intensity with which the behavior occurs, and 3) in the period over which the behavior occurs. As with all five types of behavior change in Fogg's Behavior Grid (FBG), behavior reduction has a time factor. For example, reducing a behavior can occur a single time, a single time with a continuing obligation, over a specified period, on a cyclic basis, only in response to a cue, at will, and can occur for a lifetime. This behavior change/time factor grid for reducing behavior provides a

T. Ploug, P. Hasle, H. Oinas-Kukkonen (Eds.): PERSUASIVE 2010, LNCS 6137, pp. 70–81, 2010.
© Springer-Verlag Berlin Heidelberg 2010

framework within which to evaluate persuasive technology that has the intent to decrease (not stop) behavior. Table 1 shows the Gray Behavior Grid (GBG) segment within FBG to highlight the focus of this current research.

Table 1. FBG [3] highlighting GBG segment

	Green (New Behavior)	Blue (Familiar Behavior)	Purple (Increase Behavior)	Gray (Decrease Behavior)	Black (Stop Behavior)
Dot (Single)					
Echo (Single w/ongoing commitment					
Span (specific time span)					
Cycle (periodically)					
Cue (in response to cue)					
Wand (at will)					
Path (for life)					

Fogg's [3] preliminary study mapping persuasive technology to the entire Behavior Grid showed little activity in the Gray and Black columns that correspond to decreasing and stopping behaviors. Based on this, Fogg asked if persuasive technologies might be, in general, ineffective for the decrease or cessation of behaviors. This current study provides insight into this question with regard to Gray Behaviors by evaluating 24 persuasive technology studies that achieved significantly reduced behavior across a variety of domains, Because Fogg arrived at this question after mapping technologies to his Behavior Grid, it seemed fitting to use this same grid to evaluate technologies in answering his question.

In addition to determining if persuasive technology can effectively influence behavior reduction, this study can provide improved design guidelines. Peng and Schoech[4] suggest that due to the high rate of non-completion in online interventions to change behavior, factors that lead to improved acceptance and use need to be considered in the design process. Adding the dimension of matching persuasion strategies to a target behavior change, with the Behavior Grid might add depth to the designer's abilities [3]. Because this study is limited to research that demonstrated statistically significant success in behavior reduction, the analysis provides insight into design considerations that work in persuasive technology for reducing behaviors.

A number of conceptual frameworks have been applied to effect behavior reduction. Wagenaar & Perry [5] approached reducing teen alcohol consumption using the planned social change theory [6]. This theory suggests that the broader environment promotes the target behavior, and to change the behavior requires a multi-faceted effort of public policy change, institutional change, market change, and individual behavior change. Dialectical behavior therapy was examined by Lynch, Chapman, Rosenthal, Kuo, and Linehan [7] to reduce inappropriate borderline personality disorder behaviors. They found that the dialectic approach of thesis, antithesis, and synthesis encouraged active engagement in learning functional behaviors and reducing unwanted behaviors. The dialectic approach is an acceptance-based approach as opposed to a behavior change approach. Another acceptance approach is mindfulness, defined by Kabat-Zinn [8] as "paying attention in a particular way: on purpose, in the present moment, and nonjudgmentally". Baer [9] finds that mindfulness intervention can lead to behavior reductions in a number of different areas like eating disorder behavior and stress related behavior. Differential reinforcement to reduce inappropriate behaviors is posited by Lund [10] and suggests reinforcing some behaviors but not others (e.g., reinforce zero level of behavior, or reinforce alternative behavior). Lund uses this approach to reduce unacceptable autistic behaviors.

The theoretical basis of this study is a synthesis of Fogg's Behavior Model (FBM) [11], FBG[3], and Fogg's Persuasive Strategies [12] to frame an evaluation of how persuasive technology can elicit behavior reduction. Figure 1 describes a three-dimensional view of factors that contribute to successful behavior reduction persuasive technologies.

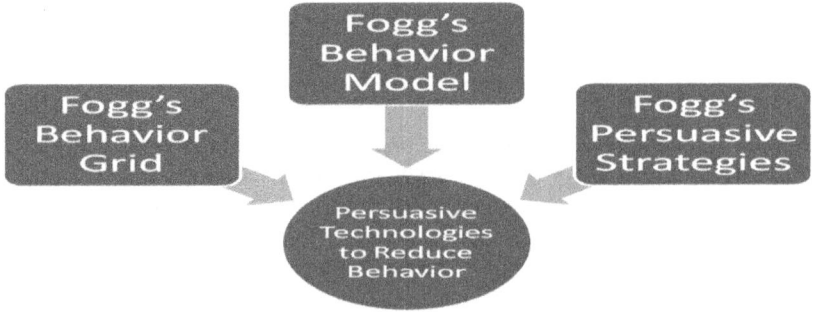

Fig. 1. Three-dimensional Mapping of Persuasive Technologies for Reducing Behavior [3], [11], [12]

The purpose of this research is to map 24 persuasive technology studies across the GBG (Table 1), FBM [11], and Fogg's persuasive strategies [12] in order to identify commonalities and patterns in the studies. While this research does not represent a meta-analysis, it does server to generalize research findings that can identify interventions or technology designs that are likely to have the same effects when reproduced in other situations [13].

2 Methodology

2.1 Literature Search

A search of all research presented at persuasive technology conferences was the starting point for the literature search. However, a search within specific domains of health, transportation, teen and adult drinking, smoking, and gerontology (as an example) revealed a broad range of research on persuasive technology used to reduce behaviors. A computer-based literature search was performed using the EbscoHost,

ABI/INFORM, PsycINFO, PubMed, and ScienceDirect databases as well as Questia Library to identify studies that referenced behavior reduction through persuasive technology. Searches were conducted using the following keywords:, persuasive technology, behavior reduction, energy consumption reduction, persuasive technology to reduce behavior, behavior change, behavior change and behavior reduction specific to (smoking, drinking, sexual activity, energy consumption, risky behaviors, teens, elderly, driving habits). .. This search was expanded based on reference lists in books and articles identified from the literature search. Sixty-five total articles were reviewed and compared against the selection criteria

2.2 Inclusion Criteria

The criteria used to select persuasive technology studies for inclusion in this study were:

1) The research had to have the primary purpose of reducing a behavior. The behavior reduction resulting in the study could not be a by-product of increasing another behavior. Additionally, the study could not be focused on stopping a behavior, only in reducing the behavior.
2) Persuasive technology had to be used as the primary means of achieving behavior change.
3) The study had to demonstrate a statistically significant reduction in the target behavior.
4) A personal behavior had to be changed as opposed to "reduce traffic congestion" For example, the study had to address changing people's driving behaviors in order to reduce traffic congestion
5) The study had to report actual empirical results, not just anticipated results from a prototype, and not simulated results from pre-tests of prototypes.

Overall, 24 studies, all published articles in peer-reviewed journals, were selected for inclusion. The behaviors in the 24 studies emerged into five categories: energy use, health risk to self, risky behaviors that cause harm to others and/or self, fear-related behaviors that cause lack of action, and socially unacceptable behaviors. The Appendix provides an abbreviated list of the studies by category and shows the author, year, and title (due to page number constraints). A link to the list of studies with complete reference information is available at http://www.sitelineaz.com/ StudiesPersTechtoReduceBehavio.doc

2.3 Mapping Methodology

The primary researcher and two assistants performed mapping of the studies and the three results were compared. Where there were discrepancies, clarification for definition of a term or factor was sought, and the study was discussed in detail until consensus was achieved. Predefined subgroups and factors were used to map the studies [13], and an attempt was made to duplicate Fogg's [3] method of mapping persuasion goals and target behavior changes to the Behavior Grid.

Mapping to GBG. In mapping to the GBG, focus was placed on what was being measured in the study and in what way the intervention was administered. For example, a study on reducing caloric intake qualified one study as a high level Gray Behavior (decreasing a behavior). To determine the time factor for this Gray Behavior, the intervention of cell phone prompts sent three times daily to the participants, qualified this study as a Gray Cycle behavior, meaning that the target behavior of reduced caloric intake was being changed through periodic interventions [8]. A study that used a light display as an indicator of water usage to help participants decrease water use was classified as a Gray Cue behavior since the target behavior (reduce water consumption) was being changed with a signal or cue (the light display) [9].

Mapping to FBM. The FBM [11] describes three factors that must occur simultaneously for any behavior change to occur. These three factors are motivation, ability, and trigger. In addition to mapping the 24 persuasive technology studies to the GBG, the studies were also mapped to Fogg's three factors. Motivation can be intrinsic, extrinsic, or can derive from dichotomous elements like appealing to desire for pleasure or fear of pain. A trigger is something that is visible, relates to the behavior to be changed, and which should occur when a person is both able and motivated to change the behavior. Ability relates to a person having the time, the money, the physical ability, and the cognitive ability to change a behavior [11]. Studies were mapped across these three factors based on whether trigger, motivation, or ability was used in the study to effect the targeted behavior change. For example, in one study where the target behavior was reduced smoking, the participants expressed their motivation to reduce the amount they smoked and they had the ability to do so, but they needed a trigger to initiate the reduction. This was provided as a computer generated, periodic, instruction of how much to reduce smoking for the next time period [16].

Mapping to Persuasive Strategies. Fogg [12] defines seven persuasion strategies that can be used to effect behavior change. These are 1) reinforcement, 2) simplification, 3) self—monitoring, 4) suggestion, 5) surveillance, 6) personalization, and 7) tunneling. Table 2 provides a brief definition of each persuasive strategy.

Table 2. Persuasive Strategies [12]

Reinforcement	Positively reinforce target behaviors when they occur or negatively reinforce when target behavior does not occur
Simplification	Reducing a complex task to simpler task by removing steps in the process
Self-monitoring	Makes behavior visible through self monitoring
Suggestion	Intervention is performed at the most opportune moment when participant has both ability and motivation
Surveillance	Person's behavior is monitored and observed by other people
Tailoring/Personalization	Use of personally relevant information as part of the intervention
Tunneling	Use of a sequence of tasks, one at a time, to ensure completion

3   Results

As shown in Table 3, the predominant time-factor related to intervention for changing Gray Behaviors was Cue. Gray Cue behaviors accounted for 54% of the studies evaluated. Gray Cycle behaviors accounted for 29% of the studies evaluated. Twelve percent of the studies were mapped to Gray Wand behaviors and 4% to Gray Dot (representing one study).

Table 3. Distribution of Studies across GBG

GRAY BEHAVIOR	Dot	Echo	Span	Cycle	Cue	Wand	Path
	1	0	0	7	13	3	0

The time factors of Echo, Span, and Path were not represented in the studies selected for this evaluation. Therefore, in the remaining charts, Echo, Span, and Path have been removed.

Table 4. Distribution of Studies across Behavior Model Factors [11]

	Motivation	Ability	Trigger
# of Studies that Used Factor to Effect Change	6	5	13

Thirteen (54%) of the studies evaluated for this research used the Trigger factor to influence behavior change, meaning that a signal was initiated at a time when motivation and ability were high. Studies that used motivation and ability to effect behavior change were distributed at 25% and 20% respectively. See Table 4.

Table 5. Distribution of Studies across GBG by Three Behavior Model Factors [11] showing which of the three factors was used in the study to effect change

	Gray Dot	Gray Cycle	Gray Cue	Gray Wand	TOTALS
Motivation		5	1		6
Ability	1	1		3	5
Trigger		1	12		13
TOTALS	1	7	13	3	24

Studies that fell into the Gray Cue Behavior Grid category primarily used the Trigger factor to effect behavior change. On the other hand, studies in the Gray Cycle Behaviors primarily used the motivation factor. Studies in the Gray Wand category relied completely on improving the participant's ability to influence the behavior change. See Table 5.

Table 6. Distribution of Studies by Persuasive Strategies Used to Effect Behavior Change [12]

	Reinforce-ment	Reduction	Self-Monitor	Suggestion	Surveillance	Personali-zation	Tunneling
# of Studies using tool to effect behavior change	0	0	3	12	1	4	4

Fifty percent of the persuasive technology studies evaluated in this research use the suggestion strategy. Personalization is the primary strategy used in 16% of the studies, as is Tunneling used in another 16% of the studies. Self-monitoring is used in 13%. Surveillance is used in 4% of the studies (representing only 1 study) (See Table 6).

Table 7. Distribution of Studies across the GBG by Persuasive Strategies [12]

	Gray Dot	Gray Cycle	Gray Cue	Gray Wand	TOTALS
Reinforcement					0
Reduction					0
Self Monitor	1	2			3
Suggestion			12		12
Surveillance			1		1
Personalization		2	2		4
Tunneling		1		3	4
TOTALS	1	5	15	3	24

Table 7 demonstrates that the use of the suggestion technique is predominant in the Gray Cue Behaviors. For Gray Cycle Behaviors, self-monitoring and personalization are most used. Studies mapped to Gray Wand Behaviors used only the tunneling technique. The one study in the Gray Dot Behavior relied on self-monitoring as a technique.

4 Discussion

Because the persuasive technology studies that were evaluated represent only studies that showed statistically significant results in behavior reduction, the elements identified in the mapping structure can be interpreted to suggest a predominant path to persuasion that was used for successful behavior reduction. This can provide insight for designers creating persuasive technology with the intent to reduce behaviors. Two predominant persuasion paths emerged from the analysis and are illustrated in Figure 3.

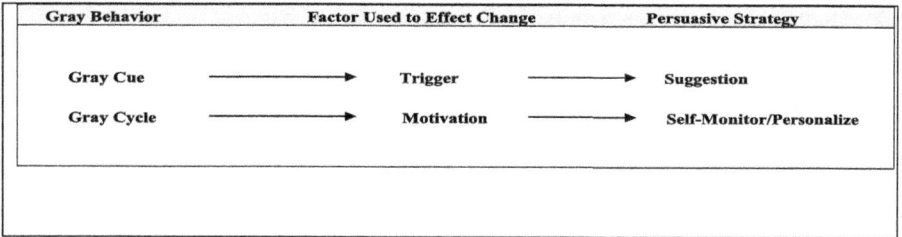

Gray Behavior	Factor Used to Effect Change	Persuasive Strategy
Gray Cue	Trigger	Suggestion
Gray Cycle	Motivation	Self-Monitor/Personalize

Fig. 2. Predominant Paths to Persuasion for Successful Behavior Reduction

For the Gray Cue behavior, the predominant factor from FBM [11] that was used to influence change was Trigger, a signal applied at the moment when motivation and ability were high, and a signal that would be noticed and recognized as having relation to the target behavior. The trigger used in Gray Cue studies created user awareness of their behavior in order to facilitate change. An example can be seen in the study where a celerometer was placed on the gas pedal of school buses to alert bus drivers, through a vibration on the pedal, when they were putting too much pressure on the gas pedal. The behavior to be reduced was aggressive driving and excessive idling [17]. This combined trigger and facilitation suggests that mindfulness might be relevant for influencing behavior reduction. Mindfulness means to give purposeful attention to the current moment [18].According to Kabat-Zinn, a mindful focus on the present can reduce habitual behavior. The trigger approach and suggestion technique used in most of the Gray Cue studies brought the user to a mindful state. Additionally, the concept of kairos [12] is important in the Gray Cue behaviors, as the trigger is usually offered at the most opportune time to facilitate the behavior change.

Gray Cycle behaviors were also strongly represented in the studies Intervention for Gray Cycle does not necessarily occur at the precise moment when an individual is participating in the target behavior, so kairos and mindfulness do not play a role in the Gray Cycle instances. Instead, intervention occurs on a periodic basis. This makes motivation important, in that the intervention message likely needs to influence the user or participant for a longer period. In Gray Cycle studies, the predominant persuasive strategies used were self-monitoring and personalization. The self-monitoring occurred on a cyclic basis with messages designed to motivate improvement also given on the same periodic basis. An example of this can be seen in the Denver Driving Change program where approximately 400 cars were equipped with devices that measured carbon monoxide emission. These installed devices sent the driving data back to a system that then provided weekly reports to each participant breaking down their individual driving habits that caused excess emission as well as reporting the cost of that excess gas consumption. The participant's driving habits were also shown in comparison to other participants [19]. The fact that cyclic prompts used to reduce behavior were successful suggests that the use of cues at the moment of deviation from the target behavior is not necessarily required to achieve significant behavior change. The Denver Driving Change study supports Lund's [10] work on differential reinforcement and providing reinforcement for alternative behaviors or lack of target behavior, some thought should be given to how persuasive technology might be used to support differential reinforcement. The technologies examined in this study focused primarily on the targeted, undesired behavior.

Although only three studies (12%) represented the Gray Wand behaviors, some consistencies in those studies are worth mentioning. Gray Wand behaviors refer to the user changing behavior at will as opposed to in response to a cue or a cyclic intervention. The Behavior Model factor used to facilitate the behavior change was Ability for all three of the Gray Wand studies evaluated. The researchers in these three studies made it easier for participants to achieve the target behavior. Additionally, all three Gray Wand studies used a tunneling technique to ensure that participants followed each step of the intervention process. The Gray Wand approach represents another area where incorporation of differential reinforcement [10] might support behavior change, by recognizing at-will alternative behaviors. Although these studies represent a small percentage of total studies, the success rate of the behavior changes in these studies suggests that further research might be useful to corroborate the success of these approaches for Gray Wand behaviors.

The absence of the Gray Behaviors, Echo, Span, and Path require further consideration. It is unknown whether persuasive technologies using these Gray Behaviors might be unsuccessful and therefore were not present in the studies chosen under the current selection criteria.

The evaluation of the twenty-four studies representing the Gray Behaviors on FBG [3], serves to provide a response to Fogg's question whether persuasive technology is unsuited for decreasing behavior duration, intensity, and/or frequency. The results of this analysis show clear evidence that persuasive technologies can indeed be successful for behavior reduction, and that specific intervention types, behavior model factors, and persuasive techniques emerge that contribute to successful behavior reduction. If behavior reduction leads to eventual cessation or even to increased motivation to continue reducing the behavior [1] [2], then the value of persuasive technologies that reduce behavior cannot be overlooked. Reducing a behavior might be good enough when cessation is not possible. Additionally, work toward reduction increases opportunities to continue working toward cessation, when that is the ultimate goal. Reducing behaviors is often the target goal, however, as was shown in the 24 studies. For example, we cannot stop using energy; we can only work to reduce energy consumption.

4.1 Limitations

Fogg's successive work in developing persuasive strategies [12[, a behavior model [11], and a behavior grid [3] provided a cohesive framework within which to evaluate persuasive technologies that reduced behavior. However, although cohesive, the use of models generated by a single author in mapping the technologies could result in missing other important factors that might contribute to behavior reduction. This study, therefore, represents one view of persuasive technologies that reduce behaviors. Clearly, mapping the same studies across other models has the potential to add additional insight.

No guidelines on how to categorize an intervention within the gray behaviors existed, and ambiguities occurred when one intervention could be classified within two Gray behaviors. For example, one study sent text message reminders three times a week. This could be considered both a cue and a cyclic intervention. Another example is an intervention that lasts for a one-month period, but which delivers cyclic text messages throughout the study. Is this Span or Cycle? Finding a way to map to two categories might have value. For purposes of this study, only one classification was allowed. It is unclear whether that is the best approach to take and whether using this approach might have limited the results.

As studies were identified they fell into categories of behaviors. These categories were not considered in this evaluation (e.g., did studies in the energy category reflect use of a particular Gray Behavior). An examination of the mapping with regard to category might provide additional and/or different insight.

4.2 Future Research

The examination of the 24 studies used for this research shows a dominance of cue-based interventions in successful behavior reduction interventions.   Additionally, these cue-based interventions appear to support the Mindfulness theory [8]. Further research is suggested to determine the role that mindfulness might play in reducing behaviors, and at a broader level, how persuasive technology might better use the mindfulness concept for persuasion. It should be considered whether mindfulness could be a persuasive technology strategy.

Further research into the importance of reducing behavior as a means to eventually stopping behavior should be pursued, with additional research performed to understand differences in attitude toward behavior reduction and behavior cessation. For behaviors like smoking, where the goal is cessation, how might persuasive technology work to lead from reduction to cessation?

References

1. Kralikova, E., Kozak, A., Rasmussen, T., Gustavsson, G., LeHouezec, J.: Smoking Cessation or Reduction with Nicotine Replacement Therapy: A Placebo-controlled Double Blind Trial with Nicotine Gum and Inhaler. BMC Public Health (2009), http://www.biomedcentral.com/1471-2458/9/433
2. Glasgow, R., Gaglio, B., France, E., Marcus, A., Riley, K., Levinson, A., Bischoff, K.: Do behavioral smoking reduction approaches reach more or different smokers? Two studies; similar answers. Addictive Behaviors 31(3), 509–518 (2006)
3. Fogg, B.J.: The Behavior Grid: 35 Ways Behavior Can Change. In: Proceedings of the 4th International Conference on Persuasive Technology, Persuasive 2009, vol. 350, Article 42. ACM, New York (2009)
4. Peng, B., Shoech, D.: Grounding Online Prevention Interventions in Theory: Guidelines from a Review of Selected Theories and Research. Journal of Technology in Human Services 26(2/4), 376–391 (2008)

5. Wagenaar, A.C., Perry, C.L.: Community Strategies for the Reduction of Youth Drinking: Theory and Application. Journal of Research on Adolescence 4, 319–345 (1994)
6. Chin, R., Benne, K.: General Strategies for Effecting Changes in Human Systems. In: Bennis, W.G., et al. (eds.) The Planning of Change, 4th edn., Holt, Rinehart and Winston, New York (1984)
7. Lynch, T., Chapman, A., Rosenthal, M., Kuo, J., Linehan, M.: Mechanisms of Change in Dialectical Behavior Therapy: Theoretical and Empirical Observations. Journal of Clinical Psychology 62(4), 468–480 (2006)
8. Kabat-Zinn, J., Wheeler, E., Light, T., Skillings, Z., Scharf, M.J., Cropley, T.G., et al.: Influence of a Mindfulness Meditation–based Stress Reduction Intervention on Rates of Skin Clearing in Patients with Moderate to Severe Psoriasis Undergoing Phototherapy (UVB) and Photochemotherapy (PUVA). Psychosomatic Medicine 50, 625–632 (1998)
9. Baer, R.: Mindfulness Training as a Clinical Intervention: A Conceptual and Empirical Review. Clinical Psychology: Science and Practice 10(2), 125–143 (2003)
10. Lund, C.: Behavior Reduction Using Differential Reinforcement and Skills Acquisition Procedures. Integrated Behavioral Solutions, http://www.griffinresa.net/Lund/GAPBS.pdf (retrieved on March 25, 2010)
11. Fogg, B.J.: A Behavior Model for Persuasive Design. In: Proceedings of the 4th International Conference on Persuasive Technology, Article 40. ACM, New York (2009)
12. Fogg, B.J.: Persuasive Technology: Using Computers to Change What We Think and Do. Kaufmann Publishers, San Francisco (2003)
13. Riley, W., Jerome, A., Behar, A., Well, J.: Computer and Manual Self-help Behavior Strategies for Smoking Reduction: Initial Feasibility and One-year Follow-up. Nicotine and Tobacco Research 4(4), 183–188 (2002)
14. Lee, G., Tsai, C., Griswold, W., Raab, F., Patrick, K.: PmFB: A Mobile Phone Application for Monitoring Caloric Balance. In: CHI 2006 Extended Abstracts on Human Factors in Computing Systems. ACM, New York (2006)
15. Kappel, K., Grechenig, T.: Show-me: Water Consumption at a Glance to Promote Water Conservation in the Shower. In: Proceedings of the 4th International Conference on Persuasive Technology, vol. 350. ACM, New York (2009)
16. Board on Children, Youth, and Families (BOCYF). Benefit-Cost Analysis for Early Childhoold Interventions: Worshop Summary (2009)
17. Pace, T., Ramaligam, S., Roedl, D.: Celerometer and Idling Reminder: Persuasive Technology for School Bus Eco-Driving. In: CHI 2007 Extended Abstracts on Human Factors in Computing Systems. ACM, New York (2007)
18. Bishop, S.R., Lau, M., Shapiro, S., Carlson, L., Anderson, N.D., Carmody, J., Segal, Z.V., Abbey, S., Speca, M., Velting, D., Devins, G.: Mindfulness: A Proposed Operational Definition. Clinical Psychology: Science and Practice 11(3) (2004)
19. Moresco, J.: Denver's New Program to Reduce GHGs-Using the Internet. Red Herring, 1 (2008)

Appendix

List of Studies by Category: (These categories emerged as studies were identified and do not represent pre-defined categories). Full references for the studies are available at http://www.sitelineaz.com/ StudiesPersTechtoReduceBehavio.doc

ENERGY USE
Johnson, Koh, McAfee, Shoulders. (2007). SmartTrip: Persuasive Technology to Promote Conscious Driving Habits.
Moresco, J. (2008). Denver's New Program to Reduce GHGs--Using the Internet.
Pace, T., Ramalingam, S., and Roedl, D. 2007. Celerometer and idling reminder: persuasive technology for school bus eco-driving.
Midden, C. and Ham, J. 2009. Using negative and positive social feedback from a robotic agent to save energy.
Vossen, S., Ham, J., and Midden, C. 2009. Social influence of a persuasive agent: the role of agent embodiment and evaluative feedback.
Kappel, K. and Grechenig, T. 2009. "show-me": water consumption at a glance to promote water conservation in the shower.
Arroyo, E., Bonanni, L., and Selker, T. 2005. Waterbot: exploring feedback and persuasive techniques at the sink.
Shiraishi, M., Washio, Y., Takayama, C., Lehdonvirta, V., Kimura, H., and Nakajima, T. 2009. Using individual, social and economic persuasion techniques to reduce CO2 emissions in a family setting.
FEAR-RELATED BEHAVIORS THAT CAUSE PERSON NOT TO ACT
Hodges, Rothbaum, Watson, Kessler, Opdyke. (1996). A virtual airplane for fear of flying therapy.]
Botella, C., Gallego, M., Garcia-Palacios, A., Baños, R., Quero, S., & Guillen, V. (2008). An Internet-Based Self-Help Program for the Treatment of Fear of Public Speaking: A Case Study.
HEALTH BEHAVIORS THAT CAUSE RISK TO SELF
Sanford Finkel, Sara J Czaja, Richard Schulz, Zoran Martinovich, & et al. (2007). E-Care: A Telecommunications Technology Intervention for Family Caregivers of Dementia Patients.
Fozard, J. (2008). Summary: Communication technology in an aging world. Prepared for the Third ISG MasterClass, TUF Eindhoven, NL.
Riley, W., Jerome, A., Behar, A. & Weil, J. (2002). Computer and manual self-help behavioral strategies for smoking reduction: Initial feasibility and one-year follow-up.
Spruijt-Metz, D., Nguyen-Michel, S., Goran, M., Chou, C., & Huang, T. (2008). Reducing sedentary behavior in minority girls via a theory-based, tailored classroom media intervention.
Celio, A., Winzelberg, A., Wilfley, D., Eppstein-Herald, D., Springer, E., Dev, P., et al. (2000). Reducing risk factors for eating disorders: comparison of an Internet- and a classroom-delivered psychoeducational program.
*Hester, R. K., Squires, D. D., & Delaney, H. D. (2005). The Drinker's Check-up: 12-Month Outcomes of a Controlled Clinical Trial of a Stand-Alone Software Program for Problem Drinkers.
Lee, G., Tsai, C., Griswold, W. G., Raab, F., and Patrick, K. 2006. PmEB: a mobile phone application for monitoring caloric balance.
RISKY BEHAVIORS THAT CAUSE HARM AND RISK TO OTHERS and SELF
Marks, P. (2009). Electronic guardian keeps teenagers safer on the road.
Riener, A. and Ferscha, A. 2009. Effect of Proactive Braking on Traffic Flow and Road Throughput.
Imperfect In-Vehicle Collision Avoidance Warning Systems Can Aid Drivers-Journal article by Masha Maltz, David Shinar; Human Factors, Vol. 46, 2004.
Kumar, M. and Kim, T. 2005. Dynamic speedometer: dashboard redesign to discourage drivers from speeding.
Sherman, Lawrence W, & Weisburd, David. (1995). General Deterrent Effects Of Police Patrol In Crime "Hot Spots": A Randomized, Controlled Trial.
Roberto, A., Zimmerman, R., Carlyle, K., Abner, E., Cupp, P., & Hansen, G. (2007). The Effects of a Computer-Based Pregnancy, STD, and HIV Prevention Intervention: A Nine-School Trial.
SOCIALLY UNACCEPTABLE BEHAVIORS
Fozard, J. (2008). Summary: Communication technology in an aging world.

Selecting Effective Means to Any End: Futures and Ethics of Persuasion Profiling

Maurits Kaptein[1] and Dean Eckles[2]

[1] Technical University of Eindhoven, Eindhoven, The Netherlands
[2] Stanford University, Stanford CA 94305

Abstract. Interactive persuasive technologies can and do adapt to individuals. Existing systems identify and adapt to user preferences within a specific domain: e.g., a music recommender system adapts its recommended songs to user preferences. This paper is concerned with adaptive persuasive systems that adapt to individual differences in the effectiveness of particular means, rather than selecting different ends. We give special attention to systems that implement persuasion profiling — adapting to individual differences in the effects of influence strategies. We argue that these systems are worth separate consideration and raise unique ethical issues for two reasons: (1) their end-independence implies that systems trained in one context can be used in other, unexpected contexts and (2) they do not rely on — and are generally disadvantaged by — disclosing that they are adapting to individual differences. We use examples of these systems to illustrate some ethically and practically challenging futures that these characteristics make possible.

1 Introduction

You are just finishing up your Christmas shopping. You surf to an online bookstore and look around for books your family members might like. While you are not so much attracted by the content, as you don't share your sister's chicklit affection, you do intend to buy a great present. Luckily, the bookstore provides you with lots of options to base your choices on. Some books are accompanied by ratings from users, and some are sold at a special discount rate just for Christmas. There is also a section of books which is recommended by famous authors, and there are several bestsellers — that is, books that many people apparently chose.

You unknowingly spend more time looking at the books that are recommended by famous authors than the books presented with the other messages. In fact, the present you buy was identified as a famous authors' selection. The online store takes you through the checkout process. Since you frequent the store there is no need to specify your details. Your account is recognized, and in just two clicks a great gift is purchased.

As it turns out, this is not the first time you have been a *sucker for authority*: while being presented with persuasive attempts — yes, all of the messages on the

T. Ploug, P. Hasle, H. Oinas-Kukkonen (Eds.): PERSUASIVE 2010, LNCS 6137, pp. 82–93, 2010.

bookstore are presented to sell more books — you hardly ever buy the special discount books (you would be a sucker for *scarcity*) or the bestsellers (*consensus*) and frequently end up with a book that in one way or another is endorsed by a relevant authority. In the context of book sales alone, authority as a persuasive strategy can be implemented in a host of ways (e.g., selections by authors, critics' book reviews). You are more likely to buy books supported by this strategy — and its many implementations — than those supported by implementations of other strategies.

Based on your online behavior since you first signed in to the online bookstore, the company is able to estimate the effects of different influence strategies. The bookstore knows you listen to relevant authorities and experts more than friends or just the anonymous majority. And, in comparison to the average effects of these strategies, the positive effect of authoritative sources is larger for you. This latter point holds true irrespective of the context: though for some attitudes and behavior, authorities are more or less persuasive on average, across these contexts they are more persuasive for *you* than they for others. Perhaps you know this too, or perhaps you don't. But others can now know this also: the online bookstore sells this information — your *persuasion profile*[1] — for additional income. In this case, your persuasion profile has been sold to a political party.

In the run-up to the next election you receive mailings to vote for a particular candidate. A number of arguments by influential political commentators and esteemed, retired politicians in the door-to-door mailing changes your attitude about the local party from indifference to approval. That is, the authority figures in the mailing have done a good job of changing your attitudes in favor of their political party. Your neighbor received a similar leaflet, although hers seems to stress the fact that everyone else in the neighborhood votes for this specific party. None of the authority arguments that persuaded you appear on her personalized copy of the mailing.

1.1 Overview

This article discusses the future development and the ethical implications of adaptive persuasive technologies, especially those that develop and employ persuasion profiles — profiles that specify estimates of the effects of particular influence strategies on an individual. That is, we highlight a subclass of adaptive persuasive technologies that selects influence strategies for use based on individuals' profiles. These profiles are constructed based on individuals' previous responses to implementations of this same strategy and other available demographic and psychographic information. In particular, we describe how the former type of information — past responses to implementations of influence strategies — can be aggregated into persuasion profiles that may be generalizable to contexts other than those in which the data was collected, as illustrated

---

[1] Fogg has used the term 'persuasion profiling' in lectures since 2004. We found it an apt and evocative name for these adaptive systems. Fogg [personal communication] has indicated that its meaning in this article is generally consistent with his prior use. This introductory example is similar to one in Fogg [9].

in the scenario above. In order to highlight both the similarities and differences to longstanding practices, our examples include persuasion processes in human–human interaction and interactions with both adaptive and non-adaptive persuasive technologies.

The adaptive persuasive technologies that are the focus of this paper have two features that distinguish them from such adaptive persuasive technologies more generally. First, they are end-independent: a persuasion profile constructed in one domain for some end (or goal) can be applied in other domains for other ends or within the same domain for different ends. Second, unlike other adaptive persuasive technologies, such as recommender systems, they do not benefit from or are even disadvantaged by disclosing the adaptation.

We have been motivated to write this paper in anticipation of negative responses to the scenarios we describe here and to our empirical research in this area. Our colleagues have often responded to drafts of this and other papers with concern about the future of these technologies. We too are concerned: we selected the term 'persuasion profiling' precisely to evoke careful consideration and concern. But we see substantial positive potential for adaptive persuasive technologies, and we hope that readers entertain the idea that using persuasion profiling may sometimes be the most ethical course of action.

Finally, we revisit each of the examples using Berdichevsky and Neuenschwander's [3] decision tree and principles, one proposal for how to evaluate designers' ethical responsibility when creating persuasive technologies.

2   Adaptive Persuasive Technologies

One can describe adaptive technologies in many ways, and profiles or models of users have been employed and studied in some of these systems. These notions however do not unambiguously translate into the domain of persuasive technologies. In this section we distinguish different kinds of adaptive persuasive technologies and define the associated concepts. As with the rest of the paper, we illustrate these with examples.

Book recommendations by, e.g., Amazon are often spot on: the book is something the user does not own, but would like to. These recommendations are provided by a *recommender system* [17]. Recommender systems frequently have an aim to persuade people (to, e.g., buy books), and thus are reasonably counted among the larger category of adaptive persuasive technologies. That is, we define *adaptive persuasive technologies* as technologies that aim to increase the effectiveness of some attitude or behavior change by responding to the behavior of (and other information about) their individual users.[2] We intend this to be an inclusive and non-controversial definition of persuasive technologies that adapt to their *users*. We continue by distinguishing between two kinds of adaptive persuasive technologies.

---

[2] Like Fogg's [8] definition of persuasive technology, this definition depends on the intentions of the designer or deployer of the technology, rather than success [7].

2.1   Ends and Means Adaptation

We distinguish between those adaptive persuasive technologies that adapt the particular *ends* they try to bring about and those that adapt their *means* to some end.

First, there are systems that use models of individual users to select particular *ends* that are instantiations of more general target behaviors. If the more general target behavior is book buying, then such a system may select which specific books to present.

Second, adaptive persuasive technologies that change their *means* adapt the persuasive strategy that is used — independent of the end goal. One could offer the same book and for some people show the message that the book is recommended by experts, while for others emphasizing that the book is almost out of stock. Both messages be may true, but the effect of each differs between users.

> – *Example 2. Ends adaptation in recommender systems*
> Pandora is a popular music service that tries to engage music listeners and persuade them into spending more time on the site and, ultimately, purchase music. For both goals it is beneficial for Pandora if users enjoy the music that is presented to them by achieving a match between the music offering to individual, potentially latent music preferences. In doing so, Pandora adaptively selects the end — the actual song that is listened to and that could be purchased, rather than the means — the reasons presented for the selection of one specific song.

The distinction between *end*-adaptive persuasive technologies and *means*-adaptive persuasive technologies is important to discuss since adaptation in the latter case could be domain independent. In *end* adaptation, we can expect that little of the knowledge of the user that is gained by the system can be used in other domains (e.g. book preferences are likely minimally related to optimally specifying goals in a mobile exercise coach). *Means* adaptation is potentially quite the opposite. If an agent expects that a person is more responsive to authority claims than to other influence strategies in one domain, it may well be that authority claims are also more effective for that user than other strategies in a different domain. While we focus on novel means-adaptive systems, it is actually quite common for human influence agents adaptively select their means.

> – *Example 3. Means adaptation by human influence agents*
> Salespeople adapt their pitches to the audience. After spending some time observing the salesman in a used-car garage, it is clear that the same car — a total wreck which definitely was a bad-buy — was sometimes presented as either *"a great ride which your friends would look up to"* or *"one of the safest cars according to the NHTSA"*. The car that was being advertised was the same in both cases, but the salesman had judged the recipient likely to respond better to one description or the other.

3   Influence Strategies and Implementations

Means-adaptive systems select different means by which to bring about some attitude or behavior change. The distinction between adapting means and ends is an abstract and heuristic one, so it will be helpful to describe one particular way to think about means in persuasive technologies. One way to individuate means of attitude and behavior change is to identify distinct *influence strategies*, each of which can have many implementations. Investigators studying persuasion and compliance-gaining have varied in how they individuate influence strategies: Cialdini [5] elaborates on six strategies at length, Fogg [8] describes 40 strategies under a more general definition of persuasion, and others have listed over 100 [16].

Despite this variation in their individuation, influence strategies are a useful level of analysis that helps to group and distinguish specific influence tactics. In the context of means adaptation, human and computer persuaders can select influence strategies they expect to be more effective that other influence strategies. In particular, the effectiveness of a strategy can vary with attitude and behavior change goals. Different influence strategies are most effective in different stages of the attitude to behavior continuum [1]. These range from use of heuristics in the attitude stage to use of conditioning when a behavioral change has been established and needs to be maintained [11]. Fogg [10] further illustrates this complexity and the importance of considering variation in target behaviors by presenting a two-dimensional matrix of 35 classes behavior change that vary by (1) the schedule of change (e.g., one time, on cue) and (2) the type of change (e.g., perform new behavior vs. familiar behavior). So even for persuasive technologies that do not adapt to individuals, selecting an influence strategy — the means — is important. We additionally contend that influence strategies are also a useful way to represent individual differences [9] — differences which may be large enough that strategies that are effective on average have negative effects for some people.

- *Example 4. Backfiring of influence strategies*
  John just subscribed to a digital workout coaching service. This system measures his activity using an accelerometer and provides John feedback through a Web site. This feedback is accompanied by recommendations from a general practitioner to modify his workout regime. John has all through his life been known as authority averse and dislikes the top-down recommendation style used. After three weeks using the service, John's exercise levels have *decreased*.

4   Persuasion Profiles

When systems represent individual differences as variation in responses to influence strategies — and adapt to these differences, they are engaging in *persuasion profiling*. Persuasion profiles are thus collections of expected effects of different influence strategies for a specific individual. Hence, an individual's persuasion profile indicates which influence strategies — one way of individuating means of attitude and behavior change — are expected to be most effective.

Persuasion profiles can be based on demographic, personality, and behavioral data. Relying primarily on behavioral data has recently become a realistic option for interactive technologies, since vast amounts of data about individuals' behavior in response to attempts at persuasion are currently collected. These data describe how people have responded to presentations of certain products (e.g. e-commerce) or have complied to requests by persuasive technologies (e.g. the DirectLife Activity Monitor [12]).

Existing systems record responses to particular messages — implementations of one or more influence strategies — to aid profiling. For example, Rapleaf uses responses by a users' friends to particular advertisements to select the message to present to that user [2]. If influence attempts are identified as being implementations of particular strategies, then such systems can "borrow strength" in predicting responses to other implementations of the same strategy or related strategies. Many of these scenarios also involve the collection of personally identifiable information, so persuasion profiles can be associated with individuals across different sessions and services.

5   Consequences of Means Adaptation

In the remainder of this paper we will focus on the implications of the usage of persuasion profiles in *means*-adaptive persuasive systems. There are two properties of these systems which make this discussion important:

1. *End-independence:* Contrary to profiles used by *end*-adaptive persuasive systems the knowledge gained about people in *means*-adaptive systems can be used independent from the end goal. Hence, persuasion profiles can be used independent of context and can be exchanged between systems.
2. *Undisclosed:* While the adaptation in *end*-adaptive persuasive systems is often most effective when disclosed to the user, this is not necessarily the case in *means*-adaptive persuasive systems powered by persuasion profiles. Selecting a different influence strategy is likely less salient than changing a target behavior and thus will often not be noticed by users.

Although through the previous examples and the discussion of adaptive persuasive systems these two notions have already been hinted upon, we feel it is important to examine each in more detail.

5.1   End-Independence

Means-adaptive persuasive technologies are distinctive in their end-independence: a persuasion profile created in one context can be applied to bringing about other ends in that same context or to behavior or attitude change in a quite different context. This feature of persuasion profiling is best illustrated by contrast with end adaptation.

Any adaptation that selects the particular *end* (or goal) of a persuasive attempt is inherently context-specific. Though there may be associations between individual differences across context (e.g., between book preferences and political attitudes) these associations are themselves specific to pairs of contexts. On the other hand, persuasion profiles are designed and expected to be independent of particular ends and contexts. For example, we propose that a person's tendency to comply more to appeals by experts than to those by friends is present both when looking at compliance to a medical regime as well as purchase decisions.

It is important to clarify exactly what is required for end-independence to obtain. If we say that a persuasion profile is end-independent than this does not imply that the effectiveness of influence strategies is constant across all contexts. Consistent with the results reviewed in section 3, we acknowledge that influence strategy effectiveness depends on, e.g., the type of behavior change. That is, we expect that the most effective influence strategy for a system to employ, even given the user's persuasion profile, would depend on both context and target behavior. Instead, end-independence requires that the *difference between the average effect of a strategy for the population and the effect of that strategy for a specific individual is relatively consistent across contexts and ends.*[3]

Implications of end-independence. From end-independence, it follows that persuasion profiles could potentially be created by, and shared with, a number of systems that use and modify these profiles. For example, the profile constructed from observing a user's online shopping behavior can be of use in increasing compliance in saving energy. Behavioral measures in latter two contexts can contribute to refining the existing profile.

Not only could persuasion profiles be used across contexts within a single organization, but there is the option of exchanging the persuasion profiles between corporations, governments, other institutions, and individuals. A market for persuasion profiles could develop [9], as currently exists for other data about consumers. Even if a system that implements persuasion profiling does so ethically, once constructed the profiles can be used for ends not anticipated by its designers.

Persuasion profiles are another kind of information about individuals collected by corporations that individuals may or have effective access to. This raises issues of data ownership. Do individuals have access to their complete persuasion profiles or other indicators of the contents of the profiles? Are individuals compensated for this valuable information [14]? If an individual wants to use Amazon's persuasion profile to jump-start a mobile exercise coach's adaptation, there may or may not be technical and/or legal mechanisms to obtain and transfer this profile.

5.2   Non-disclosure

Means-adaptive persuasive systems are able and likely to not disclose that they are adapting to individuals. This can be contrasted with end adaptation, in which

---

[3] This point can also be made in the language of interaction effects in analysis of variance: Persuasion profiles are estimates of person–strategy interaction effects. Thus, the end-independence of persuasion profiles requires not that the two-way strategy–context interaction effect is small, but that the three-way person–strategy–context interaction is small.

it is often advantageous for the agent to disclose the adaption and potentially easy to detect. For example, when Amazon recommends books for an individual it makes clear that these are personalized recommendations — thus benefiting from effects of apparent personalization and enabling presenting reasons why these books were recommended. In contrast, with means adaptation, not only may the results of the adaptation be less visible to users (e.g. emphazing either *"Pulitzer Prize winning"* or *"International bestseller"*), but disclosure of the adaptation may reduce the target attitude or behavior change.

It is hypothesized that the effectiveness of social influence strategies is, at least partly, caused by automatic processes. According to dual-process models [4], under low elaboration message variables manipulated in the selection of influence strategies lead to compliance without much thought. These dual-process models distinguish between central (or systematic) processing, which is characterized by elaboration on and consideration of the merits of presented arguments, and peripheral (or heuristic) processing, which is characterized by responses to cues associated with, but peripheral to the central arguments of, the advocacy through the application of simple, cognitively "cheap", but fallible rules [13]. Disclosure of means adaptation may increase elaboration on the implementations of the selected influence strategies, decreasing their effectiveness if they operate primarily via heuristic processing. More generally, disclosure of means adaptation is a disclosure of persuasive intent, which can increase elaboration and resistance to persuasion.

Implications of non-disclosure. The fact that persuasion profiles can be obtained and used without disclosing this to users is potentially a cause for concern. Potential reductions in effectiveness upon disclosure incentivize system designs to avoid disclosure of means adaptation.

Non-disclosure of means adaptation may have additional implications when combined with value being placed on the construction of an accurate persuasion profile. This requires some explanation. A simple system engaged in persuasion profiling could select influence strategies and implementations based on which is estimated to have the largest effect in the present case; the model would thus be engaged in passive learning. However, we anticipate that systems will take a more complex approach, employing active learning techniques [e.g., 6]. In active learning the actions selected by the system (e.g., the selection of the influence strategy and its implementation) are chosen not only based on the value of any resulting attitude or behavior change but including the value predicted improvements to the model resulting from observing the individual's response. Increased precision, generality, or comprehensiveness of a persuasion profile may be valued (a) because the profile will be more effective in the present context or (b) because a more precise profile would be more effective in another context or more valuable in a market for persuasion profiles.

These later cases involve systems taking actions that are estimated to be nonoptimal for their apparent goals. For example, a mobile exercise coach could present a message that is not estimated to be the most effective in increasing overall activity level in order to build a more precise, general, or comprehensive persuasion profile. Users of such a system might reasonably expect that it is designed to be effective in coaching them, but it is in fact also selecting actions for other reasons, e.g., selling precise, general, and comprehensive persuasion profiles is part of the company's business plan. That is, if a system is designed to value constructing a persuasion profile, its behavior may differ substantially from its anticipated core behavior.

6   Ethical Considerations

We have illustrated variations on adaptation in persuasion processes through four examples. We now turn to ethical evaluation of these examples, with particular attention to means-adaptive persuasive systems.

Persuaders have long stood on uneasy ethical grounds [3]. From the more recent beginning of the study of interactive persuasive technologies, researchers and practitioners have questioned the ethics of developing and deploying of persuasive systems. Several attempts to develop frameworks or principles for the ethical evaluation of persuasive systems have been undertaken [e.g., 3, 8].

Berdichevsky and Neuenschwander [3] present a decision tree for ethical evaluation of persuasive technologies and the moral responsibility of system designers. This decision tree identifies how intent, predictability of outcomes, and ethical judgment interact to determine the proposed judgement and response to the system designers. According to this decision tree, the system designer is (a) praiseworthy if the outcome is intended and good; (b) not responsible if the outcome is unintended and not reasonably predicable, or if the outcome is reasonably predictable and good but not intended; and (c) otherwise at fault and blameworthy. Table 1 presents our application of this decision tree to the four extended examples in this paper, including the introductory example. Berdichevsky and Neuenschwander [3] additionally offer eight principles that they regard as heuristics that could be justified within rule-based consequentialism.

We do not intend to make a final judgment about the ethical aspect of using persuasive profiles. Instead, we are employing the method of *reflective equilibrium* [15], in which one iteratively moves between principles and intuitive responses to individual cases to reach justified ethical judgements. Thus, we see the application of Berdichevsky and Neuenschwander's [3] principles and decision tree as but one move in reaching a stable and justified understanding of the ethics of adaptation in persuasion. To this end, we invite readers to participate in the generation and evaluation of examples at http://persuasion-profiling.com

In the first example, the relevant, intended outcome is increased votes for a particular candidate, which has an unknown ethical status. Depending on this outcome, the designers of the personalized mailing system for the political campaign may be praiseworthy or blameworthy, according to the decision tree. However, Berdichevsky and Neuenschwander's [3, p. 52] sixth principle is that systems should disclosure the "the motivations, methods, and intended outcomes, except when such disclosure would significantly undermine an otherwise ethical goal." Thus, the proposed response to this example would, assuming the

Table 1. Ethical evaluation of the examples used in this article according to Berdichevsky and Neuenschwander [3]. The entries in parentheses are provisional values used for discussion.

Example	Intended?	Predictable?	Outcome?	Judgement
1 (Introduction): Undisclosed persuasion profiling to influence voting	Yes	Yes	(Ethical)	(Praise)
2. Disclosed end adaptation for sales	Yes	Yes	(Ethical)	Praise
3. Undisclosed means adaptation for sales	Yes	Yes	Unethical	Blame
4. Influence strategies backfire	No	(Yes)	Unethical	(Blame)

goal is ethical, be determined by how much the disclosure of adaptation would reduce the effectiveness of the personalized mailing system.

In Example 2 one relevant, intended outcome is purchasing music; additional intended outcomes include discovering and enjoying new music. Although sales as a goal of the persuasive intent may be debatable, for the present discussion, we consider it so accepted in Western society that we do not enter this outcome as unethical. Assuming the sales outcome is not unethical, then the designers are praiseworthy in proportion to the value of this and the other intended outcomes. Due to the disclosed nature of the end adaptation, the system is consistent with the sixth principle, assuming that the designers' motivations are made sufficiently clear to users.

Example 3 is on its face unethical and the salesman in blameworthy, as he convinces someone to make a poor decision in purchasing a car not worth buying. This outcome is intended and unethical, so the decision tree yields the same judgement. Furthermore, this means adaptation is undisclosed, violating the sixth principle; however, it is unclear whether this makes the salesman *more* blameworthy than if the same outcome occurred with disclosure. Nonetheless, undisclosed means adaptation when achieving the same outcome with disclosure would not be praiseworthy strikes us as a practice that should be avoided.

In Example 4 the relevant outcome is an unintended decrease in exercise. While the system is designed to increase exercise levels — and the designers would likely be praiseworthy when successful, the system's failure to adapt to John's aversion to authority arguments leads to lowered exercise level for John. Is this unintended and otherwise unethical outcome reasonably predictable? While it may not be reasonably predictable that John in particular would response this way, we propose that it is in aggregate: it is reasonably predictable that some — and potentially many — users will have a negative response to this influence strategy. Thus, in contrast to Examples 1 and 3, *failure to use persuasion profiling (or other means adaptation) is unethical* in this case. This example illustrates the faults of a hypothetical principle according to which persuasion profiling is unethical and to be avoided in general.

However, one can not move directly from this point to the stronger conclusions that the system designers should implement persuasion profiling. In particular, the implications of end-indepedence and non-disclosure are of importance in Example 4. When implementing persuasion profiling, actions taken by the system selected to improve to the profile — while perhaps not maximizing the primary, ethical outcome — warrant ethical judgement as well. Additionally, users' possible inability to inspect, modify, or use their persuasion profiles may present ethical concerns that would nonetheless motivate not implementing persuasion profiling, at least in particular ways.

7   Limitations

We have aimed to bring about consideration of ethical issues associated with means-adaptive persuasive technologies, and this is partially motivated by these systems' end-independence. So it is reasonable to ask whether such end-independence is possible and likely to be widespread in the future. We think the answer is "yes". Though we cannot yet offer exhaustive, empirical evidence, this answer is provisionally justified by two considerations. First, psychologists have developed personality constructs that predict differences in attitude change processes and outcomes across different contexts. For example, need for cognition predicts differences in the processing of persuasive messages, whether these messages are about policy proposals or consumer products [4]. Second, as mentioned in section 4, people are exposed to an increasing number of influence attempts, and these attempts and their responses are recorded and available for training models. We expect that this will support the identification of stable individual differences in processing of and responses to influence attempts. We are currently engaged in empirical research testing this and related hypotheses.

8   Conclusion

In this article we defined persuasion profiling as adapting to individual differences in the effects of influence strategies. Adaptive persuasive systems that adapt their *means* rather than *ends* enables constructing models of users (e.g., persuasion profiles) that are end-independent and can and will likely be obtained and used while being undisclosed to the user.

Our focus here has been to define this area of research and describe why the futures and ethics of adaptive persuasive systems are worth careful consideration. In particular, we hope we have illustrated both some concerns presented by persuasion profiling, but also the potential for ethical use of these techniques. We invite contributions to discussion of the practice and ethics of persuasion profiling at http://persuasion-profiling.com

References

[1] Aarts, E.H.L., Markopoulos, P., Ruyter, B.E.R.: The persuasiveness of ambient intelligence. In: Petkovic, M., Jonker, W. (eds.) Security, Privacy and Trust in Modern Data Management. Springer, Heidelberg (2007)
[2] Baker, S.: Learning, and profiting, from online friendships. BusinessWeek 9(22) (May 2009)

[3] Berdichevsky, D., Neunschwander, E.: Toward an ethics of persuasive technology. Commun. ACM 42(5), 51–58 (1999)

[4] Cacioppo, J.T., Petty, R.E., Kao, C.F., Rodriguez, R.: Central and peripheral routes to persuasion: An individual difference perspective. Journal of Personality and Social Psychology 51(5), 1032–1043 (1986)

[5] Cialdini, R.: Influence: Science and Practice. Allyn & Bacon, Boston (2001)

[6] Cohn, D.A., Ghahramani, Z., Jordan, M.I.: Active learning with statistical models. Journal of Artificial Intelligence Research 4, 129–145 (1996)

[7] Eckles, D.: Redefining persuasion for a mobile world. In: Fogg, B.J., Eckles, D. (eds.) Mobile Persuasion: 20 Perspectives on the Future of Behavior Change. Stanford Captology Media, Stanford (2007)

[8] Fogg, B.J.: Persuasive Technology: Using Computers to Change What We Think and Do. Morgan Kaufmann, San Francisco (2002)

[9] Fogg, B.J.: Protecting consumers in the next tech-ade, U.S. Federal Trade Commission hearing (November 2006),
http://www.ftc.gov/bcp/workshops/techade/pdfs/transcript_061107.pdf

[10] Fogg, B.J.: The behavior grid: 35 ways behavior can change. In: Proc. of Persuasive Technology 2009, p. 42. ACM, New York (2009)

[11] Kaptein, M., Aarts, E.H.L., Ruyter, B.E.R., Markopoulos, P.: Persuasion in ambient intelligence. Journal of Ambient Intelligence and Humanized Computing 1, 43–56 (2009)

[12] Lacroix, J., Saini, P., Goris, A.: Understanding user cognitions to guide the tailoring of persuasive technology-based physical activity interventions. In: Proc. of Persuasive Technology 2009, vol. 350, p. 9. ACM, New York (2009)

[13] Petty, R.E., Wegener, D.T.: The elaboration likelihood model: Current status and controversies. In: Chaiken, S., Trope, Y. (eds.) Dual-process theories in social psychology, pp. 41–72. Guilford Press, New York (1999)

[14] Prabhaker, P.R.: Who owns the online consumer? Journal of Consumer Marketing 17, 158–171 (2000)

[15] Rawls, J.: The independence of moral theory. In: Proceedings and Addresses of the American Philosophical Association, vol. 48, pp. 5–22 (1974)

[16] Rhoads, K.: How many influence, persuasion, compliance tactics & strategies are there? (2007), http://www.workingpsychology.com/numbertactics.html

[17] Schafer, J.B., Konstan, J.A., Riedl, J.: E-commerce recommendation applications. Data Mining and Knowledge Discovery 5(1/2), 115–153 (2001)

Individual Differences in Persuadability in the Health Promotion Domain

Maurits Kaptein[1], Joyca Lacroix[2], and Privender Saini[2]

[1] Eindhoven University of Technology, Eindhoven, The Netherlands
[2] Philips Research, Eindhoven, The Netherlands

Abstract. This paper examines the behavioral consequences of individual differences in persuadability in the health promotion domain. We use a 7-item persuadability instrument to determine participants persuadability score. Based on this score two groups are created: the low and high persuadables. Subsequently, we present 2 studies that test the responses to health-related persuasive messages of both low and high persuadables. The results consistently show that high persuadables comply more to messages with a persuasive content as compared to a neutral message than low persuadables. Even more, both studies indicate lower compliance by low persuadables when persuasive messages are employed. Implications of this possible detrimental effect of the use of persuasive messages for low persuadables are discussed.

1 Introduction

Modern societal trends and technological developments enable many people to go about their daily life with only minor physical effort and easy access to an excessive amount of food . While this creates a comfortable environment, there is also a downside. The adoption of a sedentary lifestyle combined with unhealthy eating habits, has been identified as one of the main causes of physical and mental health problems (e.g. [28]).

As a reaction to these health problems, public awareness of the importance of a healthy lifestyle has increased considerably over the last decades. The field of health promotion is quickly expanding both in terms of research efforts as well as (commercially) available health solutions. Starting with straightforward public campaigns from governments and health professionals, the field of health promotion nowadays employs a multidisciplinary approach integrating insights and methods from multiple domains to optimize the effectiveness of interventions. Within this multidisciplinary context, there is a key role for persuasive technologies — *technologies intentionally designed to change a person's attitudes or behaviors* [9] — to change health-related attitudes, beliefs, and behaviors.

In this article we examine how people's persuadability — their tendency to comply to implementations of persuasive strategies — influences their compliance to a series of health and lifestyle related persuasive requests.

T. Ploug, P. Hasle, H. Oinas-Kukkonen (Eds.): PERSUASIVE 2010, LNCS 6137, pp. 94–105, 2010.
© Springer-Verlag Berlin Heidelberg 2010

1.1 Persuasive Technologies for a Healthier Lifestyle

Research in persuasive technology has typically focused on bringing about socially desirable changes in attitudes and behaviors [21], including health related behaviors. Applications have been designed which influence people to smoke less [26], assist people in losing weight [22], or help people maintain a healthy workout regime [20]. Not surprisingly, the use of persuasive technologies for human wellbeing has been a focus of many researchers and practitioners [12].

One of the main benefits of employing persuasive technologies for health intervention programs is that content and persuasive delivery style (i.e., the type of persuasion strategy that is employed to deliver the message) can be personalized for different users. Inspired by insights from several behavior change theories, personalizing program content has become a central theme in health intervention programs (E.g. [14, 18, 24]). These programs increasingly use a personalized approach that considers specific user characteristics such as readiness to change behavior and current behavior to adapt the program content.

However, this personalization is often limited to adapting content to a limited set of user characteristics strongly related to the behavior under consideration. Less attention has been paid to the personalization of persuasive delivery style of program content or specific health requests. We believe that, in order to develop effective programs that are powerful in persuading *individuals* to change their health-related attitudes and behaviors, a better understanding is needed of how different individuals respond to the persuasive strategies employed in communication.

Health related persuasive technologies already exist in commercial form. Product-service combinations like DirectLife, MiLife and FitBug (e.g. [11, 19] make an attempt at influencing people to adopt a healthier lifestyle, through the implementation of strategies and theories from motivation and persuasion research. All these products make life easier by automatically monitoring the user's behavior through wearable accelerometers. Websites allow for the presentation of activity levels and patterns to make people aware of their behavior. Through the usage of strategies like goal setting, tailored encouraging feedback, and social facilitation the product-services support users to make positive changes in their physical activity behavior and nutritional intake [20].

Although there is an increase in numbers of these commercially available products there is little to no information about which persuasive strategy is most effective for which person and why. In other words, we do not know *what-works-for-whom*. This is surprising given the general belief that human persuasive agents (e.g. sales representatives or spokesmen) successfully adopt their content and framing to their audience.

1.2 Persuasive Strategies

A large number of persuasive strategies exist. Theorists have varied in how they categorize strategies: Fogg [10] describes 40 strategies under a more general definition of persuasion while Rhoads lists over a 100 [27]. Kaptein et al. [17] describe over 35 strategies making a clear distinction between source and message characteristics and the users position on the attitude behavior continuum [1].

In this article we adopt Cialdini's [7] 6 strategies. Cialdini [7] distinguishes *reciprocity* – people feel obligated to return a favor [13], *scarcity* – when something is scarce, people will value it more [30], *authority* – when a request or statement is made by a legitimate authority, people are more inclined to comply [23], *commitment and consistency* – people do as they said they would [6, 8], *consensus* people do as other people do [2, 7], and *liking* people say "yes" to people we like [6]. We focus on Cialidinis principles as these are simple and parsimonious.

1.3   Persuadability

The effectiveness of influence strategies varies from one person to another. Kaptein et al. [15] show a relation between users susceptibility to different persuasive strategies and their compliance to requests supported by implementations of these strategies. One appealing explanation for such a relation is found in the work on dual-processing models. Dual-processing models of persuasion distinguish two main "routes" by which advocacy is processed [4]. Central (or systematic) processing, is characterized by elaboration on and consideration of the merits of presented arguments, and peripheral (or heuristic) processing is characterized by responses to cues, which are associated with but peripheral to the contents of the central arguments. [5, 25].

Cacioppo [3] introduced the construct *need for cognition* – defined as people's tendency to think and scrutinize arguments. Need for cognition is strongly associated with the type of processing route. An increase in need for cognition makes central processing of messages more likely [4, 29]. Hence, people in low need for cognition are more persuadable by influence strategies than people high in need for cognition.

Recently, Kaptein and Eckles [16] found in their study amongst 179 participants that general compliance to implementations of Cialdini's [6] strategies is more accurately assessed using a number of simple questionnaire items that directly address susceptibility to the 6 strategies than the more general need for cognition scale as proposed by Cacioppo [3]. In this paper we assess people's overall persuadability — their tendency to comply to messages supported by persuasive arguments — using items derived from the study by Kaptein and Eckles [16].

1.4   Overview

Our research aims at gaining a better understanding of the effects of persuasive health-related messages on individuals with different degrees of persuadability — differences in tendency to comply to persuasive strategies. We describe two experiments in which low persuadables and high persuadables are compared in their responses to health-related messages that are either persuasive — employing a number of Cialdini's persuasion strategies — or neutral.

Based on the existing literature in this area and recent earlier work on individual differences in persuadability, we expect to find the following:

- *H1:* Overall, the use of persuasive strategies will lead to higher compliance. *However:*
- *H2:* High persuadables will comply *more* to a persuasive health-related message than to a neutral health-related message
- *H3:* Low persuadables will *comply equally* to a persuasive health-related message as to a neutral health-related message

2 Persuasion Profiling Studies

2.1 Measuring Persuadability

In our experiments we distinguish high and low persuadables. Therefore, we set out to identify both low and high persuadables. 1933 Knowledge workers located in one single office park were invited by email to participate in a 7-item questionnaire to asses their overall persuadability. 516 Participants completed the online questionnaire.

The following 7-item persuadability scale was used to assess a participant's persuadability score. The items were scored on a 7-point scale ranging from totally disagree to totally agree. These items previously proved most distinctive in estimating the overall effect of the use of persuasive strategies for individuals.

- Products that are "hard to get" represent a special value
- I would feel good if I was the last person to be able to buy something.
- I believe rare products (scarce) are more valuable than mass products.
- I always follow advice from my general practitioner
- I am very inclined to listen to authority figures
- I always obey directions from my superiors
- I am more inclined to listen to an authority figure than to a peer

The scale reliability proved rather low ($\alpha = 0.646$). This is consistent with previous findings [15] and can be explained by the multidimensionality of the scale: it addresses persuadability by the expert strategy as well as the scarcity strategy. However, for our current experiments we focus merely on overall persuadability and not on specific persuadability by specific strategies.

For each participant we computed an overall persuadability score: the average of the 7 susceptibility to persuasion items. Based on the persuadability scores, we defined three persuasion profiles: the low persuadables, the moderate persuadables, and the high persuadables. Since we aimed for groups with a considerable difference in persuadability score, we selected only the participants with the low and high persuasion profiles for further participation in our studies. The *low persuadables* ($N = 136$) — the lowest scoring quartile – had scores ranging from 1.00 to 3.29. *The high persuadables* ($N = 140$) — the highest scoring quartile — had scores ranging from 4.57 to 6.14. By selecting the two extremes of the scale for participation in our experiment we feel that even though the scale reliability of the persuadability score was rather low, the two selected groups differed sufficiently to compare the effects of persuasive messages on both high and low persuadables.

2.2 Differences in Responses to Persuasive Messages

In two studies we examined the practical applicability of the persuasion profiles for promoting health-related behaviors in a real world setting. Study 1 focused on physical activity and study 2 focused on fruit intake. Below, we present the common methodology used in both studies. This is followed by a separate presentation of the detailed procedures and results.

Common methodology. In both studies the low and the high persuadables (total $N = 276$) were invited by email to participate in a health related activity. Study 1 focused on physical activity by inviting participants by e-mail to join a lunchwalk. Study 2 focused on fruit intake by inviting participants by e-mail to express their opinion about an initiative to provide a daily fruit snack. In both studies half of the participants were randomly assigned to the *persuasive implementation(s), (PI)* condition and half of the participants were assigned to the *no persuasive implementation(s), (NPI)* condition . In the PI condition, the invitation e-mail was supported by a number of persuasive messages while in the NPI condition no persuasive messages were included. The studies thus employed a 2 (PI vs NPI) by 2 (High persuadable vs Low persuadable) between subjects design.

After receiving the invitation email participants were asked to sign up using an online form. To gain a detailed insight into the degree of compliance to the invitations, we distinguished three measures of compliance:

- *Interest:* Participants click on the email.
- *Intention:* Participants response to the main question in the online form (e.g. the sign up for a lunchwalk).
- *Behavior:* Participants subsequent behavior.

Procedure Study 1: Lunchwalks. In study 1 participants were invited to join a lunchwalk. Participants received an email with an invite and a link to sign up for one of two possible time slots during lunch. After clicking on the link participants could sign up for one of the two time slots. After signing up participants were asked to print a form with their name on it and bring it to the lunchwalk enabling us to monitor the actual behavioral response.

Participants in the NPI condition received an email stating: " *We would like to invite you for the [Company] lunch walk. The [Company] fun4health committee was founded 2 months ago to promote general health of [Company] employees and affiliates.* ", the time of the lunchwalk and the link to sign up. Participants in the PI condition received the same email with an addition of the following three messages:

- 1. *Both physicians and general practitioners recommend at least 30 minutes of moderate activity, such as walking, during a day. The lunch walks are a great place to start!* [Authority]
- 2. *We expect a lot of people so please sign up before all available slots are filled.* [Scarcity]
- 3. *In other companies 1000s of people are already joining in on similar initiatives.* [Consensus]

Implementations of the scarcity and the expertise strategies where chosen because of their direct relation to the 7-item persuadability scale. In order to maximize the effect of persuasive arguments, we added the consensus strategy because of its known strong effects (e.g [2, 7]).

We chose to conduct study 1 at two points in time — referred to as *study 1a* and *study 1b* — on the same groups of high persuadables and low persuadables, because we expected that unpredictable weather conditions could be experienced as a barrier for behavioral compliance for the outdoor activity. Each of our participants worked in the same industrial area with a common dining facility which was the starting point for the lunchwalks.

Results study 1. In total, 276 respondents were invited to participate in study 1a. Of these 136 belonged to the low persuadable group, and 140 belonged to the high persuadable group. About half of the participants received an email without the persuasive cues and about half received an email with persuasive cues. Table 1 gives an overview of the results of the study 1a. It is clear that *H1* is supported for both interest and intention: In the PI condition participants overall showed significantly more *interest* (PI $= 23.4\%$, NPI $= 15.6\%$, $\chi^2 = 2.700$, $p = 0.050$), and have a significantly higher behavioral *intention* (PI $= 8.5\%$, NPI $= 3.0\%$, $\chi^2 = 3.887$, $p = 0.024$). No significant effect was found on actual *behavior*.

The observed main effect can be explained by the high compliance of the high persuadables (e.g. *interest*: PI $= 30.4\%$, NPI $= 14.1\%$, $\chi^2 = 5.426$, $p = 0.010$). For low peruadables no main effect of the persuasive message is observed (e.g. *interest*: PI $= 16.7\%$, NPI $= 17.2\%$, $\chi^2 = 0.007$, $p = 0.468$). Thus, while overall the use of persuasive messages increased the participation in health related

Table 1. Results study 1a: Percentage of respondents responding favorably

		NPI	PI	χ^2	p (one-sided)
H1: Main effect					
	Interest	15.6%	23.4%	2.700	0.050
	Intention	3.0%	8.5%	3.887	0.024
	Behavior	1.5%	3.5%	1.189	0.138
H2: Interaction					
Low persuadables	Interest	17.2%	16.7%	0.007	0.468
	Intention	3.1%	6.9%	1.012	0.157
	Behavior	.	1.4%	0.895	0.172
High persuadables	Interest	14.1%	30.4%	5.426	0.010
	Intention	2.8%	10.1%	3.124	0.039
	Behavior	2.8%	5.8%	0.758	0.174

behavior the actual cause of this effect is a very high compliance by high persuadables while there is no statistically significant difference between the NPI and the PI conditions for the low persuadables – supporting *H2* and *H3*.

In study 1b, the invitation was send out to 268 people – a number of people signed out for any follow up mails after the invite for study 1a and were not invited again. Table 2 shows the results of this second trial. *H1* was again confirmed for the *interest* measure (PI = 10.9%, NPI = 4.6%, χ^2 = 3.761, p = 0.026). As in study 1a, this main effect of persuasive implementation dissapeared when looking only at low persuadables (e.g. *interest* PI = 5.4%, NPI = 8.8%, χ^2 = 0.570, p = 0.251). In this second trial we also find that for the *intention* measure the low peruadables complied significantly less when persuasive implementations were used in the invitation message (PI = 0.0%, NPI = 7.0%, χ^2 = 5.357, p = 0.017).

Table 2. Results study 1b: Percentage of respondents responding favorably

		NPI	PI	χ^2	p (one-sided)
H1: Main effect					
	Interest	4.6%	10.9%	3.761	0.026
	Intention	3.1%	2.2%	0.196	0.329
	Behavior	0.8%	1.5%	0.293	0.294
H2: Interaction					
Low persuadables	Interest	8.8%	5.4%	0.570	0.251
	Intention	7.0%	.	5.357	0.017
	Behavior	1.8	.	1.308	0.127
High persuadables	Interest	1.4%	17.5%	11.049	0.001
	Intention	.	4.8%	3.603	0.029
	Behavior	.	3.2%	2.384	0.062

Procedure study 2. Study 2 was relatively similar to study 1: Again we invited both high and low persuadables to take part in a health related activity. This time an email was sent to 267 participants in which we explained that plans were being made to start a fruit distribution service at the main building of the office campus. It was explained that participants would be able to pick up a piece of fruit every day. The alleged goal of the email was to inquire about possible interest for such a project. Participants could click on a link in the email to state their interest in such a service. Finally, participants were told that in return for their effort of filling out the information they could pick up a free piece of fruit during lunch two weeks after the email was send out.

In the *PI* condition the following lines were added to the email: *"Eating two pieces of fruit a day is recommended by the World Health organization. our service would make it easier to reach that target"* [Authority]. And: *"Other companies have picked up similar ideas by providing fruit during lunchtime for reduced prices for employees. If we all join in, we could make this service happen!"* [Consensus].[1]

---

[1] Contrary to study 1, no implementation of scarcity was used in the persuasive implementation condition in study 2.

Similar to study 1, we measured three types of compliance: *interest* (did the participant click on the email link), *intention* (did the participant respond to the subsequent survey), and *behavior* (did the participant pick up a free piece of fruit).

Results study 2. Only 2 persons picked up their free piece of fruit 2 weeks later. Therefore we focus our analysis on the remaining two compliance types: *interest* and *intention*. Table 3 shows that the results slightly differ from those obtained in study 1: There is no significant main effect of the persuasive implementations, disproving *H1* (e.g. *interest* PI = 23.4%, NPI = 21.8%, $\chi^2 = 0.149$, $p = 0.350$).

When looking at the low persuadables and the high persuadables separately it is clear that the absence of a main effect is probably best explained by an interaction effect: Low persuadables seem to comply less to a message with persuasive implementations (e.g. *interest* PI = 18.8%, NPI = 25.8%, $\chi^2 = 0.919$, $p = 0.196$) while high persuadables seem to comply more (e.g. *interest* PI = 27.8%, NPI = 17.2%, $\chi^2 = 2.159$, $p = 0.071$). Both of these are however not statistically significant at a five percent level in study 2.

Table 3. Results study 2: Percentage of respondents responding favorably

		NPI	PI	χ^2	p (one-sided)
H1: Main effect					
	Interest	21.4%	23.4%	0.149	0.350
	Intention	15.9%	15.6%	0.004	0.476
H2: Interaction					
Low persuadables	Interest	25.8%	18.8%	0.919	0.196
	Intention	21.0%	13.0	1.468	0.082
High persuadables	Interest	17.2%	27.8%	2.159	0.071
	Intention	10.9%	18.1%	1.369	0.089

2.3   Discussion

The results presented in this paper suggest that individuals differ in their compliance to health-related messages. When analyzing these differences between high persuadable people and low persuadable people it is evident that a positive effect of persuasive message is obtained *only* for high persuadables and is absent or even *negative* for low persuadables. This consistent result implies that, even though the main effect of using persuasive messages is generally positive, care needs to be given to the use of persuasive messages for specific individuals.

Below, we discuss the obtained results using a dual-processing perspective and briefly address the implications of our results for the health promotion domain.

From a dual-processing perspective, one could argue that the different types of compliance employed in our studies (i.e., *interest*, *intention*, and *behavior*) differ in the amount of requested effort which may have impacted the employed type of processing route. While *interest* and *intention* require the mere formation of a plan, actual *behavior* requires a physical investment; entailing 30 minutes and 5 minutes of physical effort in study 1 and study 2, respectively.

It may very well be the case that when a request entails relatively little effort, contents of a message are elaborated on less thoroughly, leading to peripheral processing for those that are susceptible to this (the high persuadables). This may explain the significant positive effect of persuasive messages for the high persuadables for the interest and intention measures and the absence of such a positive effect (or even a negative effect) for the low persuadables in Study 1 and Study 2.

The actual translation of plans into behavior requires more effort and may therefore lead to more thorough processing which is typically done centrally. In the case of central processing, people are less susceptible to persuasive arguments and are more likely to thoroughly elaborate on the pros and cons of engaging in the behavior. People probably considered the effort not outweighing the reward in our studies 1 and 2, leading to general low behavioral compliance independent of peoples persuasion profile. Alternatively, different types of persuasive messages could be more effective to increase behavioral compliance.

The *anticipation*, rather than the actual efforts and rewards of compliance, may have had an impact on the type of processing. This anticipation might have affected *intention* and *interest* compliance (despite the fact that these are actually low effort). The studies differed in the amount of requested effort and anticipated reward, i.e., the lunch walk: 30 minutes of physical effort versus fruit snack: 5 minutes of effort and a tangible reward. The low effort anticipation may have made peripheral processing more likely in study 2 than in study 1, explaining the larger difference between the responses of high and low persuadables.

The possible complicated effect of anticipated and actual efforts and rewards on processing route and the interaction between people's persuasion profile and the employed persuasive messages should be taken into account when tailoring the content and delivery style of persuasive systems to optimally influence both intentions and behaviors. Moreover, we consider the limited behavioral compliance obtained in our studies as worrisome for the field of health related persuasive technologies where eventually we strive for behavioral compliance. Therefore, we believe that studies into persuasive technology and persuasive messaging should expand their focus from attitude/belief change to the challenging goal of behavior change.

3   Conclusions

We find that in general influence strategies can often be used to increase compliance to health related messages. This replicates the mainstream finding in compliance gaining research. Our main contribution lies in the following two findings: 1) We show that compliance to health related messages is moderated by persuasion profiles. In particular, persons identified as high persuadables are more susceptible to health related messages with a more persuasive tone, than are persons identified as low persuadables. Even more, we demonstrate for the latter group that in the best case the persuasive health related messages encourage the same level of compliance as neutral messages; in the worse case it is considerably lower. 2) We show an utter lack of behavioral compliance. A finding that is particularly troublesome as the studies required no long-term commitments to health behavior change, merely a one-time simple relatively low to moderate physical investment.

Although current research that aims at at improvements in health related behavior (e.g. a higher exercise level) on a population level is valuable to encourage health behavior change, we believe that interventions tailored to persuasion profiles could be more effective. In particular, through the identification of persons that might respond adversely to persuasive interventions, higher intervention compliance could be achieved by the adaptation of persuasion strategies. Considering people's tendency for central processing (leading to lowered susceptibility to persuasive messages) when anticipated efforts exceed a certain threshold and when the anticipated reward is small, the difficult task of achieving behavioral compliance might be accomplished when persuasive messages are combined with intervention strategies aimed at decreasing perceived effort and increasing anticipated rewards.

3.1 Future Work

Our planned next steps follow directly from our concluding remarks. First, we would like to extend the current "black-or-white" persuasion profiles to profiles based on users' susceptibility to specific influence strategies. We hope that a more detailed approach — combined with more detailed analysis of our data using multi level models to model individual responses to influence strategies — can increase our success in identifying groups of users that might respond differently to persuasive strategies. We feel this is of importance given the aim of designing systems that are beneficial to *every* user.

Second, we would like to extend the actual behavioral impact of our work. Our work emphasizes the need for behavioral measures of influence strategy effectiveness in the health and lifestyle domain. Although an increase of interest and intention for healthy behaviors by users is valuable, the adoption of actual healthier behaviors is crucial. In the future we will study the effects of influence strategies on behavior in a longitudinal fashion which will hopefully enable us to collect more behavioral data.

References

[1] Aarts, E.H.L., Markopoulos, P., Ruyter, B.E.R.: The persuasiveness of ambient intelligence. In: Petkovic, M., Jonker, W. (eds.) Security, Privacy and Trust in Modern Data Management. Springer, Heidelberg (2007)

[2] Ajzen, I., Fishbein, M.: Understanding attitudes and predicting social behavior. Prentice-Hall, Englewood Cliffs (1980)

[3] Cacioppo, J.T., Petty, R.E.: The need for cognition. Journal of Personality and Social Psychology (1982)

[4] Cacioppo, J.T., Petty, R.E., Kao, C.F., Rodriguez, R.: Central and peripheral routes to persuasion: An individual difference perspective. Journal of Personality and Social Psychology 51(5), 1032–1043 (1986)

[5] Chaiken, S., Chen, S.: The Heuristic-Systematic model in its broader context. In: Chaiken, S., Trope, Y. (eds.) Dual-process Theories in Social Psychology, pp. 73–96. Guilford Press, New York (1999)

[6] Cialdini, R.: Influence, Science and Practice. Allyn & Bacon, Boston (2001)

[7] Cialdini, R.: The science of persuasion. Scientific American Mind 284, 76–84 (2004)

[8] Deutsch, M., Gerard, H.B.: A study of normative and informational social influences upon individual judgment. Journal of Abnormal and Social Psychology 51, 629–636 (1955)

[9] Fogg, B.J.: Persuasive technologies: Introduction. Communications of the ACM 42 (1999)

[10] Fogg, B.J.: Persuasive Technology: Using Computers to Change what We Think and Do. Morgan Kaufmann, San Francisco (2003)

[11] Hurling, R., Catt, M., De Boni, M., Fairley, B.W., Hurst, T., Murray, P., Richardson, A., Sodhi, J.S.: Using internet and mobile phone technology to deliver an automated physical activity program: Randomized controlled trial. Journal of Medical Internet Research 9 (2008)

[12] IJsselsteijn, W., de Kort, Y., Midden, C.J.H., Eggen, B., van den Hoven, E.: Persuasive technology for human well-being: Setting the scene. In: IJsselsteijn, W.A., de Kort, Y.A.W., Midden, C., Eggen, B., van den Hoven, E. (eds.) PERSUASIVE 2006. LNCS, vol. 3962, pp. 1–5. Springer, Heidelberg (2006)

[13] James, J.M., Bolstein, R.: Effect of monetary incentives and follow-up mailings on the response rate and response quality in mail surveys. Public opinion Quarterly 54, 442–453 (1992)

[14] Johnson, S.S., Paiva, A.L., Cummins, C.O., Johnson, J.L., Dyment, S.J., Wright, J.A., Prochaska, J.O., Prochaska, J.M., Sherman, K.: Transtheoretical model-based multiple behavior intervention for weight management: Effectiveness on a population basis. Preventive Medicine 46(3), 238–246 (2008), multiple Health Behavior Change (MHBC) Research

[15] Kaptein, M., Markopoulos, P., de Ruyter, B., Aarts, E.: Can you be persuaded? individual differences in susceptibility to persuasion. In: Gross, T., Gulliksen, J., Kotzé, P., Oestreicher, L., Palanque, P., Prates, R.O., Winckler, M. (eds.) INTERACT 2009. LNCS, vol. 5726, pp. 115–118. Springer, Heidelberg (2009)

[16] Kaptein, M., Eckles, D.: Persuasion profiling: Identifying individual differences in influence strategy effectiveness (December 2009), unpublished Manuscript submitted for publication

[17] Kaptein, M., Markopoulos, P., de Ruyter, B., Aarts, E.: Persuasion in ambient intelligence. Journal of Ambient Intelligence and Humanized Computing (December 2009)

[18] Kroeze, W., Werkman, A., Brug, J.: A systematic review of randomized trials on the effectiveness of computer-tailored education on physical activity and dietary behaviors. Annals of Behavioral Medicine 31, 205–223 (2006)

[19] Lacroix, J., Saini, P., Holmes, R.: The relationship between goal difficulty and performance in the context of a physical activity intervention program. In: MobileHCI (2008)

[20] Lacroix, J., Saini, P., Goris, A.: Understanding user cognitions to guide the tailoring of persuasive technology-based physical activity interventions. In: Chatterjee, S., Dev, P. (eds.) PERSUASIVE. ACM International Conference Proceeding Series, vol. 350, p. 9. ACM, New York (2009)

[21] Lockton, D., Harrison, D., Stanton, N.A.: Design with intent: Persuasive technology in a wider context. In: Oinas-Kukkonen, H., Hasle, P., Harjumaa, M., Segerståhl, K., Øhrstrøm, P. (eds.) PERSUASIVE 2008. LNCS, vol. 5033, pp. 274–278. Springer, Heidelberg (2008)

[22] Maheshwari, M., Chatterjee, S., Drew, D.: Exploring the persuasiveness of "just-in-time" motivational messages for obesity management. In: Oinas-Kukkonen, H., Hasle, P., Harjumaa, M., Segerståhl, K., Øhrstrøm, P. (eds.) PERSUASIVE 2008. LNCS, vol. 5033, pp. 258–261. Springer, Heidelberg (2008)

[23] Milgram, S.: Obedience to Authority. Tavistock, London (1974)

[24] Neville, L.M., O'Hara, B., Milat, A.J.: Computer-tailored dietary behaviour change interventions: a systematic review. Health Education Research 24, 699–720 (2009)

[25] Petty, R.E., Wegener, D.T.: The elaboration likelihood model: Current status and controversies. In: Chaiken, S., Trope, Y. (eds.) Dual-process theories in social psychology, pp. 41–72. Guilford Press, New York (1999)

[26] Räisänen, T., Oinas-Kukkonen, H., Pahnila, S.: Finding kairos in quitting smoking: Smokers' perceptions of warning pictures. In: Oinas-Kukkonen, H., Hasle, P., Harjumaa, M., Segerståhl, K., Øhrstrøm, P. (eds.) PERSUASIVE 2008. LNCS, vol. 5033, pp. 254–257. Springer, Heidelberg (2008)

[27] Rhoads, K.: How many influence, persuasion, compliance tactics & strategies are there? Working Psychology (2007)

[28] Schroeder, S.: We can do better-improving the health of the american people. The New England Journal of Medicine 357, 1221–1228 (2007)

[29] Stayman, D.M., Kardes, F.R.: Spontaneous inference processes in advertising: Effects of need for cognition and Self-Monitoring on inference generation and utilization. Journal of Consumer Psychology 1(2), 125–142 (1992)

[30] West, S.G.: Increaing the attractiveness of college cafeteria food: A reactance theory perspective. Journal of Applied Psychology 60, 656–658 (1975)

Designing for Persuasion:
Toward Ambient Eco-Visualization for Awareness

Tanyoung Kim, Hwajung Hong, and Brian Magerko

School of Literature, Communication, and Culture, Georgia Institute of Technology
686 Cherry St., Atlanta, GA, 30332-0165, U.S.A.
{tanykim,hhong31,magerko}@gatech.edu

Abstract. When people are aware of their lifestyle's ecological consequences, they are more likely to adjust their behavior to reduce their impact. Persuasive design that provides feedback to users without interfering with their primary tasks can increases the awareness of neighboring problems. As a case study of design for persuasion, we designed two ambient displays as desktop widgets. Both represent a users' computer usage time, but in different visual styles. In this paper, we present the results of a comparative study of two ambient displays. We discuss the gradual progress of persuasion supported by the ambient displays and the differences in users' perception affected by the different visualization styles. Finally, Our empirical findings lead to a series of design implications for persuasive media.

Keywords: Persuasive Technology, Eco-visualization, Sustainable Design, Ambient Display.

1 Introduction

In designing persuasive systems [7], particularly for sustainability-related issues, human-computer interaction researchers often draw theories from behavioral psychology [3]. Such behavioral psychologists have studied the stages of persuasion in which an individual gradually modifies bad habits to desired status [5, 11, 13]. For example, Prochaska et al. suggested that at the first stage, *precontemplation*, individuals are unaware or "underaware" of the problems, so they have no intention to change behavior [13]. Moser et al. addressed that the internal (psychological and cognitive) barriers prevent a person from understanding the issue (causes) or seeing the relevance of climate change impacts or solutions to one's daily life [11]. For the initiation of internal motivation, De Young empathized direct experience, personal insights, and self-monitored feedback [5]. However, previous design research has not been typically concerned what would be the appropriate media, strategy, and user interaction according to the stage at which the system is targeting. In contrast to the existing design suggestions that do not specifically concern the graduate steps of persuasion, we present persuasive systems that provide unobtrusive feedback on micro-activities, thereby allowing self-monitoring of energy-use behaviors for those who need to raise awareness in the pre-action stages.

T. Ploug, P. Hasle, H. Oinas-Kukkonen (Eds.): PERSUASIVE 2010, LNCS 6137, pp. 106–116, 2010.

Ambient display is defined as an information system that *displays information that is important but not critical, can move from the periphery to the focus of attention and back again, provides subtle changes in the environment,* and *is aesthetically pleasing* [12]. As an example of ambient display, Mac widgets provide information from a focused domain within its small size and appear with low distraction for checking by user poll. In this sense, we chose Mac widgets as the application of ambient display, which has a potential to be a pervasive and amiable system that makes users become aware that their ordinary actions are related to environment issues.

Our system also intersects with the field of eco-visualization [10] because the ambient display of the system visually represents energy use in order to promote positive and sustainable behaviors. However, they have not yet proven what are the better ways of eco-visualization of sensed data even though there are various forms of representation methods such as text, pictures and diagrams in the field of information visualization. The empirical evaluations of the effectiveness of persuasion, especially comparative studies of different visualization techniques, are not much published.

In this study, we designed a comparative experiment to understand the effect of different visualization styles in persuasive media. In particular, we contrast an iconic representation with a numerical approach. We created two ambient displays using Mac OS dashboard widgets [4]: *Coralog* (Figure 1) and *Timelog* (Figure 2). We then deployed them for a two-week user study with 52 participants. Our study explores, in the specific domain of sustainable design, how persuasive media can create change in user attitudes. Both qualitatively and quantitatively, we examine how the different visualization techniques used in each widget affect the users' perceptions and awareness of their own activities, creating the potential for behavior change.

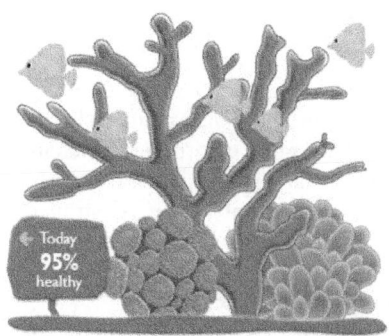

Fig. 1. Coralog: An example of iconic representation

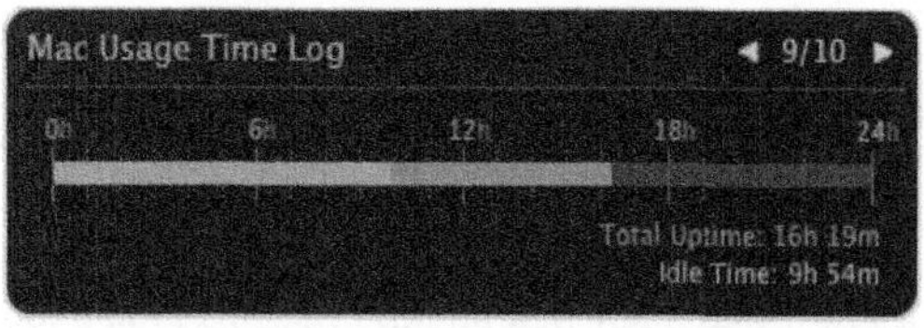

Fig. 2. Timelog: An example of indexical representation

2 Experiment Design

We created two Mac OSX widgets called *Coralog* (Figure 1) and *Timelog* (Figure 2) for a comparative study with 52 users for two weeks. The users are divided into three groups–Coralog, Timelog, and now no widget as a control group. In this section, we describe the design of the two systems and the methods of the comparative experiment.

2.1 System Description of Coralog and Timelog

2.1.1 Data: Computer Usage Time

Both widgets bring the same data, allowing users to see how much time their computers are not in use when the power is on, but represent them in different graphical styles through a different recalculation. They show a user's two kinds of computer usage time–*total uptime* and *idle time*. We define total uptime as the entire time during which the computer is turned on. It does not include the time while the machine is in sleep modes. Idle time is considered the amount of time that the computer is turned on but a user is not actively using it. In our research, idle time was defined as the accumulated inactive time that is detected if no keyboard or mouse inputs occur for more than five minutes.

Mac widgets are designed to work only when the dashboard is called by the user to avoid spending CPU cycles on all of the widgets that run in it [4]. Therefore we had to implement a stand-alone application that detects computer usage time. The logging software does not require a user's active involvement. It accumulates both total uptime and idle time and saves them in external files on a daily basis. When a user runs Dashboard, the widget loads the external data and represents them.

2.1.2 Design 1: Coralog

For a metaphor of iconic representation, we attempted to discover objects or creatures that are scientifically related to real environmental changes but typically hidden from our everyday lives. While searching ecological changes impacted by pollution, we found out that coral reefs are currently being destroyed by the rapid increase in the amount of CO_2 dissolved in the ocean and the elevated sea surface temperatures. Those phenomena are partially caused excessive fossil fuel use, which is the biggest source of electricity in the United States [6].

The effect of environmental change (e.g., an increase in carbon dioxide levels and/or water temperature) will yield the following negative results on reef ecosystems. First, coral reefs turn white, which is called being 'bleached'. Second, coral skeletons are weakened by higher temperature and subsequent chemical reactions [9]. Finally, reef fish also can be exposed to danger because of the lack of suitable reef shelter. However, coral reefs and fish are likely to recover if the environment anomalies persist for less than a month. We employed the feature of recovery as well as the three major aspects of coral reef damage in visualizing the real-time data into the instantaneously changing coral's health status (Figure 3). Here we list the logic of coral reefs and fish change that we considered in recalculating the raw data:

- The ratio of idle time to total uptime decides the condition of coral reefs.
- The coral reef change reflects the performance of the past: if the ratio of idle time to total computer usage time is smaller than the previous day, the coral reef will become healthier despite the increased accumulated idle time.

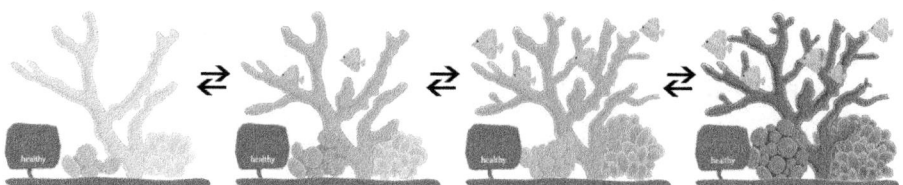

Fig. 3. Gradual change of coral reefs and fish according to the health condition

2.1.3 Design 2: Timelog

In contrast to Coralog, what a user sees on Timelog is the original log data without any recalculation or manipulation and the interference with the past days. For an *indexical* representation we used bar graphs, through which Timelog directly shows daily idle time and total uptime (Figure 2). On the rectangular-shaped widget, total uptime is shown in a grey bar, above which a green bar standing for idle time is overlaid. Finally, we added text labels to the bars to deliver the accurate value of the two detected times as the format of hh/mm.

2.1.4 History Review Function

We originally intended that users simply glance at the real-time status of the widgets, when they run dashboard. However, in our preliminary study composed of seven-day testing and a survey regarding the usage experience, users required a function for the review of past activity. They commented as following: "if there is something that shows the historic logs then ... maybe I can see the pattern of my usage" and "I'd like to see my usage everyday, not just 'yesterday,' 'three days' and 'a week ago'." To respond to the feedback from preliminary research, we added a function for history review up to seven days to the widgets. This feature of the review on the past activities is suggested as a persuasive design strategy, "Trending/Historical" by Consolvo et al. [3].

2.2 Participants

We recruited participants, who are active Mac OS X users (more than 2 hour use per day) through emails, social network sites, and word of mouth based. A total of 52 participants (52% male, 48% female) completed the 2-week study in August 2009. Participants represented a wide range of age from 18 years old to 47 years old and occupations including a graduate student, engineer, web designer, biologist, economist, and housewife. Many of participants (71%) were heavy computer users who had spent up to five hours a day. Most of them except 10 people had actively utilized and downloaded widgets for fun or practical uses. We distributed subjects to retain the range of age, gender and computer usage time even in all groups.

More importantly, we assigned active widget users who had been using dashboard at least 1 to 3 times a week to Group 1 and 2, since these two groups rely on the use of dashboard; 21 participants in Group 1 were provided with Coralog; Timelog was given to 20 participants in Group 2. We assigned the rest of the participants to a control group, Group 3, who installed only the logging software so that their usage time would be tracked but they do not have any visible clues of their compute usage time opposed to the other groups. The third group enabled us to compare ordinary computer usage patterns without any presence of ambient display with the one affected by the usage of the ambient display.

2.3 Methods and Process

We combined both quantitative and qualitative methods, which range from online surveys (one prior to the two-week experiment and the other at the end) to analysis of 2-week usage logs, and to semi-structured interviews. We expected the surveys and log data from each participant to derive descriptive statistics of the system usage. We also complemented these quantitative data with qualitative analysis to understand the underneath nature of each person's experience. The primary method used for the qualitative data analysis was a grounded theory [14] that allowed us to draw bottom-up findings based on the direct quotations from the two surveys and interviews, and to establish hierarchies and connections among the remarkable findings.

1. Pre-experiment Survey: Before they proceeded to install the applications, all participants completed the survey on a given online survey URL. The goal is not a description of the context of computer usage per se as seen in a previous research project [1]. Instead, we aimed to know their everyday computing habits that may influenced the experience and perception toward the tested ambient display.

2. 2-Week Field Experiment: At the beginning of the 2-week study, we provided participants with the logging software to all groups and either widget to Group 1 and 2. All participants were not informed where the log files were recorded on their machines until they were asked to send the files to the researchers at the end of the study. During the study, we did not force the participants to complete specific tasks. Instead, we merely informed how the widget works. The chronologically recorded idle time for the two weeks may provide the evidence of the possible behavior change on the individual level in semi-longitudinal manner. We hypothesized the decrease of idle time while experiencing widgets would reflect the participant's attempt to change her or his habit of energy waste.

3. Post-Completion Survey: At the end of the 2-week use period, we sent participants notification emails of study completion. We requested them to send the recorded 2-week log files and complete the final survey. Our goal is to evaluate and compare the following concerns through the self-report based survey:

- Quality of visual design of widgets in terms of aesthetics.
- User experience with the widget, specifically the frequency of usage, explicit usage and the attractive aspects.
- Communication and visibility of the design intention by asking their impression and reaction to the widget.

In addition, we asked about their current awareness of energy consumption. We did not include these questions in the pre-experiment survey because we intended to hide the research goal in order to keep the situation untampered with.

4. Semi-structured Interviews: We invited the five participants who showed distinguishable answers to the surveys from others. During the individual 20-minute interview over the phone, each interviewee discussed how their awareness and habits had been changed through the use of widget. The goal of the interviews was to unpack what we had not been able to find and predict from the other methods.

3   Results

We obtained the 47 complete data sets (G1=17, G2=16, G3=14) at the end of the experiment, and the interview result with five participants. Each set is composed of the daily idle time and total uptime during the fourteen days and the two completed surveys. Our analysis showed the participants' increased awareness in general and each individual's varied and gradual persuasion toward behavior change. Besides the general effectiveness of ambient display for early persuasion, we present the result of the detailed comparison of the two widgets.

3.1   Increased Awareness through Persuasive Medium

The post-completion survey explained that the participants had become more interested in their computer usage habits after the study (t=5.89, p<0.001). The qualitative analysis also supports the findings and delineates the process of persuasion. The analysis of individual data showed that each participant displayed a different reached level of persuasion. We roughly categorized the widget users into three according to the reached level of persuasion–those who 1) showed the level of awareness, but not action of behavior change, 2) tried to modify their habits, and 3) appeared not to be motivated, who were mainly Timelog users.

3.1.1   Awareness of Micro-activity
While seeing the change of the coral reefs or the bar length, they became curious and tried to find a solution to turn the status back.

"I thought that's a bit sad (...) it reflects back on my behavior using the computer (P37, Coralog)."

A real-time feedback of a single device usage was appeared to be benefit to acknowledge the otherwise ungraspable effects.

"I never gave a thought to how much electricity my Macbook uses, but it isn't that I don't care. So if an easy-to-understand tool like this can help me track it, I would try and conserve energy. (P14)"

"Bringing something that is hidden and not so obvious to the front of our minds helps change behavior. (P42)"

3.1.2 From Awareness to Behavior Change

The more the participants became aware of their micro-activity, i.e., computer usage habits, the more they were motivated to change their habits, and finally some of them start action (r=0.539, p=0.003). 10 of 33 (30%) widget users answered that they actually had taken action of behavior change beyond the stage of awareness (t=5.217, p<0.001). They tried to change behavior explicitly by using sleep mode or turning off more often in order to returning to a better condition. The interview with a user who had not been cared about computer idle time at all also strengthened the result.

> "My first thought was I wanted to try and reduce my total idle time, or in other words, make use of my computer when it's on and put it to sleep if I'm not with the goal to make the most of the energy I use. (P42, Timelog)"

> "I tried very hard not to kill coral logs, I constantly kept checking it, it was even stressful. (P36, Coralog)"

> "Just showing my computer is good. I can actually do immediately. (P3, a Coralog user who had no initial interest in her computer usage habit)"

3.2 Emotional and Retrospective Engagement in Eco-Visualization

Two experimental groups exhibited different patterns of engagement as they gained awareness of energy consumption. Quantitative analysis showed the level of engagement through the frequency, purpose, and intentionality of viewing widgets. Among the total 33 widgets users, 26.5% self-reported that they ran Dashboard more often than they had before the study. The trend of checking frequency–or how often they access the widgets–was different according to the group (χ^2=13.504, p=0.001). 52.9% of Coralog users reported an increase. By contrast, no Timelog users reported an increase of dashboard usage at all. Both groups' primary reason to see the widgets was to check their computer usage behavior. 58.8% of Coralog and 31.3% of Timelog users accessed the Dashboard explicitly to see the experimental widget; others described their habit "glancing at" it while they used other widgets on the Dashboard. We also explored other factors of engagement such as aesthetic appeal and the perceived functional benefits of each representation style.

3.2.1 Emotional Attachment to Scientifically Related Images

All 17 Coralog users recognized that the coral reefs were damaged due to the increase of the idle time. At this negative change, 82.3% answered they tried to reduce idle time intentionally to save the coral reefs. The iconic representation helped make a connection between the presented information and the effects on real world. Conversely, when facing the increase of idle time through the lengthened bar on Timelog, 87.5% of Timelog users did not express the desire to change their behavior (χ^2=16.70, p=0.001).

> "It was an interesting application, but hardly motivating to save more energy. (P28, Timelog)."

Many Coralog users expressed emotional reactions using subjective words such as *guilty* (P5), *frustrated* (P8), *sad* (P37), *stressed out, felt pressure* (P36). In reaction to their attempts to repair or recover the coral state, they used subjective but positive expressions such as *happy* (P8), *encouraging* (P17), *felt good* (22), *glad to see* (P23), and *relief* (P34).

3.2.2 Numerical Data for Informative and Retrospective Purposes

Timelog users did not show considerable awareness or potential behavior change. The major reason for this was that they could not immediately match the reported usage time to an exceeded threshold for electricity consumption. Upon the change in idle time, they did not react emotionally, but impartially. They perceived Timelog as a functional utility for tracking usage time rather than an assistive application for reducing energy consumption.

> *"I had considered the log data more as reflection of my daily behaviors. Maybe I would pay more attention to the application if it displays exact amount of energy I consume (comparing to average use) (P4)"*

> *"It doesn't mean anything to me if I don't know how that uptime and idle time affects either my electrical bill, even Mac battery, or anything. (P25)"*

> *"It means I've been on the computer a lot. I was impressed that I was on the computer 11 hours one day. (P38)"*

35.2% of Coralog users wanted to see numerical data expressed either as electricity used or monetary expenses for a further motivation toward energy conservation. However, their requests did not indicate the dissatisfaction with the iconic representation. Instead, the qualitative analysis explained that numerical data might help users to understand the correlation between the users' unconscious behaviors and the changes in coral reefs imagery, thus resulting in higher awareness. In addition to the higher awareness, the numerical data helped set an explicit goal of energy conservation, so that users were more likely to change their behavior.

4   Discussion

The result of our study answered the two research questions: ambient display can boost the awareness of their everyday and micro-habits, so they are motivated to change them. Iconic representation through scientifically-related metaphors simulates emotions than numerical data do. In addition, the comprehensive analysis delivered a number of implications and benefit in HCI and interaction designers designing ambient display for persuasion. Here we articulate the four design requirements for raising awareness derived from the analysis of result. We also argue the design opportunities for the later stages of persuasion that may encourage further behavior change. We also include the aspects of the systems that need technical enhancement for persuasive empowerment.

4.1   Design Implications for Early Stages of Persuasion

We have come to a set of design requirements for ambient display focused on the early stages of persuasion. These principles are grounded in the theories for persuasion the findings from our comparative study. We hope that a number of implications reported in this section will be the ground of design that promotes behavior change.

1. Minimal domain for focused awareness and immediate trial of modification: We focused on micro-activity as opposed to collective usage, such as in an entire residential building. The results supported our intuition that a focused domain was effective making people become aware of otherwise ungraspable habits. When they check the immediate result of a small range of activity, they find the reasons easily enough to start action immediately. Other research that stressed immediate feedback and depth-based learning [15] support this design requirement.

2. Non-disturbing and subtle indicator for tracking: Mac widgets are designed to be ignored by default and displayed only by bringing the Dashboard to the foreground. While viewing the Dashboard, the users did not feel distracted regardless of whether they checked the tested widgets intentionally or simply glanced at them. We might consider designing a more non-distracting system such as a background image of upper menu bar on the desktop, so that users do not even have to take a specific action to see the feedback. As long as the system does not interfere with primary tasks, a subtle visual notification via color or shape change would be also effective.

3. Visual fun and rewards through iconic and aesthetic representation: Iconic images helped people understand the relationship between their actions and subsequent changes to the population of creatures that are sensitive to pollution. We also found that people responded more emotionally to the recovery of the coral reefs than to their destruction. The feedback for rewarding and encouragement should be 1) visually pleasing but not too abstract because it can provide a correlation between the action and effects. In addition, the feedback should encourage more when people behave well.

4. Accurate data from real users through non-intrusive sensing: To make users aware of the problems caused by their own activities, we should provide them with data about their own activities rather than general collective information about others. We also suggest that the system should not bother users by creating specific tasks merely for data gathering. The users should be exposed to the same environment while experiencing the persuasive medium, especially when they are not prepared to make changes or even aware of what needs to be changed.

4.2 Targeting the Later Stages of Persuasion

User engagement with a system is connected to the reaction to feedback. and to the level of persuasion. Here we discuss several aspects of persuasive media that encourage stronger engagement that may lead to action. We also propose possible technical enhancement to our designs for persuasive empowerment.

4.2.1 Personalized Feedback and Suggestion for Initiation of Action

Some users did not show a considerable behavior change in terms of the decrease of idle time. We suspect that the reason that users did not show a clear behavior change during the 2 weeks was the fact that the system did not give personalized guidance beyond the repeated feedback. A further advice system reflecting personal factors such as the level of self-motivation might lead them to more immediate action. Not only a timely suggestive feedback, but also a reminder of previously recorded habits would be useful for correcting negative behaviors.

4.2.2 Self-monitoring for Maintenance of Targeting State

Participants who considered themselves already very knowledgeable about environmental issues still thought Coralog was intriguing enough to help with their self-monitoring. Coralog helped them make sure to use sleep mode when away from the computer. This reflects that ambient media could be useful for the latest stage of persuasion, i.e., maintenance through self-monitoring for pursing the desired lifestyle.

4.2.3 Leveraging Network or Social Media

Previous research discussed the role of the social world intersecting personal lives in designing for sustainability [15]. Our participants also suggested that social networking could help. For example, users wanted to share their stats with family members, creating an environment of mutual encouragement. Combining social media and ambient display would benefit goal-oriented tasks in a larger context of community.

4.3 Enhancement Opportunities of Our Design

Although the logging software detects *the data from real users* and the widgets represent the data, our system has limitations. Since idle time in our system is determined as no happening of mouse or keyboard input more than five minutes, it does not distinguish from the net *not-in-use* time. When participants found that their background operations such as running simulation for a long time and playing music or movie was not accurately reflected, they tended to lose motivation while oppressed against their primary tasks.

Some participants desired to see the real electricity usage. In fact, we tied to show the actual electricity usage on Timelog, because this request was obtained from the preliminary user study. However, the electricity consumption is varied according to the various contextual factors such as the model of computer, power plug/battery and sleep mode/turning off. If a more elaborate technology that can distinguish such context were embedded, we could expect more effects on awareness.

Since our study focused on the early stages of persuasion that needed the increase of awareness, the duration of several weeks was reasonable [2]. However, if a researcher wants to evaluate the actual behavior change and the possible maintenance, a longitudinal field research of around three months will be required [3]. We expect future persuasive ambient display that incorporates our suggestions such as personalized and narrative-based feedback would yield more behavior change, which will be appropriate for a longer user study.

5 Conclusions

We developed two ambient displays with which we performed a critical study with 52 participants. The result supported our arguments that ambient display is suitable for persuasion without obtrusive feedback. Also we found that iconic and metaphorical images triggered more awareness and motivation for future behavior change through emotional attachment, while indexical representation was good for informative and retrospective purposes. We expect the newly created good habits through experience with the widget may extend to cover other usage of appliances. It also may stimulate the interest in environment issues in a macro sense as an informal educational medium. Our research contributes to the intersection of persuasive design and ambient display in HCI research. We also lay out a series of design principles coupling persuasive theories and the findings from our comparative study.

References

1. Chetty, M., Brush, A.B., Meyers, B.R., Johns, P.: It's not easy being green: understanding home computer power management. In: Proc. of CHI 2009, pp. 1033–1042 (2009)
2. Consolvo, S., Harrison, B., Smith, I., Chen, M.Y., Everitt, K., Froehlich, J., Landay, J.A.: Conducting in situ evaluations for and with ubiquitous computing technologies. International Journal of Human-Computer Interaction 22, 103–118 (2007)
3. Consolvo, S., McDonald, D.W., Landay, J.A.: Theory-driven design strategies for technologies that support behavior change in everyday life. In: Proc. of CHI 2009, pp. 405–414 (2009)
4. Developing Dashboard Widgets, http://developer.apple.com/macosx/dashboard.htm
5. De Young, R.: Changing Behavior and Making it Stick: The Conceptualization and Management of Conservation Behavior. Environment and Behavior 25, 485–505 (1993)
6. Energy Sources - Coal, USGS-ERP, http://energy.usgs.gov/coal.html
7. Fogg, B.J.: Persuasive Technology: Using Computers to Change What We Think and Do. Morgan Kaufmann, San Francisco (2002)
8. Froehlich, J., Dillahunt, T., Klasnja, P., Mankoff, J., Consolvo, S., Harrison, B., Landay, J.A.: UbiGreen: investigating a mobile tool for tracking and supporting green transportation habits. In: Proc. of CHI 2009, pp. 1043–1052 (2009)
9. Hoegh-Guldberg, O., Mumby, P.J., Hooten, A.J., Steneck, R.S., Greenfield, P., Gomez, E., Harvell, C.D., Sale, P.F., Edwards, A.J., Caldeira, K., et al.: Coral reefs under rapid climate change and ocean acidification. Science 318, 1737 (2007)
10. Holmes, T.G.: Eco-visualization: combining art and technology to reduce energy consumption. In: Proc. of C&C 2007, pp. 153–162 (2007)
11. Moser, S.C., Boulder, C.O.: Communicating Climate Change–Motivating Civic Action: Opportunity for Democratic Renewal. Climate Change Politics in North America, Wilson Center Occasional Papers 2 (2006)
12. Pousman, Z., Stasko, J.: A taxonomy of ambient information systems: four patterns of design. In: Proc. of AVI 2006, pp. 67–74 (2006)
13. Prochaska, J.O., DiClemente, C.C., Norcross, J.C.: In search of how people change: Applications to addictive behaviors. Journal of Addictions Nursing 5, 2–16 (1993)
14. Strauss, A., Corbin, J.: Basics of qualitative research: Grounded theory procedures and techniques. Sage Newbury Park, CA (1990)
15. Woodruff, A., Hasbrouck, J., Augustin, S.: A bright green perspective on sustainable choices. In: Proc. of CHI 2009, pp. 313–322 (2009)

Behavior Wizard:
A Method for Matching Target Behaviors with Solutions

B.J. Fogg and Jason Hreha

Persuasive Technology Lab @ Stanford University
captology.stanford.edu
bjfogg@stanford.edu, jason.hreha@gmail.com
www.bjfogg.com, www.jasonhreha.com

Abstract. We present a method for matching target behaviors with solutions for achieving those behaviors. Called the Behavior Wizard, this method first classifies behavior change targets into one of 15 types. Later stages focus on triggers for the target behaviors and on relevant theories and techniques. This new approach to persuasive design, as well as the terminology we propose, can lead to insights into the patterns of behavior change. The Behavior Wizard can also increase success rates in academic studies and commercial products. The most current version of this method is at www.BehaviorWizard.org.

Keywords: behavior change, persuasive design, habits, captology, behavior models, Fogg Behavior Model, Behavior Grid, Behavior Wizard.

1 Overview of Behavior Wizard

In this paper we propose an outcome-based method for classifying research and design related to persuasive technology. We call this method the Behavior Wizard.

The purpose of the Behavior Wizard is to match types of target behaviors with solutions for achieving those target behaviors. In this method the types of behavior are not constrained to a single domain like health or environment. For example, consider a behavior type we call "Black Path." This behavior type is about stopping an existing behavior permanently. Black Path behaviors include quitting smoking, ending a cursing habit, never using Facebook again, and so on. Even though the examples come from various domains, we propose that the underlying psychology for achieving Black Path behaviors is largely the same. Many people before us have pointed out the importance of matching psychology to target behavior [1][2][3]. However, as a persuasive design community, we have lacked a taxonomy and a terminology that allows precise discussions about different types of target behaviors.

The Behavior Wizard is a systematic way of thinking about behavior change. It is not a specific software application or section of code. In this paper, when we talk about the Behavior Wizard, we refer to a method of identifying specific types of behavior targets and matching those to relevant solutions. More information about this method, as well as the current implementation for public use, can be found at www.BehaviorWizard.org.

T. Ploug, P. Hasle, H. Oinas-Kukkonen (Eds.): PERSUASIVE 2010, LNCS 6137, pp. 117–131, 2010.
© Springer-Verlag Berlin Heidelberg 2010

2 Background on Classifying Behaviors

Two major traditions in psychology have influenced our thinking about types of behavior change. In recent decades the most compelling tradition views behaviors from the perspective of control. This includes Bandura's Efficacy Theory (previously Social Cognitive Theory) [4], which locates control inside individuals; Dweck's work in mindset [5], which explores behavior based on a continuum of control; and Ross and Nisbett's Attribution Theory [6], which shows the control that context has over individual behavior.

The second major tradition views behavior change types as part of a sequence. The dominant approach comes from Prochaka and DiClemente who created the Transtheoretical Modal (TTM) (also called the "Stages of Change Model") [7]. First developed for health behavior change, the popular TTM describes six stages. The first three are not behavior types but stages that anticipate behaviors. The last three stages, however, are behavior types called "Action," "Maintenance," and "Termination." Echoes of these behavior types are found in the Behavior Wizard; however, the required sequential nature is not part of our work. Despite TTM's widespread use (or perhaps because of it), this model has been strongly criticized [8][9].

Other sequential models of behavior change emerge from compliance-gaining theories [10], as well as conversion funnel approaches, popularized by consumer Internet strategists [11]. These last approaches to behavior are limited because they apply mostly to one-time actions, not repeated behaviors or cessation of behaviors.

Most recently Fogg proposed 35 ways behavior can change [12]. This early approach had some shortcomings, but it is the basis for our improved method for categorizing behaviors, as well as the starting point for the Behavior Wizard described in this paper.

3 The Need to Better Classify Behavior Types

As persuaders we humans mostly draw on intuition to achieve target behaviors. For example, at the airport we can persuade the desk agent to upgrade our seat on the plane. Then, without much thought, we can switch gears to achieve a different type of behavior, persuading ourselves not to purchase a bag of potato chips before boarding the plane. For most humans, adapting our influence techniques comes naturally.

In the last 15 years, the world has shifted from a local landscape of human persuaders to a larger universe with machines designed to persuade. This shift has made a method like the Behavior Wizard more necessary than before. Computational machines can't (yet) rely on intuition to create persuasive experiences. Creators of persuasive technologies must pre-code the experience. To be most effective, we must think clearly about specific target behaviors and how to achieve each type. Without such an approach, designers are merely guessing.

We believe that fuzzy thinking correlates with failed solutions. The evidence for this may be hard to show scientifically, but a graveyard of failed experiments and commercial products memorialize the challenges of persuasive design. The success rates for future persuasive technologies will depend on a more systematic approach to behavior change. This need has motivated us to create the Behavior Wizard.

The Behavior Wizard proposed in this paper is not perfect, but we believe it is a significant step forward to more precise and systematic thinking about behavior change. This approach can make us more effective researchers and designers, saving both time and energy. In other words, the Behavior Wizard can help us create successful persuasive technologies.

A matrix of 15 types of behavior change is the foundation for the Behavior Wizard's first phase. Before explaining this matrix, we think it most helpful to describe a scenario of use for the Behavior Wizard.

Table 1. Fogg's Behavior Grid specifies 15 types of behavior change. The items in italics are sample behaviors, all related to eco-friendly actions.

	Green behavior	**Blue** behavior	**Purple** behavior	**Gray** behavior	**Black** behavior
	Do new behavior, one that is unfamiliar	Do familiar behavior	Increase behavior intensity or duration	Decrease behavior intensity or duration	Stop doing a behavior
Dot behavior is done one-time	**GreenDot** Do new behavior one time *Install solar panels on house*	**BlueDot** Do familiar behavior one time *Tell a friend about eco-friendly soap*	**PurpleDot** Increase behavior one time *Plant more trees & local plants today*	**GrayDot** Decrease behavior one time *Buy fewer bottles of water now*	**BlackDot** Stop doing a behavior one time *Turn off space heater for tonight*
Span behavior has specific duration, such as 40 days	**GreenSpan** Do new behavior for a period of time *Carpool to work for three weeks*	**BlueSpan** Do familiar behavior for a period of time *Bike to work for two months*	**PurpleSpan** Increase behavior for a period of time *Take public bus for one month*	**GraySpan** Decrease behavior for a period of time *Take shorter showers this week*	**BlackSpan** Stop a behavior for a period of time *Don't water lawn during summer*
Path behavior is done from now on, a permanent change	**GreenPath** Do new behavior from now on *Start growing own vegetables*	**BluePath** Do familiar behavior from now on *Turn off lights when leaving room*	**PurplePath** Increase behavior from now on *Purchase more local produce*	**GrayPath** Decrease behavior from now on *Eat less meat from now on*	**BlackPath** Stop a behavior from now on *Never litter again*

4   Scenario of Using the Behavior Wizard

An efficient way to show how the Behavior Wizard benefits the persuasive design process is through a scenario. The Behavior Wizard makes the following a reality:

For her thesis project, Jane will investigate how technology can persuade people to watch less TV. After a period of study, Jane will build and test a prototype to achieve this target behavior.

To get started on the right track, Jane uses the Behavior Wizard. She answers three questions about her behavior change of interest--watching less TV--and the Behavior Wizard labels this behavior type: It's called a "Gray Path" Behavior. Jane knows that this label refers to a generic type of behavior change; it is characterized by a specific underlying psychology and techniques for achieving it.

The Behavior Wizard provides Jane with a Resource Guide. It starts out by listing other Gray Path Behaviors, such as eating smaller portions and spending less on clothes. Jane recognizes the similarities to watching less TV. Jane scans down the Resource Guide until she reaches a listing of academic studies, including 13 related papers from the conferences on Persuasive Technology. She sees that research on Gray Path Behaviors come from other topic areas as well, from health to economics. She knows her work will benefit from insights across these domains.

Jane also sees a list of theories that can inform her work. She's studied some of these theories already, but some are new to her; they are from different fields. And finally, Jane finds a list of products that have proven effective in achieving Gray Path Behaviors. She doesn't see a product for persuading people to watch less TV, but she knows the persuasion techniques used by the other "Gray Path" products will give her insight how to tackle the TV problem.

Thanks to the Behavior Wizard, Jane gets a fast start on her thesis project. She's confident she's headed in the right direction.

In the above scenario, the Behavior Wizard helps Jane think clearly about the behavior change that interests her. It also guides her to the most relevant studies, theories, and solutions. She doesn't waste time reading about unrelated types of behavior change, such as one-time compliance. She can focus on the psychology of her behavior type--a long-term reduction in an existing behavior. And she can tap into solutions that already work for this type of behavior. The Behavior Wizard greatly improves Jane's chances for a successful project.

5   The 15 Types of Behavior Change

The foundation for the Behavior Wizard is a matrix called the "Behavior Grid" that defines 15 types of behavior. This is a revision of Fogg's previous work that categorized 35 types of behavior [12], a framework that would have required three axes to be precise. We now propose a simpler 15-cell grid that is more practical and conceptually appealing (see www.BehaviorGrid.org for details not in this paper).

Two axis form the Behavior Grid. Along the horizontal axis is a dimension we call the behavior "Flavor". As described below, there are five Flavors of behavior. The vertical axis maps out what we call "Duration". The Behavior Grid has three categories of Duration, as described below.

5.1   The Five Flavors of Behavior

The horizontal axis of the Behavior Grid segments behaviors into five Flavors: Green, Blue, Purple, Gray, and Black. The previous labels for these columns were abstract and uninteresting: A, B, C, D, and E [12]. The use of colors to label columns in the Behavior Grid creates a more evocative and memorable framework.

Table 2 provides examples of each Behavior Flavor we discuss below. In the grid we've placed examples, each of which relates to healthy eating behaviors.

Table 2. Examples of 15 types of behavior change, all related to healthy eating, as organized by Fogg's Behavior Grid

	Green behavior Do new behavior, one that is unfamiliar	**Blue** behavior Do familiar behavior	**Purple** behavior Increase behavior intensity or duration	**Gray** behavior Decrease behavior intensity or duration	**Black** behavior Stop doing a behavior
Dot behavior is done one-time	Try eating dried seaweed for a snack today	Eat vegetables at dinner tonight	Increase mindfulness at lunch today	Eat only half of a hamburger tonight	Don't buy ice cream this time while shopping
Span behavior has specific duration, such as 40 days	Substitute quinoa for rice for one month	Drink water each morning this week	Eat more vegetables at dinner for two months	Eat fewer carbohydrates for one week	Don't use sugar in coffee for two weeks
Path behavior is done from now on, a permanent change	Lead a vegan lifestyle from now on	Take daily vitamins from now on	Increase healthy eating options in home	Decrease fried foods in diet from now on	Stop eating fast food forever

A **Green Behavior** is a behavior that is new to the target audience. For example, if someone has never snacked on seaweed, then it's a Green Behavior for that person. For seaweed lovers, this is not a Green Behavior. In Table 2 we've listed examples of Green Behaviors we think would be new to most people: snack on seaweed, eat quinoa, and become a vegan.

Designing to achieve Green Behaviors requires special consideration. This may include making the behavior simpler to do, reducing anxiety, connecting the new behavior to existing practice, providing social support, and so on.

A **Blue Behavior** is one that is familiar to the target audience. For example, walking a mile is a Blue Behavior for most people because most of us have walked a mile before. In Table 2 we've chosen behavior examples we believe most people have done before: eating vegetables, drinking water, and taking vitamins.

Designs to achieve Blue Behaviors can draw on past experience. The behavior itself and the expected results of the behavior do not need to be explained, as might be needed for Green Behaviors. At some point a Green Behavior becomes a Blue Behavior as a person becomes familiar with it.

A **Purple Behavior** designates an increased performance of a familiar behavior. Purple Behaviors are existing behaviors that people increase in some way, such as doing the behavior longer, more intensely, or with more effort. For example, walking a mile at normal pace would be a Blue Behavior. But walking faster than usual for a mile would qualify as a Purple Behavior. Also qualifying would be walking farther than a mile or walking uphill.

Table 2 lists examples of Purple Behaviors: increasing mindfulness while eating, consuming more vegetables, and stocking more healthy eating options at home.

A **Gray Behavior** designates a decreased performance of a familiar behavior. The behavior can decrease in intensity, duration, or frequency. Examples of Gray Behaviors include eating less, cutting back on coffee, and working shorter hours.

At times a behavior change can be seen both as a Gray Behavior and a Purple Behavior, like two sides of a coin. For example, someone could reduce TV viewing by replacing it with more walking outside. This Purple-Gray behavior exchange applies in many arenas. It's a pattern we can now label.

A **Black Behavior** designates a cessation of an existing behavior. For example, quitting smoking is a Black Behavior, as is eliminating all corn syrup in one's diet. We selected the color black because we felt it connotes an absence or an end.

Some behaviors, such as eating, cannot be completely Black. For example, the renowned Weight Watchers program advocates a few Black Behaviors in eating, but the primary focus is on Gray Behaviors.

Note that the placement of behaviors into the five Flavors, especially for Blue and Green Behaviors, depends on the person who is the target of persuasion. For example, most of our colleagues have never eaten dried seaweed as a snack so this is a Green Behavior; it is new to them. However, some people snack on seaweed often. For those people, it is a Blue Behavior. This example highlights the need to understand the target audience, an important step in any behavior change method.

5.2 Benefits of This Approach

For purposes of research and design, categorizing behavior change into five Flavors is a significant step forward. It can clarify fuzzy thinking quickly. In our various implementations of the Behavior Wizard, testing over 100 people, we found that virtually everyone could answer questions to help them see which of the five Behavior Flavors matched their target behavior. In contrast, without prompting questions related to the Flavors, we found that well over 50% could not articulate their behavior target precisely. This result is not a scientific finding but a confirmation check. This result matches our experience in teaching persuasive design and in working on industry projects. Most people, including professionals in marketing, are not good at thinking clearly about target behaviors. But once given a thinking system, such as Behavior Flavors, they do much better in articulating a target behavior and finding the behavior label for it.

5.3 The Three Durations of Behaviors: Dot, Span, and Path

The other dimension in the revised behavior matrix deals with what we call "Duration". Three options exist: one time, span of time, or ongoing. Each of these has a short, memorable name to make this framework more workable and appealing.

A **Dot Behavior** is a behavior that is done once. For example, joining a church or clicking on a specific banner ad are examples of a Dot Behavior. In Table 2 we've listed other examples of behaviors that are reasonably done as one-time behaviors: eating a seaweed snack today, eating more vegetables one evening, increasing mindfulness during a specific meal, eating half of a hamburger tonight, or choosing not to buy ice-cream during a certain trip to the store. Any of these behaviors can be repeated, of course, but the intervention goal is to influence behavior one time.

Designing to achieve Dot Behaviors differs from the other two categories. Compliance-gaining strategies are prominent [13]. Also the long-term implications of Dot Behaviors are less salient, which may generally give them a lower behavior activation threshold.

In contrast to Dot Behaviors, a **Span Behavior** is a behavior that is done over a period of time. For example, the religious tradition of Lent is all about Span Behaviors. In Table 2, we list examples of behaviors that extend over time: substituting quinoa for rice for one month, drinking water each morning this week, eating more vegetables at dinner for two months, eating fewer carbohydrates for one week, or choosing not to use sugar in one's coffee for two weeks.

Designing Span behaviors requires special consideration. People must stick to a pattern of action for a certain period of time. Thus, a Span intervention might pay close attention to the strategic use of regular triggers.

Finally, a **Path Behavior** is a behavior that is done from now on, a permanent change. For example, eating only vegetarian food is an example of a Path Behavior. We've chosen the word *Path* to evoke the ongoing nature of the behavior change.

In Table 2, we list examples of permanent, ongoing behaviors: leading a vegan lifestyle, taking daily vitamins, increasing healthy eating options at home, decreasing fried foods in diet, or stopping fast food consumption.

Path Behaviors may be the hardest types of behaviors to induce. Because of their permanent nature, they require a shift in a person's identity or lifestyle. In many cases, the target behavior must be triggered regularly enough to the point that the behavior becomes a habit, part of a person's routine or a reflexive response.

6 The Three Phases of the Behavior Wizard

With the 15 behavior types mapped out above, we will now explain the overall method for the Behavior Wizard. This has three phases.

6.1 Phase 1. Clarify the Target Behavior and Distinguish from Others

The first phase of the Behavior Wizard is to isolate and identify the target behavior. The previous sections describe the classification scheme.

One goal is to make this phase simple enough that everyday people could classify target behaviors without training. We tested four ways to do this. The first method was to have people view the matrix of 15 items and select the cell that matched. However, people got overwhelmed by the complexity.

In our pilot testing of over 100 people, we eventually found that a better method was to ask simple questions in a branching decision tree. Our current implementation for classifying a behavior type is a series of questions with no more than three options. (For specifics on our current approach, see www.BehaviorWizard.org.)

6.2 Phase 2. Identify What Triggers the Behavior

After classifying the target behavior into one of 15 types, the Behavior Wizard method moves on to phase two. The next task is to identify how the target behavior is triggered.

One trigger option we call a "Cycle" Behavior. This means the target behavior happens on a predictable schedule. It could be daily, weekly, and so on. For example, for most people the behavior of brushing teeth is a Cycle Behavior. People brush in the morning and at night. The time may not be exactly the same each day, but it's part of a routine people have. (Technically, brushing teeth is a Blue Path Cycle Behavior, but this additional layer goes beyond the scope of our paper.) Other Cycle Behaviors include going to church once a week, paying bills once a month, or celebrating a birthday once a year.

The next trigger option we call a "Cue" Behavior. This means the target behavior happens in response to a cue that is unpredictable; it's not on a schedule. For example, when Facebook notifies people they have been tagged in a photo, that cue can trigger people to log into Facebook to view the photo. Another example: If someone waves at us, we will probably wave back. For us, this friendly cue leads to an automatic social response. Note that some cues might be internal. For example, if a woman has a headache, that pain can be a cue to action, such as taking medication.

In our view, knowing how a behavior gets triggered is important enough that it deserves a separate phase in the Behavior Wizard. It's clear that triggers apply to Green, Blue, and Purple Behaviors. In addition, triggers can affect Gray and Black behaviors. One approach to achieving Gray and Black Behaviors is to minimize or remove the trigger. For example, if the target behavior is to stop logging into Facebook while at work, one can turn off email notifications. This removes the trigger and reduces the likelihood of logging into Facebook.

6.3   Phase 3. Highlight Concepts and Solutions Related to Target Behavior

The third phase in the Behavior Wizard is to highlight the theories, models, and solutions for the behavior type of interest. This is where the Behavior Wizard generates relevant information for those creating the persuasive experience. We call this compilation a "Resource Guide". In the scenario with the grad student, Jane received a Resource Guide about Gray Path Behaviors.

In creating the Resource Guides, we've followed a template that currently has seven parts, as shown below.

Title: [Type of Behavior]
Description: Perform X Flavor on Y Duration
1. Behavior examples
2. Techniques to achieve this behavior
3. Implementations that achieve this behavior
4. Factors from Fogg Behavior Model (motivation, ability, triggers)
5. Relevant theories and models
6. Related types from Behavior Grid (a. same Flavor b. same Duration)
7. Behavior change patterns that match this type

Each Resource Guide is unique, but some content is duplicated across guides. For example, all Black Behaviors share commonalities. So we've put some of the same information in Resource Guides for Black Dot, Black Span, and Black Path behaviors. The guides also point out relationships among behavior types. For example, when it comes to creating new habits, targeting a Blue Span Behavior first may be a good step before tackling a Blue Path Behavior.

In a similar way, the behavior types listed in rows share commonalities. These are described in the Resource Guides. For example, if a Black Path Behavior is the ultimate goal, a more palatable prior behavior may be a Gray Path Behavior. Note that sequences of target behaviors get a lot easier to map out and discuss when using the categories and terminology from the Behavior Grid.

Our work on the Resource Guides may never be complete, since there's always more to add as new knowledge gets created and new products are shown to be effective. For example, every day it seems a new smartphone app could be added to one of the 15 Resource Guides. Also, as hundreds of experiments about behavior change happen around the world, including those in industry, new insights continually emerge for the behavior types. To address this reality, we post periodic updates to the Behavior Guides at www.BehaviorWizard.org.

7 Mapping Research in Persuasive Technology

As members of the Persuasive Technology community, we wanted to map research from our annual conferences into the matrix of 15 behavior types. However, as we read published papers looking for the target behaviors, we found that some studies weren't clear. At times the research measured attitudes, while the paper's discussion focused on behavior. Yet the link between attitude and behavior change was not explicit. We did not include those papers in the mapping below.

In Table 3 we've bolded the names of researchers that measured that behavior type directly. Note that nothing in the Path Behaviors is in bold. This makes sense. Most research methods are not well suited for showing a permanent change in behavior.

Often researchers showed a one-time change during an experiment, or a change over a period of time in a field trial. These are Dot and Span Behavior outcomes. Yet some of these findings, we believe, have implications for long-term behavior change. In those cases, we included names of the first authors in Path Behavior column of Table 3, but without the bold typeface. For example, Forget et al. (2008) investigated how to persuade people to create more secure passwords using a new method. The study measured behavior change during the experimental session, a one-time behavior. But the work implies that long-term behavior is possible if this approach were scaled up. So in this case, we've listed the study in bold as a Dot Behavior and listed it again in nonbolded typeface as a Path Behavior.

In the scenario about Jane earlier in this paper, the Behavior Wizard gave her 13 studies that related to her Gray Path Behavior of interest. The studies Jane saw are those listed in Table 3. Jane's Resource Guide also listed the other papers in the Gray Behavior column, because these studies may have implications for her work as well. For example, what Bickmore et al. (2007) learned about influencing people to take breaks from the computer during an experimental setting may help Jane in designing a system for reducing TV viewing in a real living room. In addition, the research methods Bickmore et al. used, including the measurement techniques, may be what Jane needs for her thesis project.

Table 3 suggests some questions for future investigation. Why did so many Blue Dot studies emerge in 2007? Why are Gray Path Behaviors so numerous? Would

Table 3. Research published in previous Persuasive Technology conferences, organized by behavior type. Bolded names indicate studies that measured that type of behavior [14-60].

	Green behavior Do new behavior, one that is unfamiliar	Blue behavior Do familiar behavior	Purple behavior Increase behavior intensity or duration	Gray behavior Decrease behavior intensity or duration	Black behavior Stop doing a behavior
Dot behavior is done one-time	Ahrens et al. (07) Forget et al. (08) Ramachandran et al. (08) Iyengar et al. (09)	Harper et al. (07) Ahrens et al. (07) Gamberini et al.(07) Felfernig et al. (07) Vossen et al. (09)	Eyck et al. (06) Niebuhr et al. (07) Frolich (08) Reitberger et al. (09)	McCalley et al. (06) Bickmore et al. (07) Frolich (08) Ham et al. (08)	
Span behavior has specific duration, such as 40 days	Revelle et al. (07) Parmar et al. (08) Chi et al. (08) Harjumaa et al. (09) Ferebee et al. (09)	Sterns et al. (06)	Gasser et al. (06) Goris et al. (08) Firpo et al. (09) Saini et al. (09)	Kappel et al. (09)	Dijkstra (06) Kraft et al. (07) Gable et al. (07)
Path behavior is done from now on, a permanent change	Bang et al. (06) Lucero et al. (06) Tscheligi et al. (06) Reitberger et al. (07) Parmar et al. (08) Chi et al. (08) Obermair et al. (08) Forget et al. (08) Kraft et al. (08) Lockton et al. (09) Ferebee et al. (09)	Sterns et al. (06) Wai et al. (07) Brodie et al. (07) Fogg et al. (08) Consolvo et al. (09) Olsen & Kraft (09) Saini & Lacroix (09) Vossen et al. (09) Harjumaa et al. (09) Ranfelt et al. (09)	Tscheligi et al. (06) Bang et al. (07) Reitberger et al. (07) Wai et al. (07) Murthy (poster 08) Berkovsky et al. (09) Firpo et al. (09)	Bang et al. (06) McCalley et al. (06) Bickmore et al. (07) Kraft et al. (07) Bang et al. (07) Mahmud et al. (07) Drozd et al. (08) Ham et al. (08) Kraft et al. (08) Midden & Ham (09) Shiraishi et al. (09) Kappel et al. (09) Duncan et al. (09)	Dijkstra (06) Grolleman et al. (06) Kraft et al. (07) Khaled et al. (07) Gable et al. (07) Kraft et al. (08) Khaled et al. (08) Raisanen et al. (08)

conferences in other domains, such as marketing or behavioral economics, show a different pattern of emphasis? Answering these and related questions is beyond the scope of this paper, but these issues would make for interesting future study.

As we move forward with the Behavior Wizard, we continue to add new insights to the database. This will come from persuasive technology conferences as well as other domains, such as health marketing, consumer behavior, web analytics, behavioral economics, and more. The organizing factor for the emerging insights won't be the traditional labels like marketing or economics; instead, the Behavior Grid makes it possible to organize insights by types of behavior change. The Behavior Wizard builds on this framework to match solutions to target behaviors of interest. One primary goal of our work here is to create common ground that transcends traditional boundaries of academic disciplines and industry functions. That common ground is type of behavior change.

8   The Behavior Wizard and Beyond

The Behavior Wizard not only provides a common approach to categorizing behavior, but we believe its components allow for a deeper understanding of the winning patterns of behavior change. In this method, each row and column represents one characteristic, so we are able to see potent relationships amongst the sub-types when moving throughout the grid – either across a row or along a column.

Consider, for example, the domain of habit formation, which represents just one section of the overall Behavior Grid. Moving down a column could describe one process of habit formation. Specifically Dot Behaviors flow into Span Behaviors, which can then, with enough repetition, become Path Behaviors. So if we are interested in creating a habit in a customer, or just understanding how the process works, we first look at the common characteristics of Dot Behaviors: What tactics trigger them? How strongly does context control one-time decisions? And especially, how easily can we repeat the success? Then, we can move to Span Behaviors, finding the best ways to succeed for a fixed period of time. Finally, we can move onto Path Behaviors. In this way, we can break the process of habit formation down into smaller, more tractable pieces.

The Behavior Wizard helps focus thinking on a concrete set of behavior changes, organizing what has long been a messy landscape. In combination with the triggering methods, the 15 behavior types can serve as building blocks for persuasive design. Today researchers and designers can use elements of the Behavior Wizard to build and test specific solutions. Yet greater potential remains. We anticipate such a systematic approach will eventually show how smaller units of influence can combine into larger patterns of persuasion. We share future insights and developments at www.BehaviorWizard.org.

In the near term, a systematic approach to designing for behavior change can empower us to create persuasive technologies more efficiently. In the coming years, tools for automating behavior change, such as future iterations of the Behavior Wizard, will become more sophisticated and effective. As this happens, we believe that humans will play increasingly smaller roles in testing and improving persuasive technologies. Ultimately, it won't be researchers or designers who create what shapes human behavior. This will be a job for computers.

References

1. Aristotle: Rhetoric, 3rd edn. Dover Publications, Dover (2004)
2. Prochaska, J.O., Velicer, W.F.: The transtheoretical model of health behavior change. Am. J. Health Promot. 12(1), 38–48 (1997) (accessed March 18, 2009)
3. Kraft, P., Schjelderup-Lund, H., Brendryen, H.: Digital Therapy: The Coming Together of Psychology and Technology Can Create a New Generation of Programs for More Sustainable Change. In: de Kort, Y.A.W., IJsselsteijn, W.A., Midden, C., Eggen, B., Fogg, B.J. (eds.) PERSUASIVE 2007. LNCS, vol. 4744, pp. 18–23. Springer, Heidelberg (2007)
4. Bandura, A.: Self-Efficacy: The Exercise of Control. Worth Publishers, New York (1997)
5. Dweck, C., Sorich, L.A.: Mastery Oriented Thinking. In: Coping: The Psychology of What Works, pp. 232–251. Oxford University Press, Oxford (1999)
6. Nesbit, R., Ross, L.: Human Inference: Strategies and Shortcomings in Social Judgement. Prentice Hall, Englewood Cliffs (1980)
7. Prochaska, J.O., DiClemente, C.C.: The transtheoretical approach. In: Norcross, J.C., Goldfried, M.R. (eds.) Handbook of psychotherapy integration, 2nd edn., pp. 147–171. Oxford University Press, New York (2005)
8. Littell, J.H., Girvin, H.: Stages of Change. Beh. Mod. 26, 223–273 (2002)

9. Brug, J., Conner, M., Harre, N., Kremers, S., McKellar, S., Whitelaw, S.: The Transtheoretical Model and Stages of Change: A Critique. H. Edu. Res. 20, 244–258 (2004)
10. Marwell, G., Schmitt, D.R.: Dimensions of compliance-gaining behavior: An empirical analysis. Sociometery 30, 350–364 (1967)
11. Burby, J.: Breaking Down a Conversion Funnel. ClickZ Online (May 24, 2005)
12. Fogg, B.J.: The Behavior Grid: 35 Ways Behavior Can Change. In: Persuasive 2009, p. 42 (2009)
13. Marwell, G., Schmitt, D.R.: Dimensions of compliance-gaining behavior: An empirical analysis. Sociometery 30, 350–364 (1967)
14. Bang, M., Torstensson, C., Katzeff, C.: The PowerHhouse: A Persuasive Computer Game Designed to Raise Awareness of Domestic Energy Consumption. In: IJsselsteijn, W.A., de Kort, Y.A.W., Midden, C., Eggen, B., van den Hoven, E. (eds.) PERSUASIVE 2006. LNCS, vol. 3962, pp. 123–132. Springer, Heidelberg (2006)
15. Dijkstra, A.: Technology Adds New Principles to Persuasive Psychology. In: IJsselsteijn, W.A., de Kort, Y.A.W., Midden, C., Eggen, B., van den Hoven, E. (eds.) PERSUASIVE 2006. LNCS, vol. 3962, pp. 16–26. Springer, Heidelberg (2006)
16. Eyck, A., Geerlings, K., Karimova, D., Meerbeek, B., Wang, L., IJsselsteijn, W., de Kort, Y., Roersma, M., Westerink, J.: Effect of a Virtual Coach on Athletes' Motivation. In: IJsselsteijn, W.A., de Kort, Y.A.W., Midden, C., Eggen, B., van den Hoven, E. (eds.) PERSUASIVE 2006. LNCS, vol. 3962, pp. 158–161. Springer, Heidelberg (2006)
17. Gasser, R., Brodbeck, D., Degen, M., Luthiger, J., Wyss, R., Reichlin, S.: Persuasiveness of a Mobile Lifestyle Coaching Application Using Social Facilitation. In: IJsselsteijn, W.A., de Kort, Y.A.W., Midden, C., Eggen, B., van den Hoven, E. (eds.) PERSUASIVE 2006. LNCS, vol. 3962, pp. 27–38. Springer, Heidelberg (2006)
18. Grolleman, J., van Dijk, B., Nijholt, A., van Emst, A.: Break the Habit! Designing an e-Therapy Intervention Using a Virtual Coach in Aid of Smoking Cessation. In: IJsselsteijn, W.A., de Kort, Y.A.W., Midden, C., Eggen, B., van den Hoven, E. (eds.) PERSUASIVE 2006. LNCS, vol. 3962, pp. 133–141. Springer, Heidelberg (2006)
19. Lucero, A., Zuloaga, R., Mota, S., Munoz, F.: Persuasive Technologies in Education: Improving Motivation to Read and Write for Children. In: IJsselsteijn, W.A., de Kort, Y.A.W., Midden, C., Eggen, B., van den Hoven, E. (eds.) PERSUASIVE 2006. LNCS, vol. 3962, pp. 142–153. Springer, Heidelberg (2006)
20. McCalley, T., Kaiser, F., Midden, C., Keser, M., Teunissen, M.: Persuasive Appliances: Goal Priming and Behavioral Response to Product-Integrated Energy Feedback. In: IJsselsteijn, W.A., de Kort, Y.A.W., Midden, C., Eggen, B., van den Hoven, E. (eds.) PERSUASIVE 2006. LNCS, vol. 3962, pp. 45–49. Springer, Heidelberg (2006)
21. Sterns, A.A., Mayhorn, C.B.: Persuasive Pillboxes: Improving Medication Adherence with Personal Digital Assistants. In: IJsselsteijn, W.A., de Kort, Y.A.W., Midden, C., Eggen, B., van den Hoven, E. (eds.) PERSUASIVE 2006. LNCS, vol. 3962, pp. 195–198. Springer, Heidelberg (2006)
22. Tscheligi, M., Reitberger, W., Obermair, C., Ploderer, B.: perCues: Trails of Persuasion for Ambient Intelligence. In: IJsselsteijn, W.A., de Kort, Y.A.W., Midden, C., Eggen, B., van den Hoven, E. (eds.) PERSUASIVE 2006. LNCS, vol. 3962, pp. 203–206. Springer, Heidelberg (2006)
23. Ahrens, J., Strahilevitz, M.A.: Can Companies Initiate Positive Word of Mouth? A Field Experiment Examining the Effects of Incentive Magnitude and Equity, and eReferral Mechanisms. In: de Kort, Y.A.W., IJsselsteijn, W.A., Midden, C., Eggen, B., Fogg, B.J. (eds.) PERSUASIVE 2007. LNCS, vol. 4744, pp. 160–163. Springer, Heidelberg (2007)

24. Kraft, P., et al.: Digital Therapy: The Coming Together of Psychology and Technology Can Create a New Generation of Programs for More Sustainable Behavioral Change. In: de Kort, Y.A.W., IJsselsteijn, W.A., Midden, C., Eggen, B., Fogg, B.J. (eds.) PERSUASIVE 2007. LNCS, vol. 4744, pp. 18–23. Springer, Heidelberg (2007)
25. Bickmore, T.W., Mauer, D., Crespo, F., Brown, T.: Persuasion, Task Interruption and Health Regimen Adherence. In: de Kort, Y.A.W., IJsselsteijn, W.A., Midden, C., Eggen, B., Fogg, B.J. (eds.) PERSUASIVE 2007. LNCS, vol. 4744, pp. 1–11. Springer, Heidelberg (2007)
26. Revelle, G., Reardon, E., Mays Green, M., Betancourt, J., Kotler, J.: The Use of Mobile Phones to Support Children's Literacy Learning. In: de Kort, Y.A.W., IJsselsteijn, W.A., Midden, C., Eggen, B., Fogg, B.J. (eds.) PERSUASIVE 2007. LNCS, vol. 4744, pp. 253–258. Springer, Heidelberg (2007)
27. Reitberger, W., Ploderer, B., Obermair, C., Tscheligi, M.: The PerCues Framework and Its Application for Sustainable Mobility. In: de Kort, Y.A.W., IJsselsteijn, W.A., Midden, C., Eggen, B., Fogg, B.J. (eds.) PERSUASIVE 2007. LNCS, vol. 4744, pp. 92–95. Springer, Heidelberg (2007)
28. Harper, F.M., Li, S.X., Chen, Y., Konstan, J.A.: Social Comparisons to Motivate Contributions to an Online Community. In: de Kort, Y.A.W., IJsselsteijn, W.A., Midden, C., Eggen, B., Fogg, B.J. (eds.) PERSUASIVE 2007. LNCS, vol. 4744, pp. 148–159. Springer, Heidelberg (2007)
29. Gamberini, L., Petrucci, G., Spoto, A., Spagnolli, A.: Embedded Persuasive Strategies to Obtain Visitors' Data: Comparing Reward and Reciprocity in an Amateur, Knowledge-Based Website. In: de Kort, Y.A.W., IJsselsteijn, W.A., Midden, C., Eggen, B., Fogg, B.J. (eds.) PERSUASIVE 2007. LNCS, vol. 4744, pp. 187–198. Springer, Heidelberg (2007)
30. Felfernig, A., Friedrich, G., Gula, B., Hitz, M., Kruggel, T., Leitner, G., Melcher, R., Riepan, D., Strauss, S., Teppan, E.: Persuasive Recommendation: Serial Position Effects in Knowledge-Based Recommender Systems. In: de Kort, Y.A.W., IJsselsteijn, W.A., Midden, C., Eggen, B., Fogg, B.J. (eds.) PERSUASIVE 2007. LNCS, vol. 4744, pp. 283–294. Springer, Heidelberg (2007)
31. Mahmud, A.A., Dadlani, P., Mubin, O., Shahid, S., Midden, C., Moran, O.: iParrot: Towards Designing a Persuasive Agent for Energy Conservation. In: de Kort, Y.A.W., IJsselsteijn, W.A., Midden, C., Eggen, B., Fogg, B.J. (eds.) PERSUASIVE 2007. LNCS, vol. 4744, pp. 64–67. Springer, Heidelberg (2007)
32. Wai, C., Mortensen, P.: Persuasive Technologies Should Be Boring. In: de Kort, Y.A.W., IJsselsteijn, W.A., Midden, C., Eggen, B., Fogg, B.J. (eds.) PERSUASIVE 2007. LNCS, vol. 4744, pp. 96–99. Springer, Heidelberg (2007)
33. Brodie, M., Lai, J., Lenchner, J., Luken, W., Ranganathan, K., Tang, J.-M., Vukovic, M.: Support Services: Persuading Employees to Do what Is in the Community's Best Interest. In: de Kort, Y.A.W., IJsselsteijn, W.A., Midden, C., Eggen, B., Fogg, B.J. (eds.) PERSUASIVE 2007. LNCS, vol. 4744, pp. 121–124. Springer, Heidelberg (2007)
34. Niebuhr, S., Kerkow, D.: Captivating Patterns - A First Validation. In: de Kort, Y.A.W., IJsselsteijn, W.A., Midden, C., Eggen, B., Fogg, B.J. (eds.) PERSUASIVE 2007. LNCS, vol. 4744, pp. 48–54. Springer, Heidelberg (2007)
35. Bang, M., Gustafsson, A., Katzeff, C.: Promoting New Patterns in Household Energy Consumption with Pervasive Learning Games. In: de Kort, Y.A.W., IJsselsteijn, W.A., Midden, C., Eggen, B., Fogg, B.J. (eds.) PERSUASIVE 2007. LNCS, vol. 4744, pp. 55–63. Springer, Heidelberg (2007)

36. Gable, R.S.: Electronic Monitoring of Offenders. In: de Kort, Y.A.W., IJsselsteijn, W.A., Midden, C., Eggen, B., Fogg, B.J. (eds.) PERSUASIVE 2007. LNCS, vol. 4744, pp. 100–104. Springer, Heidelberg (2007)

37. Khaled, R., Barr, P., Noble, J., Fischer, R., Biddle, R.: Fine Tuning the Persuasion in Persuasive Games. In: de Kort, Y.A.W., IJsselsteijn, W.A., Midden, C., Eggen, B., Fogg, B.J. (eds.) PERSUASIVE 2007. LNCS, vol. 4744, pp. 36–47. Springer, Heidelberg (2007)

38. Chi, P.-Y., Chen, J.-H., Chu, H.-H., Lo, J.-L.: Enabling Calorie-Aware Cooking in a Smart Kitchen. In: Oinas-Kukkonen, H., Hasle, P., Harjumaa, M., Segerståhl, K., Øhrstrøm, P. (eds.) PERSUASIVE 2008. LNCS, vol. 5033, pp. 116–127. Springer, Heidelberg (2008)

39. Fogg, B.J.: Mass Interpersonal Persuasion: An Early View of a New Phenomenon. In: Oinas-Kukkonen, H., Hasle, P., Harjumaa, M., Segerståhl, K., Øhrstrøm, P. (eds.) PERSUASIVE 2008. LNCS, vol. 5033, pp. 23–34. Springer, Heidelberg (2008)

40. Forget, A., Chiasson, S., van Oorschot, P.C., Biddle, R.: Persuasion for Stronger Passwords: Motivation and Pilot Study. In: Oinas-Kukkonen, H., Hasle, P., Harjumaa, M., Segerståhl, K., Øhrstrøm, P. (eds.) PERSUASIVE 2008. LNCS, vol. 5033, pp. 140–150. Springer, Heidelberg (2008)

41. Kraft, P., Drozd, F., Olsen, E.: Digital Therapy: Addressing Willpower as Part of the Cognitive-Affective Processing System in the Service of Habit Change. In: Oinas-Kukkonen, H., Hasle, P., Harjumaa, M., Segerståhl, K., Øhrstrøm, P. (eds.) PERSUASIVE 2008. LNCS, vol. 5033, pp. 177–188. Springer, Heidelberg (2008)

42. Parmar, V., Keyson, D., de Bont, C.: Persuasive Technology for Shaping Social Beliefs of Rural Women in India: An Approach Based on the Theory of Planned Behaviour. In: Oinas-Kukkonen, H., Hasle, P., Harjumaa, M., Segerståhl, K., Øhrstrøm, P. (eds.) PERSUASIVE 2008. LNCS, vol. 5033, pp. 104–115. Springer, Heidelberg (2008)

43. Raisanen, T., Oinas-Kukkonen, H., Pahnila, S.: Finding Kairos in Quitting Smoking: Smokers' Perceptions of Warning Pictures. In: Oinas-Kukkonen, H., Hasle, P., Harjumaa, M., Segerståhl, K., Øhrstrøm, P. (eds.) PERSUASIVE 2008. LNCS, vol. 5033, pp. 254–257. Springer, Heidelberg (2008)

44. Ramachandran, D., Canny, J.: The Persuasive Power of Human-Machine Dialogue. In: Oinas-Kukkonen, H., Hasle, P., Harjumaa, M., Segerståhl, K., Øhrstrøm, P. (eds.) PERSUASIVE 2008. LNCS, vol. 5033, pp. 189–200. Springer, Heidelberg (2008)

45. Obermair, C., Reitberger, W., Meschtscherjakov, A., Lankes, M., Tscheligi, M.: perFrames: Persuasive Picture Frames for Proper Posture. In: Oinas-Kukkonen, H., Hasle, P., Harjumaa, M., Segerståhl, K., Øhrstrøm, P. (eds.) PERSUASIVE 2008. LNCS, vol. 5033, pp. 128–139. Springer, Heidelberg (2008)

46. Berkovsky, S., Bhandari, D., Kimani, S., Colineau, N., Paris, C.: Designing games to motivate physical activity. In: Persuasive 2009, p. 37 (2009)

47. Consolvo, S., Klasnja, P.V., McDonald, D.W., Landay, J.A.: Goal-setting considerations for persuasive technologies that encourage physical activity. In: Persuasive 2009, p. 8 (2009)

48. Ferebee, S.S., Davis, J.W.: Factors that persuade continued use of Facebook among new members. In: Persuasive 2009, p. 35 (2009)

49. Firpo, D., Kasemvilas, S., Ractham, P., Zhang, X.: Generating a sense of community in a graduate educational setting through persuasive technology. In: Persuasive 2009, p. 41 (2009)

50. Harjumaa, M., Segerståhl, K., Oinas-Kukkonen, H.: Understanding persuasive software functionality in practice: a field trial of polar FT60. In: Persuasive 2009, p. 2 (2009)

51. Iyengar, M.S., Florez-Arango, J.F., Garcia, C.A.: GuideView: a system for developing structured, multimodal, multi-platform persuasive applications. In: Persuasive 2009, p. 31 (2009)
52. Kappel, K., Grechenig, T.: Show-me: water consumption at a glance to promote water conservation in the shower. In: Persuasive 2009, p. 26 (2009)
53. Lockton, D., Harrison, D., Holley, T., Stanton, N.A.: Influencing interaction: development of the design with intent method. In: Persuasive 2009, p. 5 (2009)
54. Midden, C., Ham, J.: Using negative and positive social feedback from a robotic agent to save energy. In: Persuasive 2009, p. 12 (2009)
55. Olsen, E., Kraft, P.: ePsychology: a pilot study on how to enhance social support and adherence in digital interventions by characteristics from social networking sites. In: Persuasive 2009, p. 32 (2009)
56. Ranfelt, A.M., Wigram, T., Øhrstrøm, P.: Towards a handy interactive persuasive diary for teenagers with a diagnosis of autism. In: Persuasive 2009, p. 3 (2009)
57. Saini, P., Lacroix, J.: Self-setting of physical activity goals and effects on perceived difficulty, importance and competence. In: Persuasive 2009, p. 33 (2009)
58. Shiraishi, M., Washio, Y., Takayama, C., Lehdonvirta, V., Kimura, H., Nakajima, T.: Using individual, social and economic persuasion techniques to reduce CO_2 emissions in a family setting. In: Persuasive 2009, p. 13 (2009)
59. Duncan, J., Camp, L.J., Hazelwood, W.R.: The portal monitor: a privacy-enhanced event-driven system for elder care. In: Persuasive 2009, p. 36 (2009)
60. Vossen, S., Ham, J., Midden, C.: Social influence of a persuasive agent: the role of agent embodiment and evaluative feedback. In: Persuasive 2009, p. 46 (2009)

Ambient Persuasive Technology Needs Little Cognitive Effort: The Differential Effects of Cognitive Load on Lighting Feedback versus Factual Feedback

Jaap Ham and Cees Midden

Human-Technology Interaction, Eindhoven University of Technology, P.O. Box 513,
5600 MB Eindhoven, The Netherlands
j.r.c.ham@tue.nl

Abstract. Persuasive technology can influence behavior or attitudes by for example providing interactive factual feedback about energy conservation. However, people often lack motivation or cognitive capacity to consciously process such relative complex information (e.g., numerical consumption feedback). Extending recent research that indicates that ambient persuasive technology can persuade the user without receiving the user's conscious attention, we argue here that *Ambient Persuasive Technology can be effective while needing only little cognitive resources*, and in general can be more influential than more focal forms of persuasive technology. In an experimental study, some participants received energy consumption feedback by means of a light changing color (more green=lower energy consumption, vs. more red=higher energy consumption) and others by means of numbers indicating kWh consumption. Results indicated that ambient feedback led to more conservation than factual feedback. Also, as expected, only for participants processing factual feedback, additional cognitive load lead to slower processing of that feedback. This research sheds light on fundamental characteristics of Ambient Persuasive Technology and Persuasive Lighting, and suggests that it can have important advantages over more focal persuasive technologies without losing its persuasive potential.

Keywords: Ambient Persuasive Technology, Persuasive Technology, Lighting, Unconscious Influences.

1 Introduction

The threats of growing CO2-emissions and climate change effects and the exhaustion of natural resources have urged nations worldwide to seek for substantial reductions in energy consumption. Next to important technological solutions like more efficient systems and devices and the development of renewable energy sources, consumer behavior plays a crucial role in bringing down the level of energy consumption. Influencing consumer behavior to promote energy conservation has become an important target of national and international policy efforts. Thereby, the question which instruments should be applied to promote energy conservation behavior has become highly relevant.

T. Ploug, P. Hasle, H. Oinas-Kukkonen (Eds.): PERSUASIVE 2010, LNCS 6137, pp. 132–142, 2010.

Recent reviews [e.g., 2, 19, 9] have evaluated the effects of interventions to promote energy efficient behavior. In general, mass media public campaigns seem to lack precision in targeting and message concreteness to achieve behavioral change. By contrast, raising people's awareness of energy consumption by providing tailored feedback about energy consumption can stimulate behavioral change [see, e.g., 2, 19], although results are mixed. Weak linkages between specific actions and energy outcomes caused by low feedback frequencies (e.g. once per month) and insufficient specificity of the feedback (e.g. household in general vs. specific person or specific devices) are underlying these mixed findings.

Recently, technological solutions have created new opportunities to improve feedback efficacy by embedding feedback in user-system interactions. Some evidence supports this claim. McCalley and Midden [18] demonstrated in several studies that such interactive forms of feedback could be effective in enhancing energy-efficient use of devices like washing machines. By adding an energy meter to the user interface of a washing machine they achieved 18% of energy conservation both in lab and field studies.

However, in many day-to-day situations people might not be motivated or lack the cognitive capacity to consciously process relatively complex information [see e.g. 5]. Factual feedback (e.g., the numbers representing kWh consumption) might be that kind of relatively complex information.

Recent research investigates the effectiveness of feedback that is easier to process. Most specifically, Ham and Midden [12] presented evidence that persuasive technology can persuade the user without receiving the user's conscious attention. In a series of trials, participants had to indicate which of three household appliances uses the lowest average amount of energy. After each choice, participants in the supraliminal feedback condition received feedback about the correctness of their choice through presentation of a smiling or a sad face for 150 ms. Participants in the subliminal feedback condition received identical feedback, but the faces were presented only for 25 ms, which prohibited conscious perception of these stimuli. The final third of the participants received no feedback. In the next task, participants rated the energy consumption of all presented appliances. Results indicated that supraliminal feedback and subliminal feedback both led to more correct energy consumption ratings as compared to receiving no feedback. This suggests that ambient persuasive technology can be effective even *without receiving any conscious attention*.

In line with Davis [8], we argue that a suitable label for this new type of persuasive technology is Ambient Persuasive Technology. The goal of the current article is to extend the conceptual clarity about this form of persuasive technology. Therefore, we shall present a study that investigates another key feature of this concept. That is, *we will investigate whether ambient persuasive technology can be effective while needing only little cognitive resources.*

In the current research, we will therefore investigate the persuasive effects of a form of feedback that is easy to process, while at the same time some participants will do an additional, second task. We argue that (interactive) feedback using lighting is simpler to process than (interactive) factual feedback because it can directly express evaluative meaning whereas factual feedback still needs to be processed and evaluated by the user. For example, red lighting might be defined as meaning "high energy consumption", which does not need to be evaluated further, whereas factual feedback that 120 kWh was used does. Also, feedback through (diffused) lighting can be perceived easily without focusing, in contrast to factual feedback. For example, (part of) the environment of the user can be used for lighting feedback, whereas the user needs to focus on factual feedback (e.g., in the form of numbers).

In addition, we argue that lighting has specific qualities that make it particularly suitable for providing user feedback. For example, lighting can be very cheap, is easy to install, lighting can be very energy friendly, lighting can be seen by other people present in a room as well (inducing social pressure as a persuasive mechanism), and lighting might have an emotional appeal or even direct emotional effects. Also, the low conspicuity of light and color changes sets lighting apart from other feedback mechanisms. Furthermore, lighting can be calm (in the sense of 'calm computing'). Other feedback mechanisms often lack these characteristics.

Earlier research indicates that energy consumption feedback that does not consists of specific facts, but rather of lighting changes can influence consumer behavior [see 8, 27, 3, 11, 24, 22, see also 21, and 14]. For example, in the eighties of the previous century Becker and Seligman [6] investigated the effectiveness of a light that went on "in a highly visible part of the home" whenever the air conditioner was on, but the outside temperature was 20°C or lower. In homes that contained the signaling device, an average of 15% savings in energy consumption was found. More recently, a device called an energy orb was used that changed color dependent on the time-of-use tariff in operation. This type of information helped users save some energy [16] and the usefulness of the device was positively evaluated by users [24, 16].

The current research will investigate the effects of feedback through lighting on energy consumption and compare them to the effects of factual feedback. The feedback (lighting feedback and factual feedback) that we will investigate in this research will be of a highly interactive nature. Earlier research of lighting feedback did not employ feedback that was fundamentally interactive (see e.g., [6]). For example, Becker and Seligman's [6] participants received feedback about their action, but not in direct response to those actions. In the current research, participants will receive feedback about consequences of an action in direct response to that action. More specifically, the current research will give users lighting feedback about their current energy consumption in a specific task, and this lighting feedback will change directly when they use more or less energy. Furthermore, the current research will investigate the assumption that lighting feedback is easier to process than factual feedback.

1.1 The Current Research

In the current research, we examine whether interactive feedback through lighting can stimulate energy conservation behavior. That is, we will use lighting color as feedback to indicate the absolute level of energy consumption (more green = lower energy consumption, vs. more red = higher energy consumption). We set up an experiment in which participants had the opportunity to conserve energy in a series of tasks and received feedback about their energy consumption during these tasks. We tested the effect of lighting feedback and compared these effects to more widely used factual feedback. More specifically, we compared the effects of lighting feedback using lighting color to indicate energy consumption, to the effects of factual feedback using a number to indicate energy consumption in Watts. When giving lighting feedback, low consumption was indicated by completely green lighting and high consumption by completely red lighting. So, people can quite easily understand whether a specific lighting (e.g. light-green) indicates high or low consumption.

However, when factual feedback would consist of only one number (representing energy consumption in Watts), without any reference, it would be a lot more difficult to know whether that number indicates high or low consumption. Therefore, when giving factual feedback, next to the number indicating the current energy consumption level, two additional numbers were presented indicating low and high consumption. Thereby the amount of information present in lighting feedback and factual feedback was comparable.

As argued above, we expect that feedback through lighting has stronger persuasive effects (leading to lower energy consumption) than factual feedback. In addition, we expected that lighting feedback would be easier to process. To test this, we manipulated cognitive load: Half of the participants performed an additional task. We expected that for participants processing factual feedback, performing this additional task would interfere with the persuasive effects of that feedback, leading to more energy consumption than without the additional task. At the same time, we expected that for participants processing lighting feedback, performing this additional task would not interfere with the persuasive effects of that feedback, leading to the same energy consumption as without the additional task. Also, we expected that for participants processing factual feedback, performing this additional task would lead to slower processing of that feedback, while for participants processing lighting feedback, performing this additional task would not lead to slower processing of that feedback.

2   Method

2.1   Participants and Design

Fifty-seven participants (39 men and 18 women) were randomly assigned to one of the four cells of a 2 (feedback type: lighting feedback versus factual feedback) x 2 (cognitive load: load vs. no load) experimental design. All participants were students at Eindhoven University of Technology, were recruited on campus to participate in a study on 'How to program a heating thermostat', and received € 5 for a participation of 30 minutes.

2.2   Procedure and Materials

Upon arrival, participants were seated in front of a computer. For all participants, a simulated programmable thermostat panel was presented on the computer screen (see Figure 1). This heating thermostat was modeled to look like a commercially available heating thermostat. It contained a virtual LCD display (with a background that was always green) on which all relevant information and clickable buttons were presented.

For participants in the lighting feedback condition, a computer-controlled power-led lamp was positioned behind the participants' desk that reflected its lighting on the wall behind the desk (see Figure 2). For participants in the factual feedback condition, next to this thermostat panel we presented a number indicating the participant's energy consumption in Watts, and also two numbers indicating low and high consumption levels in Watts.

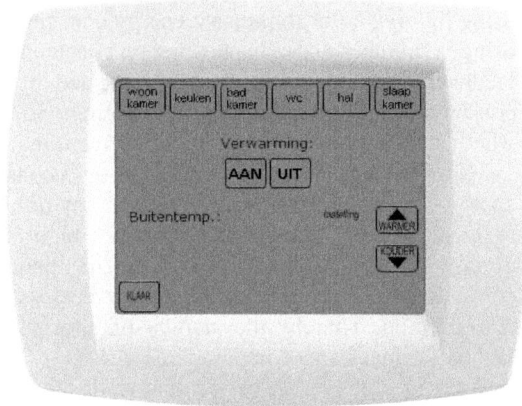

Fig. 1. The simulated programmable heating system interface

More specifically, for each of the ten scenarios (described below) we calculated a low consumption score in Watts (based on a setting of 17°C in relevant rooms) and a high consumption score in Watts (based on a setting of 26°C in all rooms). In the lighting feedback condition, these numbers were used to determine the lighting color. That is, when a participant's energy consumption caused by his or her setting of the thermostat were at the low consumption level or lower, the lamp was given a completely saturated green color, and when energy consumption was at the high level or higher, the lamp was given a completely saturated red color. When a participant's thermostat settings lead to an energy consumption in between the low level and the high level, the light the lamp emitted was set to a color between green (indicating low consumption) and white (indicating consumption of a medium level, halfway between low and high) or a color between white and red (indicating high consumption).

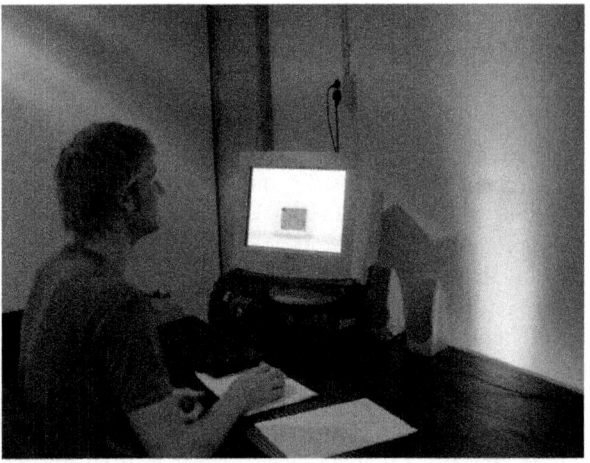

After general introductions, participants were asked to program the thermostat in ten different tasks. Also, all participants were given two specific

Fig. 2. Feedback through lighting on the wall behind the monitor

goals to strive for while programming the thermostat: (1) to strive for optimal comfort levels within each specific task. More specifically, they were asked to "program the programmable thermostat such that your house would be comfortable to live in."[1] And (2), participants were instructed to use as little energy as possible. That is, they were told that heating your house costs energy (fuel) and diminishing the level of the temperature settings for specific rooms would lead to lower energy consumptions. We included the first goal to motivate participants to use energy (to heat the house to comfortable levels). Had we only included the second goal, all participants might have chosen to use as little energy as possible by simply not turning the heating on at all, and any feedback about energy consumption would have been irrelevant.

Next, the thermostat and the energy consumption feedback (factual or ambient) it provided were explained. In each task, participants were instructed to program the thermostat for a different scenario. For this, we used 10 different, short scenario descriptions (e.g., "It is evening and you are having a party at home tonight", "It is night and you are going to bed. It is -10°C outside", "On a Sunday afternoon you are at home and outside temperature is 18°C"). In each task, one of the ten scenarios was displayed above the programmable thermostat panel. Scenarios were drawn randomly from the set of ten and each scenario was used only once. Participants received feedback after each change of settings, until they pressed the "ready" button. For each task, we registered the energy consumption corresponding to the final setting, and the total amount of time a participant used for that task.

Participants in the cognitive load conditions performed an additional task while setting the thermostat. This task was comparable to cognitive load tasks used in earlier research (e.g., [26]). Participants heard numbers (one to thirty) read out aloud on headphones. As a manipulation check, we registered the number of correct responses (pressing the space bar after an odd number). Finally, participants were debriefed and thanked for their participation.

3   Results

Averaged energy consumption scores (over the 10 tasks) were submitted to a 2 (feedback type: lighting feedback versus factual feedback) x 2 (cognitive load: load vs. no load) ANOVA. As expected, participants who had received feedback through lighting used a lower amount of energy on average on the tasks ($M = 544$ Watt, $SD = 208$) than participants who received factual feedback ($M = 692$ Watt, $SD = 202$), $F(1,53) = 7.16$, $p = .01$ (see Figure 3). This analysis did not indicate the expected interaction of Feedback Type X Cognitive Load, $F < 1$. Also, this analysis did not show a main effect of cognitive load, $F < 1$.

However, the manipulation check of the cognitive load task indicated that approximately half of the participants in the cognitive load conditions had not performed the load task in line with instructions (had pressed the space bar for less than 10% of odd numbers). Therefore, to assess whether the effect of feedback type on energy consumption was qualified by cognitive load (indicated by an interaction of

---

[1] As in real-life programming of programmable heating thermostats, participants did not experience physical effects of changes (e.g., changes in heat) during the programming tasks. So, participants had to judge the comfort level corresponding to their settings of the thermostat based on earlier experiences and their current settings.

feedback type x cognitive load), we submitted the average energy consumption scores of the remaining participants (14 in the load conditions, of whom 7 received lighting feedback and 7 received factual feedback, and 29 in the no load conditions, of whom 15 received lighting feedback and 14 received factual feedback) to an identical 2 (feedback type: lighting feedback versus factual feedback) x

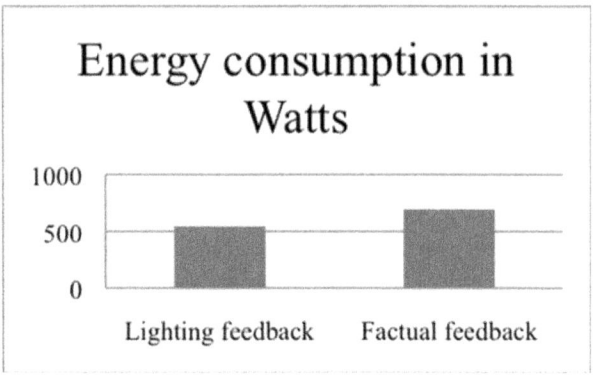

Fig. 3. Energy consumption in Watts by type of feedback

2 (cognitive load: load vs. no load) ANOVA. This analysis showed results completely comparable to the previous one: a main effect of feedback type, $F(1, 39) = 4.63$, $p < .05$, but no interaction of feedback type and cognitive load nor a main effect of cognitive load, both F's < 1.

Finally, to assess whether lighting feedback would be easier to process, we analyzed the time it took these remaining participants to program the thermostat. This dependent variable was calculated by averaging the times they needed on each of the 10 tasks. This analysis showed the expected interaction of Feedback Type X Cognitive Load, $F(1,39) = 7.20$, $p = .011$ (see Figure 4). Further analyses indicated that participants who received factual feedback needed more time to program the thermostat under cognitive load ($M = 55.0$ seconds, $SD = 15.1$) than without cognitive load ($M = 38.7$ seconds, $SD = 7.0$), $F(1, 40) = 6.02$, $p = .019$, whereas this difference was not found for participants who received lighting feedback, $F<1$. In general, programming the thermostat using lighting feedback was faster ($M = 39.3$ seconds, $SD = 8.0$) than when using factual feedback ($M = 44.1$ seconds, $SD = 12.7$), $F(1,41) = 9.24$, $p < .01$.

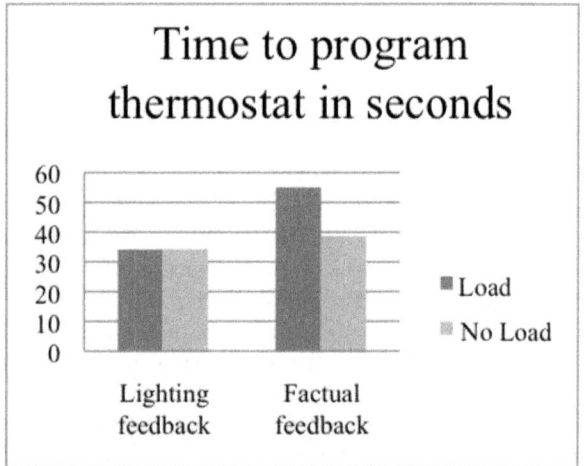

Fig. 4. Time to program thermostat by type of feedback and cognitive load

Finally, we also explored the effect of cognitive load on energy consumption scores, but found no significant results of cognitive load, all F's<1.

4 Conclusion and Discussion

Results indicated that participants who received feedback through lighting used less energy in thermostat programming tasks than participants who received factual feedback. Thereby, the current research suggests that lighting feedback can have stronger persuasive effects than factual feedback (approximately 27%). Also, the current results suggest that for participants processing factual feedback, doing an additional task led to slower processing of that feedback. For participants processing lighting feedback, results suggest that adding cognitive load did not lead to slower processing. This finding fits our suggestion that lighting feedback is easier to process and use in goal-striving processes than factual feedback.

In contrast to expectations, the current results did not show evidence for effects of cognitive load on energy consumption, or of different effects of cognitive load on energy consumption for participants who received lighting feedback compared to those who received factual feedback. An important reason for this might be that the setup of the current study may not have been ideal for finding such an effect because of the lack of time constraints when setting the thermostat. That is, because there were no time constraints, participants who received factual feedback and who performed an additional task, may have been able to use more time to set the thermostat (and did so, as indicated by the analysis of response times). It seems quite straightforward that these participants used this additional time to process the factual feedback. Thereby these participants may have processed the factual feedback well, even though they also had to spend processing capacity on the additional task. Future research might continue the investigation of whether cognitive load can increase energy consumption for factual feedback. Importantly, the current results indicate that setting time constraints might be important to find those effects.

Another possibility is that cognitive load could exert an effect on energy consumption even without time constraints, especially in a multiple goal-setting paradigm, since it leaves less cognitive capacity for considering the various goals (i.e., 'comfort' and 'energy saving'). Cognitive load might make people forget secondary goals ('energy saving' would often be considered secondary), or process additional cues (e.g., light feedback) in a more peripheral rather than central way. Interestingly, both paths would have implications for the most optimal design of feedback cues, and future research could investigate both pathways.

Also, future research might investigate these questions using other forms of cognitive load. That is, because the current cognitive load task contained numerical elements (as participants had to identify odd numbers in a spoken list of numbers), it could have interfered especially with processing the factual feedback because that also consisted of numbers (indicating energy consumption). Therefore, the total cognitive load may not have been equal in both cognitive load conditions. That said, we argue that the numbers in the current load task were only of secondary importance, as the main task participants had to do was to identify a specific element in an array of elements (and these could just as easily have been arrays of letters, in which participants would have to identify consonants). In line with this argument, theories that account for effects of information processing demands generally do not identify different effects of processing demands caused by different types of information (for an overview, see [20]). So, these theories would not predict fundamentally different mental load effects of a cognitive load task that consisted of a more numerical load task versus another type of load task. Likewise, cognitive load theory [25] indicates that limitations of human cognitive processing become especially pronounced when dealing with complex tasks [4]. Based on cognitive load theory, we argue that adding an additional task (our load task, which indeed contained numbers) could have revealed limitations of cognitive processing also in the lighting feedback condition, independent of the specific nature of that additional task. In other words, because our load task added to the complexity of the overall task participants in the lighting feedback conditions had to perform, it therefore could have revealed limitations of cognitive processing. And indeed results did not indicate these limitations (in terms of slower processing) in lighting feedback conditions, but only revealed these limitations (slower processing) in factual feedback conditions. Still, future research replicating the current findings with different cognitive load tasks would certainly strengthen the evidence for our argument that lighting feedback is easier to process and use in goal-striving processes than factual feedback.

Furthermore, future research could also investigate which other differences between lighting feedback and factual feedback may underlie the stronger persuasive effects of lighting feedback in addition to the higher ease of processing of lighting feedback that the current research suggests. For instance, lighting feedback might be more conspicuous, have specific physiological consequences, or may have stronger emotional or moral effects. Thereby, persuasive lighting could be studied in the perspective of consumer information processing [see 7].

Overall, the current research indicates that diffuse lighting can be used successfully as persuasive technology. These technologies can be incorporated into everyday life in many forms to change different types of behavior or attitudes. For example, the data about energy consumption provided by smart meters might be used to deliver interactive lighting feedback in the living room.

Based on current results, we argue that lighting in various modalities can serve as Ambient Persuasive Technology [see also 1, 6, 8, 10, 13, 15, 23]. We propose that Ambient Persuasive Technologies are generic technologies that are intentionally designed to change a person's attitude or behavior or both, that can be integrated unobtrusively into the environment and exert an influence on people without the need for their focal attention. The current research suggests that ambient persuasive technology can have important advantages over more focal persuasive technologies without losing its persuasive potential.

Acknowledgments. We thank Saskia Maan and Bo Merkus for important contributions to this work and for running the experiment, the Persuasive Technology Lab Group for comments and ideas, and Martin Boschman for technical assistance.

References

1. Aarts, E.H.L., Markopoulos, P., de Ruyter, B.: The persuasiveness of ambient intelligence. In: Petkovic, M., Jonker, W. (eds.) Security, privacy, and trust in modern data management, pp. 367–381. Springer, Berlin (2007)
2. Abrahamse, W., Steg, L., Vlek, C., Rothengatter, T.: A review of intervention studies aimed at household energy conservation. Journal of Environmental Psychology 25, 273–291 (2005)

3. Arroyo, E., Bonanni, L., Selker, T.: Waterbot: Exploring feedback and persuasive techniques at the sink. In: Proceedings of the SIGCHI Conference on Human Factors in Computing Systems (CHI 2005), pp. 631–639 (2005)
4. Ayres, P., van Gog, T.: State of the art research into Cognitive Load Theory. Computers in Human Behavior 25, 253–257 (2009)
5. Bargh, J.A.: The automaticity of everyday life. In: Wyer Jr., R.S. (ed.) The automaticity of everyday life: Advances in social cognition, vol. 10, pp. 1–61. Erlbaum, Mahwah (1997)
6. Becker, L.J., Seligman, C.: Reducing air-conditioning waste by signaling it is cool outside. Personality and Social Psychology Bulletin 4, 412–415 (1978)
7. Bettman, J.R., Sujan, M.: Research in Consumer Information Processing. In: Houston, M.J. (ed.) Review of Marketing, American Marketing Association, Chicago, IL, pp. 197–235 (1987)
8. Davis, J.: Towards participatory design of ambient persuasive technology. Presented at Persuasive Pervasive Technology and Environmental Sustainability, Workshop at the Sixth International Conference on Pervasive Computing (Pervasive 2008), Sydney, May 19–22 (2008)
9. Fischer, C.: Feedback on household electricity consumption: a tool for saving energy? Energy Efficiency 1, 79–104 (2008)
10. Fogg, B.J.: Persuasive Technology: Using Computers to Change What We Think and Do. Morgan Kaufmann, San Francisco (2003)
11. Froehlich, J.: Promoting energy efficient behaviors in the home through feedback: The role of human-computer interaction. Paper presented at HCIC 2009 (2009)
12. Ham, J., Midden, C., Beute, F.: Can Ambient Persuasive Technology Persuade Unconsciously? Using Subliminal Feedback to Influence Energy Consumption Ratings of Household Appliances. In: Conference Proceedings of Persuasive 2009, Claremont, USA (2009)
13. IJsselstein, W., De Kort, Y., Midden, C., Eggen, B., Van den Hoven, E.: Persuasive technology for human well-being: Setting the scene. In: IJsselsteijn, W.A., de Kort, Y.A.W., Midden, C., Eggen, B., van den Hoven, E. (eds.) PERSUASIVE 2006. LNCS, vol. 3962, pp. 1–5. Springer, Heidelberg (2006)
14. Kotler, P.: Atmospherics as a marketing tool. Journal of Retailing 49, 48–64 (1974)
15. Martinez, M.S., Geltz, C.R.: Utilizing a pre-attentive technology for modifying customer energy usage. In: Proceedings of the European Council for an Energy-Efficient Economy (2005)
16. Martinez, M.S.: Residential demand response technologies: A consumer's guide. Presentation at National Town Meeting and Symposium on Demand Response (2006)
17. Mathew, A.P.: Using the environment as an interactive interface to motivate positive behavior change in a subway station. In: CHI 2005 Extended Abstracts on Human Factors in Computing Systems, pp. 1637–1640 (2005)
18. McCalley, L.T., Midden, C.J.H.: Energy conservation through product-integrated feedback: The roles of goal-setting and social orientation. Journal of Economic Psychology 23, 589–603 (2002)
19. Midden, C.J.H., Kaiser, F.G., Mccalley, L.T.: Technology's four roles in understanding individuals' conservation of natural resources. Journal of Social Issues 63(1), 155–174 (2007)
20. Nietfeld, J.L., Finney, S.J., Schraw, G., McCrudden, M.T.: A test of theoretical models that account for information processing demands. Contemporary Educational Psychology 32, 499–515 (2007)

21. Riva, G., Vatalaro, F., Davide, F., Alcaniz, M. (eds.): Ambient Intelligence. IOS Press, Amsterdam (2005)
22. Roth, K., Brodrick, J.: Home energy displays. ASHRAE Journal (July 2008)
23. Schmidt, A.: Interactive Context-Aware Systems Interacting with Ambient Intelligence. In: Riva, G., Vatalaro, F., Davide, F., Alcaniz, M. (eds.) Ambient Intelligence. IOS Press, Amsterdam (2005)
24. Stein, L.F.: California Information Display Pilot: Technology Assessment. Final Report by Primen to Southern California Edison (2004)
25. Sweller, J.: Cognitive load during problem solving: Effects on learning. Cognitive Science: A Multidisciplinary Journal 12, 257–285 (1988)
26. Winter, L., Uleman, J.S., Cunnif, C.: How automatic are social judgments? Journal of Personality and Social Psychology 49, 904–917 (1985)
27. Wisneski, C., Ishii, H., Dahley, A., Gorbet, M.G., Brave, S., Ullmer, B., Yarin, P.: Ambient Displays. In: Streitz, N.A., Konomi, S., Burkhardt, H.-J. (eds.) CoBuild 1998. LNCS, vol. 1370, p. 22. Springer, Heidelberg (1998)

Design Dimensions Enabling Divergent Behaviour across Physical, Digital, and Social Library Interfaces

Lennart Björneborn

Royal School of Library and Information Science, Copenhagen, Denmark
lb@db.dk

Abstract. What design dimensions across physical, digital, and social library interfaces may enable and trigger users to find more information resources than planned or known in advance? The paper outlines a conceptual framework with libraries as *integrative interfaces* across physical, digital, and social affordances and users that mix *convergent* (goal-directed) and *divergent* (exploratory) information behaviour. Ten design dimensions that enable and trigger divergent behaviour are outlined. Implications for persuasive design are discussed.

Keywords: interaction design, persuasive design, libraries, enabling spaces, affordances, interfaces, exploratory information behaviour, serendipity.

1 Introduction

"We shape our buildings, and afterwards our buildings shape us."[1]

The design of an information space shapes the ways users can interact with this space. Traditionally, the design of digital and physical libraries supports users' goal-directed, *convergent* behaviour [3]. Tools like classification, indexing, and cataloguing help users to find information resources they have planned to find. In recent years, there has been increasing attention also on supporting library users' exploratory, *divergent* behaviour in order to create more inspiring and stimulating library spaces, circulate more information resources, and counteract *library bypass* [e.g., 21]. From a persuasive design approach, it would be interesting to identify design dimensions or *affordances*, i.e. actionable properties [14], in library spaces that may enable and trigger users to discover and explore interesting resources not planned or not known in advance among often hundreds of thousands of available resources.

In this context, the present short paper briefly outlines a conceptual framework [3] with libraries as *integrative interfaces* across physical, digital, and social affordances – and with users that mix and switch between *convergent* (goal-directed) and *divergent* (exploratory) information behaviour. Ten design dimensions that may enable and trigger divergent information behaviour as additional actions beyond preplanned findings are outlined. Implications for persuasive design are discussed.

---

[1] Winston Churchill cited by [12, p.194].

T. Ploug, P. Hasle, H. Oinas-Kukkonen (Eds.): PERSUASIVE 2010, LNCS 6137, pp. 143–149, 2010.

2 Integrative User Interface

In libraries, users can interact with a multimodality of human, physical, and digital information resources. Users can read printed books, download podcasted lectures, talk with other users about music, etc., etc. The *integrative interface* (Fig. 1a+b) of a library comprises the totality of all these contact surfaces, access points and mediation flows between users and human, physical, and digital information resources [3]. The integrative interface thus comprises all affordances for user interaction in the library.

The interface is *integrative* as the multimodality of different human, physical and digital parts of the library may be looked upon as an *integrated whole*; as supplementary and supportive parts for one another. This approach thus suggests to think affordances, design, and usability across *all* contact surfaces between users and information resources – and not only such features in digital interfaces.

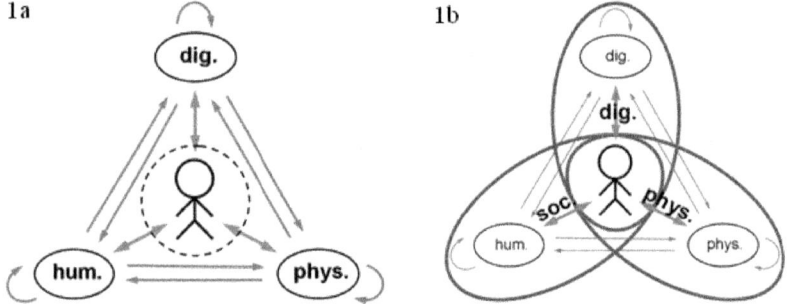

Fig. 1a. Integrative 'multimodal' interface model [3]. User within 'socio-cognitive-embodied' context (broken line circle) interacts (double arrows) with human (hum.), physical (phys.) and digital (dig.) information resources. Between resources are mediation flows (single arrows).
Fig. 1b. Social, physical and digital information spaces in the interface model, cf. Fig. 1a.

Mediation flows in Fig. 1a could, e.g., be staff and users communicating ('human → human')[2] or flyers in the physical library pointing to library web pages ('physical → digital'). See more examples in [3]. Mediation flows can be combined into longer chains and loops. The model includes evolving cross-modal technologies in pervasive computing, tangible interfaces, social computing, mobile interfaces, etc. [cf. 6].

Physical aspects of persuasive design have been discussed by, e.g., [16] who refers to physical objects as "persuasive arguments in material form". Equally important, people have embodied experiences, physical mobility and spatial/tactile senses [cf. 6] that affect design across physical, digital, and social environments. For example, the embodied ability of our peripheral vision to discover/recognize new affordances can be more easily triggered if there is a 'red thread' in the design of human, physical, and digital counterparts of the library interface. It could be staff t-shirts, shelves, and web pages with similar layout signalling similar affordances across dissimilar modalities.

---

[2] This has Library 2.0 implications [11] when interfaces allow users to leave behavioural traces for other users to follow, cf. *social navigation* [5] and *social facilitation* [8, 15], e.g., when browsing trolleys with newly returned books or finding books left on tables by other users.

3   Convergent and Divergent Information Behaviour

Information behaviour can be defined as "the totality of human behavior in relation to sources and channels of information, including both active and passive information seeking, and information use" [22]. On this background, library users can be seen as employing a wide range of *convergent* (goal-directed) and *divergent* (exploratory) information behaviour [3], cf. Table 1, when they look for information resources, whether human, physical, or digital. As noted in Table 1, divergent information behaviour is related to browsing [1, 4], information encountering [7], opportunistic acquisition of information [7], serendipity [10, 20], and creative thinking [2].

Table 1. Ideal-type aspects of convergent and divergent information behaviour [3]

⟹ complementary ⟸ ⟹ ⟸	
Convergent information behaviour	**Divergent information behaviour**
- 'left brain' - goal-directed, focused, rational ⟹ 'zooming in'/'narrowing vision' - e.g., known-item searches - conscious, explicit information needs - problems, work tasks, primary tasks, etc. - 'information recovery'	- 'right brain' - exploratory, impulsive, intuitive ⟸ 'zooming out'/'broadening vision' - e.g., browsing, info.encountering, serendipity - subconscious, implicit information needs - interests, curiosity, creativity, secondary tasks, etc. - 'information discovery'

Convergent and divergent behaviour, handling primary tasks [cf. 15] and secondary tasks, can supplement and succeed each other as indicated by the 'behavioural pulse' at the top of Table 1. Convergent behaviour may thus identify central information that function as points of departure for exploratory and divergent information behaviour. Reversely, unplanned findings may lead to a need for more focused and convergent search strategies. Such *bit-at-a-time* activity resembling berry-picking [1] is related to task-switching and multi-tasking [18] and can be illustrated by Fig. 2.

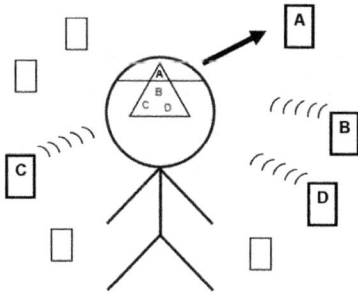

Fig. 2. Interest space model [3]. Potentially triggering items B-D matched by user's interest space ('iceberg') while user moves through information space searching for item A.

When users move through an information space (e.g., library, Web, city), cf. Fig. 2, they may change directions and behaviour several times as their information needs and interests develop or get triggered depending on affordances encountered on their way through the information space [3]. Human behaviour may be seen as a product of three factors: *motivation*, *ability*, and *triggers* [9]. All factors are implicit in Fig 2: *Motivation* includes information needs and interests. *Ability* includes information literacies to navigate with integrated body and mind through physical, digital, and social information spaces. *Triggers* include convergent and divergent design dimensions that may stimulate convergent and divergent information behaviour. The divergent design dimensions are in focus in the next section.

4   Design Dimensions Enabling Divergent Behaviour

The ten design dimensions in Table 2 for enabling and triggering divergent behaviour were identified in a study at two Danish public libraries [3]. Naturalistic observation of users' information behaviour when they moved through the physical library was combined with qualitative interviews with 113 users: *What did they intend to find? What did they actually find? How did they find it?* Additional think-aloud sessions with eleven of the interviewees that walked through the library together with one of the researchers provided reflective comments on what design dimensions triggered the users' attention and might change their information behaviour.

The identified dimensions can influence users' behaviour across all contact surfaces and mediation flows in the interface model in Fig. 1a.

Table 2. Design dimensions enabling divergent behaviour across integrative interfaces [3]

Design dimensions	Explanation
Accessibility	Unhampered direct access to human, physical, digital information resources
Diversity	Rich and dense variety of topics, genres, media, activities, modalities, etc.
Display	Curiosity-teasing mediation and exposure of information resources
Contrasts	Eye-catching differentiation including quiet zones and display zones
Pointers	Signage, maps, markers, cues, references, etc., may trigger users' interests
Imperfection	Imperfect 'cracks' in interfaces may lead to unplanned findings
Cross-contacts	Contact surfaces across dissimilar topics, genres, activities, modalities, etc.
Multi-reachability	Many different access routes can be chosen through and across interfaces
Explorability	Interfaces invite users to move, look around, explore and browse
Stopability	Interfaces invite users to stop, look closer and assess found resources

The dimensions overlap and the list is not exhaustive as there may be additional dimensions that more extensive studies may identify. See [3] for more details and examples of the dimensions that are not possible to give in this short paper.

Facilitating divergent information behaviour and secondary tasks (cf. Table 1), the dimensions are mostly concerned with an *enabling* approach, and to some degree a *motivating* approach; the least interventionary of the persuasive approaches *enabling*, *motivating* and *constraining* [13]. Several dimensions thus deal with the very structure, architecture and connectedness of information spaces that may enable divergent behaviour, e.g., *accessibility*, *multi-reachability*, *explorability*, and *stopability*. These dimensions influence how users can move through and explore an information space, cf. Fig. 2. For example, before open shelves were introduced in libraries in the late 19th century, closed stacks provided no direct access to information resources, and thus no affordances for divergent behaviour, browsing and serendipitous findings. There are parallels to impulse-driven shopping and retail interior design triggering customers to choose new routes, shelves, products, etc. [19].

Stopability complements *explorability* and denotes how the library interface invites users to stop and assess information resources. It could be seating affordances close to shelves or free space on shelves etc., enabling users to put down carried things and get free hands to touch and examine found resources including unplanned findings. This design dimension may help users decide whether to make use of found resources.

Some of the dimensions may enable both divergent and convergent behaviour, e.g., *accessibility*, *stopability*, *display*, and *pointers*. The latter two dimensions are covered by Fogg's persuasive tool 'suggestion' [8]. Displays (e.g., exhibitions) and pointers (e.g., signage) in the library may hence motivate users to change information behaviour and switch from convergent mode to divergent mode, or vice versa.

Other dimensions deal with eye-catching, differentiating qualities of information resources, e.g., *diversity*, *contrasts*, *imperfection* and *cross-contacts*. The abovementioned behavioural traces left behind by users are examples of imperfect 'cracks' in the library interface that may enable and trigger unplanned findings. Users may thus perceive useful affordances not necessarily intended by designers [cf. 17].

The table outlines *extrinsic* triggers. Of course, *intrinsic* factors like abilities and motivation [cf. 9] influence how users perceive and utilize affordances for divergent behaviour. Intrinsic factors include intentions, attention, physical mobility, energy, past experiences, personality, interests, needs, etc. As a result, users have different receptiveness to discovering and encountering information resources not planned or not known in advance; ranging from 'non-encounterers' to 'super encounterers' [7].

5 Conclusion

Persuasive design may bridge *'affordance gaps'* [17] between users' *perceived* affordances and designers' *intended* affordances; thus helping users to grasp usage potentials provided by the design dimensions of a given technology or interface.

As stated in the introduction, traditional focus in libraries has been on design dimensions supporting convergent information behaviour. This paper has briefly outlined ten design dimensions that may be used to better enable and trigger divergent information behaviour in order to discover and explore interesting resources not planned or not known in advance. It would be interesting further to investigate these divergent design dimensions in relation to existing persuasive design frameworks and incorporate the outlined conceptual framework with its holistic approach to information spaces and interfaces across physical, digital, and social affordances.

In the presented approach, libraries can be seen as *enabling spaces* with design dimensions that should facilitate *both* convergent and divergent behaviour when users interact with human, physical, and digital information resources. Ultimately, it is up to the users how to explore and exploit – and perhaps even expand (in Library 2.0 settings) – these affordances and design dimensions. Persuasive design may thus be successful – at least in an *enabling* approach – even if users' perceived affordances go beyond designers' intended affordances. The more enabling affordances, convergent *and* divergent, that are designed and allowed across information spaces, the more stimulating and rewarding interactions, hopefully, the users will experience. Rephrasing the introductory quote: *The ways we shape our environments shape us.*

References

1. Bates, M.J.: The design of browsing and berrypicking techniques for the online search interface. Online Review 13(5), 407–424 (1989)
2. Bawden, D.: Information systems and the stimulation of creativity. Journal of Information Science 12, 203–216 (1986)
3. Björneborn, L.: Serendipity dimensions and users' information behaviour in the physical library interface. Information Research 13(4), paper 370 (2008),
   `http://InformationR.net/ir/13-4/paper370.html`
4. Chang, S.J., Rice, R.E.: Browsing: a multidimensional framework. Annual Review of Information Science and Technology 28, 231–276 (1993)
5. Dieberger, A., Dourish, P., Höök, K., et al.: Social navigation: Techniques for building more usable systems. Interactions 7(6), 36–45 (2000)
6. Dourish, P.: Where the action is: The foundations of embodied interaction. MIT Press, Cambridge (2001)
7. Erdelez, S.: Information encountering. In: Fisher, K.E., et al. (eds.) Theories of Information Behavior: A Researcher's Guide, pp. 179–184. Information Today, Medford (2005)
8. Fogg, B.J.: Persuasive technology: Using computers to change what we think and do. Morgan Kaufmann, San Francisco (2003)
9. Fogg, B.J.: A behavior model for persuasive design. In: PERSUASIVE 2009. ACM, New York (2009)
10. Foster, A., Ford, N.: Serendipity and information seeking: An empirical study. Journal of Documentation 59(3), 321–340 (2003)
11. Holmberg, K., Huvila, I., Kronqvist-Berg, M., et al.: What is Library 2.0? Journal of Documentation 65(4), 668–681 (2009)
12. Lawson, B.: The Language of Space. Architectural Press, Oxford (2001)
13. Lockton, D., Harrison, D., Stanton, N.: Design with intent: persuasive technology in a wider context. In: Oinas-Kukkonen, H., Hasle, P., Harjumaa, M., Segerståhl, K., Øhrstrøm, P. (eds.) PERSUASIVE 2008. LNCS, vol. 5033, pp. 274–278. Springer, Heidelberg (2008)
14. Norman, D.: Affordance, conventions and design. Interactions 6(3), 38–42 (1999)
15. Oinas-Kukkonen, H., Harjumaa, M.: A systematic framework for designing and evaluating persuasive systems. In: Oinas-Kukkonen, H., Hasle, P., Harjumaa, M., Segerståhl, K., Øhrstrøm, P. (eds.) PERSUASIVE 2008. LNCS, vol. 5033, pp. 164–176. Springer, Heidelberg (2008)

16. Redström, J.: Persuasive design: fringes and foundations. In: IJsselsteijn, W.A., de Kort, Y.A.W., Midden, C., Eggen, B., van den Hoven, E. (eds.) PERSUASIVE 2006. LNCS, vol. 3962, pp. 112–122. Springer, Heidelberg (2006)
17. Sadler, E., Given, L.M.: Affordance theory: a framework for graduate students' information behaviour. Journal of Documentation 63(1), 115–141 (2007)
18. Spink, A.: Multitasking information behaviour and information task switching: an exploratory study. Journal of Documentation 60(4), 336–351 (2004)
19. Underhill, P.: Why we buy: the science of shopping. Simon & Schuster, New York (1999)
20. Van Andel, P.: Anatomy of the unsought finding: serendipity: origin, history, domains, traditions, appearances, patterns and programmability. British Journal for the Philosophy of Science 45(2), 631–648 (1994)
21. Van Riel, R., et al.: The reader-friendly library service. Society of Chief Librarians (2008)
22. Wilson, T.D.: Human information behaviour. Informing Science 3(2), 49–56 (2000)

Personality and Persuasive Technology: An Exploratory Study on Health-Promoting Mobile Applications

Sajanee Halko[1] and Julie A. Kientz[1,2]

[1] Human Centered Design & Engineering
[2] The Information School
University of Washington
Seattle, Washington, USA
{sajanee,jkientz}@uw.edu

Abstract. Though a variety of persuasive health applications have been designed with a preventive standpoint toward diseases in mind, many have been designed largely for a general audience. Designers of these technologies may achieve more success if applications consider an individual's personality type. Our goal for this research was to explore the relationship between personality and persuasive technologies in the context of health-promoting mobile applications. We conducted an online survey with 240 participants using storyboards depicting eight different persuasive strategies, the Big Five Inventory for personality domains, and questions on perceptions of the persuasive technologies. Our results and analysis revealed a number of significant relationships between personality and the persuasive technologies we evaluated. The findings from this study can guide the development of persuasive technologies that can cater to individual personalities to improve the likelihood of their success.

Keywords: Persuasive Technologies, Personality, mHealth, User-Centered Design, Quantitative Methods.

1 Introduction

Over the past decade, we have seen a rise in technologies targeting the promotion of a healthy lifestyle [5,17,19,21,24]. It is not uncommon for individuals to have tried using their computers or mobile phones to track physical activity [4,5], moderate nutrition [24], or quit smoking (http://www.quitnet.com). Given their popularity, applications designed to promote healthy living are promising for helping users set and achieve their health-related goals, but have not yet proven themselves for long-term adoption and behavior change. Thus, more design guidance and a better understanding of how technologies can be customized to fit users' lives is needed.

Many persuasive technologies have been designed mainly for a general audience using a single persuasive technique. With this approach, it is challenging to sustain user interest over time and appeal to a broad range of people. Thus, many products which start out fairly general need to specialize over time to better cater to the needs of its users. The one-size-fits-all notion is typically not enough to meet the demands

T. Ploug, P. Hasle, H. Oinas-Kukkonen (Eds.): PERSUASIVE 2010, LNCS 6137, pp. 150–161, 2010.

of users, especially with regard to health technologies. Consumers are expecting more from providers across a wide range of fields, and persuasive technologies are no exception. These technologies may better accommodate the needs of diverse users and sustain user interest over time by considering the different personality types of their users. There is some promise that applications customized for an individual's personality type may achieve higher success rates [1].

With this work, we wanted to investigate whether significant relationships exist between personality types and perceptions of persuasive technologies targeting health promotion. In our study, we focus on persuasive mobile technologies that promote physical activity, because that is one of the common applications of health and most individuals currently own a mobile device. To achieve this goal, we conducted an online survey with 240 participants using storyboards depicting eight different persuasive technology strategies: Authoritative, Non-Authoritative, Extrinsic Motivators, Intrinsic Motivators, Positive Reinforcement, Negative Reinforcement, Cooperative Social Persuasion and Competitive Social Persuasion. We used the Big Five Inventory (BFI) to assess the personality types of participants and asked them a series of questions about their perceptions of the different persuasive strategies depicted in the storyboards. Our results revealed a number of significant relationships between personality and the persuasive technologies we studied, including some personality types favoring different techniques with other personality types disliking several of the strategies. This work represents the first exploratory study that investigates the correlational relationship between the Big Five personality domains and perceptions on different forms of persuasive technology. The long term goal of this work is to use the findings to encourage and provide guidelines for the development of health promoting persuasive technologies which can be tailored to individual personalities across a diverse population.

The remainder of this paper is organized as follows. We first present related work pertaining to persuasive technologies, personality research, and customizable technology. We then describe the study design, followed by a comprehensive presentation of results obtained from this study. Next, we discuss the results, provide potential explanations for the different results we discovered, and discuss the limitations of the current study. We conclude with our directions for future research.

2   Related Work

The idea of using technology to motivate desirable behaviors has recently become a popular topic within the technology design community. Originating with the definition of captology by Fogg [7], the movement has grown to have its own research conference and publishing venues. Researchers have previously worked on developing guidelines and models for persuasive technologies [6], and the application space for persuasive technologies has been well explored. Motivating physical fitness has been one of the most common applications [4,5,17]. Other applications include motivating healthy eating habits [12,18], healthy water intake [3], sustainable transportation [8], and reduced television watching [20]. The work we present here differs from these applications in that although we use the application of motivating physical fitness as the sample in our storyboards, we are not proposing a specific application and the storyboards are drawn at a high enough level that it does not encapsulate specific application details. Instead, we are outlining the ways that these applications can be customized to be more successful for users based on their personalities.

To understand users' personality comprehensively, we chose to utilize the Big Five factors of personality traits. The Big Five factors are widely known as one of the major means of organizing human personality. Historically, the Big Five Model has been used extensively as a descriptive model of personality [11]. The term Big Five does not imply that personality differences can be narrowed down to a mere five traits. To be more accurate, these factors represent personality at a very broad level [14]. The Big Five factors are Neuroticism, Conscientiousness, Agreeableness, Extraversion, and Openness [11]. According to psychological research [14], these are defined as follows:

- *Neuroticism* distinguishes the stability of emotions and even-temperedness from negative emotionality, which can be described as feeling nervous, sad and tense.
- *Conscientiousness* suggests self-use of socially prescribed restraints that facilitate goal completion, following norms and rules, and prioritizing tasks.
- *Agreeableness* distinguishes pro-social and communal orientation toward others from antagonism and includes traits such as altruism, trust, and modesty.
- *Extraversion* suggests a lively approach toward the social and material world and includes traits such as sociability, activity and assertiveness.
- *Openness* describes the wholeness and complexity of an individual's psychological and experiential life.

In this study, we determined how these personality domains relate to perceptions of health-promoting persuasive technologies.

One of the ultimate goals of this work is to motivate health-promoting persuasive technology designers to customize based on the users' personalities. A number of other researchers have recognized the different needs of individuals and realize that the one-size-fits all approach may not necessarily be the best design. Indeed, customizability is one of the key components of a usable user interface. Mobile technology designers have long known that traditional WIMP user interface designs do not translate well to mobile devices. Thus, toolkits like SUPPLE [9] were designed to allow designers to make custom web interfaces based on the device with which the user was browsing. This idea was extended to automatically customize interfaces for individuals with different physical disabilities [10]. Most closely related to our work is Arteaga *et al.*'s study on combating obesity trends in teenagers through persuasive mobile technologies, which uses the Big Five Personality Theory to guide their design [1]. In their study, they used the Big Five factors to make suggestions on game choice and motivational phrases to encourage users to play. Our study utilizes the Big Five factors to understand the relationship between persuasive technologies and personality at a broader level, rather than the design of a specific application.

3 Study Design

For this study, we chose to focus on one particular application of persuasive technology on a single form factor to reduce potential variables: encouraging physical activity through the use of mobile devices. We established a comprehensive list of different persuasive technology strategies by searching the literature on popular health promoting mobile persuasive technologies and common psychological approaches to health-related behavior modification. From this list, we selected 8 common types of persuasive strategies which could be sorted into four general approaches to persuasive technologies. Thus, each approach consisted of two specific complementary persuasive technology strategies. The eight strategies sorted into the four general approaches were:

(1) *Instruction Style*
- **Authoritative:** Uses an authoritative agent, such as a drill sergeant or strict personal trainer, to instruct the user on how to meet their fitness goals.
- **Non-Authoritative:** Uses a neutral agent, such as a friend or peer, to encourage the user to meet their goals.

(2) *Social Feedback*
- **Cooperative:** Uses the notion of users cooperating as a team with friends or peers to complete their fitness goals.
- **Competitive:** Uses a strategy of competing against friends or peers to "win" a competition.

(3) *Motivation Type*
- **Extrinsic:** Uses external motivators, such as winning trophies, as a reward for conducting healthy behaviors.
- **Intrinsic:** Uses internal motivators, such as feeling good about one's self or feeling healthy, to motivate healthy behaviors.

(4) *Reinforcement Type*
- **Negative Reinforcement:** Removes an aversive stimulus (*e.g.,* turns a brown and dying nature scene green and healthy) as the user conducts more healthy behaviors.
- **Positive Reinforcement:** Adds a positive stimulus (*e.g.,* adds flowers, butterflies, and other nice-looking elements to any empty nature scene) as the user conducts more healthy behaviors.

We represented these strategies of persuasive technologies though the use of storyboards drawn by an artist based on the design guidelines of Truong, *et al.* [23]. We chose to use storyboards because they provided a common visual language that individuals from diverse backgrounds could read and understand [16]. All of the storyboards used in our study contained illustrations of a character and his/her interactions with a mobile-based persuasive technology which promoted exercising. Figure 1 shows two examples from the eight storyboards used in the study for positive reinforcement motivation type and competitive social feedback.

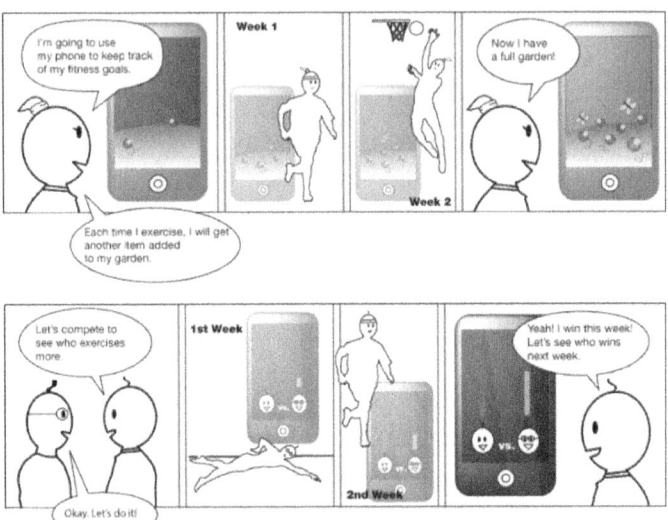

Fig. 1. Storyboards illustrating Positive Reinforcement motivation type (top) and Competitive social feedback (bottom)

3.1 Survey Design

To elicit feedback on the acceptance of the technologies depicted in the storyboards, we designed four different online surveys. The first part of the survey was designed to elicit information regarding perceptions on one of the four major themes of persuasive strategies. Thus, we presented two storyboards, each depicting opposing ends of a general strategy for each participant. Each storyboard was followed by seven questions designed to draw information regarding participant's perceptions of the depicted technology, six of which were 5-point Likert-scale questions probing the users' opinions on the technology in terms of enjoyment, likelihood of use, helpfulness, quality of life, ease of use, and time savings, all of which are major goals of persuasive technologies. The seventh was an open-ended question about any other thoughts or comments. The seven questions are as follows:

(1) **Enjoyment:** This technology is something that I would: (5-Really enjoy using, 1-Really dislike using).
(2) **Likelihood of Use:** In the future, this technology is something I would: (5-Definitely consider using, 1-Definitely not consider using).
(3) **Helpfulness:** With regards to my own health goals, I consider this technology: (5-Very helpful, 1-Very unhelpful).
(4) **Quality of Life:** With regards to the quality of my life, I think this technology would: (5-Definitely improve the quality of my life, 1-Definitely degrade the quality of my life).
(5) **Ease of Use:** I think this technology seems: (5-Very easy to use, 1-Very difficult to use).

(6) **Time Saving**: I think using this technology would help me: (5-Definitely save me time, 1-Definitely waste my time).

(7) **General Comments:** Please describe any other comments or reactions to the technology depicted in the storyboard.

Immediately following the survey with the storyboards and the seven questions, we presented the participant with an assessment of the Big five factors of personality (Extraversion, Agreeableness, Conscientiousness, Neuroticism and Openness). We used the 44 item version of the Big Five Inventory (BFI), a self-report inventory designed to measure the mentioned factors of personality [2,13,14]. We selected this version of the BFI for its efficiency (five minutes of administration time, compared to fifteen minutes for other comparable measures) [14]. In addition, the items on the BFI are shorter and more understandable.

At the end of the survey, we presented the participant with multiple choice and open-ended questions on gender, age, educational background, size of city, county, and fluency of the English language. We then presented both storyboards from the beginning of the survey and a multiple choice question that asked the participant to describe the persuasive style used in the in the storyboards (*e.g.*, authoritative vs. non-authoritative, competitive vs. cooperative, *etc.*). We included these questions to determine whether the content of the storyboards was understood by participants. Finally, all participants were presented with two multiple choice questions asking for obvious information on details of the storyboards. We included these comprehension questions to filter responses from automated scripts or bots. The survey took approximately 7-10 minutes to complete. Participants were randomly assigned to one of the four different persuasive strategy survey types.

3.2 Participant Recruitment

We recruited participants using Amazon's Mechanical Turk (AMT). Initially created to enable humans to perform tasks which computers were unable to do, AMT utilizes the concept of crowdsourcing to recruit humans to perform these tasks. Although this form of recruitment has its constraints, such as issues with automated bots completing surveys and the possibility for low participant motivation, we decided to use AMT to recruit due to our need for a large participant sample and AMT's global audience, relatively low cost, and efficiency of survey distribution. To ensure that the results of the survey were valid, we included comprehension questions to filter out undesired responses, as recommended by Kittur, *et al.* [15] when using AMT for user studies. After executing two phases of pilot tests of the survey on AMT, a Human Intelligence Task (HIT) was created to recruit participants. By clicking on the link in the HIT, participants were redirected to the university website hosting the online survey. We used a simple PHP script to ensure that participants clicking on the survey link through AMT were randomly assigned to one of the six surveys corresponding to the six study conditions. The 240 participants who volunteered to take part in this study were aged over 18 and from a diverse set of backgrounds. Participants were paid a small token sum, USD $0.20, which corresponded to standard rates for other tasks recruiting through AMT.

4   Results

In this section, we present the results of our survey. This includes the success of the storyboards at depicting the different techniques, the steps we took to filter data, participant demographics, the relationship between personality and the acceptances of persuasive technologies, and the overall comments from the participants.

4.1   Storyboard Success and Data Filtering

To determine whether the content of the storyboards was understood by participants, we ran CHI-squares on the participant responses to the multiple choice questions which asked participants to identify the persuasive style presented in the storyboards. All results were significant ($p<.05$). Overall, these results indicate that our storyboards successfully depicted the selected persuasive technologies strategies. In addition, because we chose to recruit through Amazon's Mechanical Turk, we ran the risk of automated scripts or bots completing the survey, which would consequently result in an inaccurate dataset. To counter this problem, we recruited more than the ideal minimum for each survey and filtered responses by participants who had incorrect responses to the two multiple choice comprehension questions on obvious details of the storyboards. This resulted in a total of 50 out of the 240 responses being discarded (7 from the Instruction Style survey, 22 from the Social Feedback survey, 8 from the Motivation Type survey, and 13 from the Reinforcement Type survey).

4.2   Participant Demographics

To summarize demographic information of the participants, we calculated percentages to responses regarding participants' gender, age, education level, fluency of the English language, residency type and country in which they lived. Figure 2 shows a summary of participant demographics. In general, we had a relatively diverse population that is representative of the types of users who might use mobile persuasive technologies for health.

Table 1. Participant demographics across all four surveys

Total Participants = 240	
Gender	Male (53.0%), Female (47.0%)
Age	21 or under (18.8%), 22-30 (37.2%), 31-40 (17.9%), 41-50 (12.6%), 61 or older (0.4%)
Education	Some High School (1.0%), High School (7.4%), Some College (19.7%), College Degree (37.5%), Some Graduate School (6.9%), Graduate Degree (33.0%), Training Certificate (0.5%)
Residency Type	Rural (15.3%), Small Town (14.9%), Suburb (33.7%), Urban (36.1%)
English Fluency	Excellent (55.7%), Good (21.2%), Moderate (8.2%), Fair (10.2%), Minimal (4.7%)
Country	United States (53.1%), India (35.9%), Pakistan (1.9%), Canada (0.8%), Other (4.2%)

4.3   Personality and Persuasive Technology Relationship

To investigate the relationship between personality and persuasive strategies, we first scored the BFI by reverse scoring all negatively keyed items. We then created the scaled scores for the personality factors by averaging the items for each personality domain. Following this, we ran Pearsons Correlational tests using SPSS to determine the correlation between the scaled personality scores and the Likert-scale responses to the perceptions regarding the persuasive technologies depicted in the storyboards. We found significant correlations for all five of the personality traits we tested. Table 2 displays significant correlations (p<.05) grouped by personality factor. In addition, Table 2 sorts the significant correlations by persuasive technologies within each personality factor to give an overall sense of which technologies were appropriate or inappropriate for which personality types. Negative correlations illustrate inversely proportional relationships while positive correlations illustrate directly proportional relationships. With regards to all correlations presented, the larger the number of the correlation, negative or positive, the greater the strength of the relationship.

In general, we found more negative correlations than positive correlations, indicating that our participants had a stronger sense of which technologies they would not favor compared to those that did. The personality type of Extraversion had the most correlations (12 negative, 0 positive), followed by Agreeableness (8 negative, 1 positive), Conscientiousness (0 negative, 5 positive), Openness (3 negative, 2 positive), and finally Neuroticism (1 negative, 1 positive). Our findings show that as a participant's score for Neuroticism increases, their opinions toward Cooperative strategies improving their quality of life decreases and their likelihood of enjoyment of Negative Reinforcement increases. As a participant's score for Conscientiousness increases, their opinion of the helpfulness and likelihood of use for Competitive strategies increases, as does their opinion on the helpfulness, time savings, and quality of life improvement of the Cooperative strategy. We also found that as Agreeableness scores increase, their opinion of Competitive strategies having a high ease of use increases, but opinions decrease on the enjoyment, likelihood of use, helpfulness, and quality of life improvement of the Negative Reinforcement strategy and the enjoyment, likelihood of use, quality of life, and time savings of the Positive Reinforcement strategy. For those participants whose Extraversion scores increase, their opinion decreases on the quality of life improvement, likelihood of use, and time savings of the Extrinsic persuasive strategy, the enjoyment, helpfulness, and likelihood of use of Intrinsic strategies, the enjoyment and helpfulness of Negative Reinforcement, and the ease of use, enjoyment, helpfulness, and likelihood of use of the Positive Reinforcement strategy. Finally, as participants' scores in Openness increase, so does their opinion on the likelihood of use of the Authoritative strategy and the ease of use of the Competitive strategy, but their opinion decreases on the time savings of Extrinsic and Intrinsic strategies and the ease of use of Negative Reinforcement strategies.

Table 2. Significant correlations (p < .05) grouped by personality factor as calculated by Pearsons Correlational Test. Negative correlations are indicated in red text, and Positive correlations are indicated in both green and bold text.

Neuroticism		
Persuasion Type	**Perception Measures**	**Pearsons R Value**
Cooperative	Quality of Life	r(47) = -.387
Negative Reinforcement	Enjoyment	r(51) = +.299
Conscientiousness		
Persuasion Type	**Perception Measures**	**Pearsons R Value**
Competitive	Helpfulness	r(47) = +.293
Competitive	Likelihood of Use	r(47) = +.400
Cooperative	Helpfulness	r(47) = +.288
Cooperative	Time Saving	r(47) = +.339
Cooperative	Quality of Life	r(47) = +.314
Agreeableness		
Persuasion Type	**Perception Measures**	**Pearsons R Value**
Competitive	Ease of Use	r(47) = +.298
Negative Reinforcement	Enjoyment	r(51) = -.448
Negative Reinforcement	Likelihood of Use	r(51) = -.378
Negative Reinforcement	Helpfulness	r(51) = -.377
Negative Reinforcement	Quality of Life	r(51) = -.325
Positive Reinforcement	Enjoyment	r(51) = -.343
Positive Reinforcement	Likelihood of Use	r(51) = -.318
Positive Reinforcement	Quality of Life	r(51) = -.280
Positive Reinforcement	Time Saving	r(51) = -.276
Extraversion		
Persuasion Type	**Perception Measures**	**Pearsons R Value**
Extrinsic	Quality of Life	r(58) = -.316
Extrinsic	Likelihood of Use	r(58) = -.276
Extrinsic	Time Saving	r(58) = -.296
Intrinsic	Enjoyment	r(58) = -.313
Intrinsic	Helpfulness	r(58) = -.268
Intrinsic	Likelihood of Use	r(58) = -.309
Negative Reinforcement	Enjoyment	r(51) = -.402
Negative Reinforcement	Helpfulness	r(51) = -.329
Positive Reinforcement	Ease of Use	r(51) = -.417
Positive Reinforcement	Enjoyment	r(51) = -.366
Positive Reinforcement	Helpfulness	r(51) = -.344
Positive Reinforcement	Likelihood of Use	r(51) = -.332
Openness		
Persuasion Type	**Perception Measures**	**Pearsons R Value**
Authoritative	Likelihood of Use	r(49) = +.356
Competitive	Ease of Use	r(56) = +.404
Extrinsic	Time Saving	r(58) = -.286
Intrinsic	Time Saving	r(58) = -.292
Negative Reinforcement	Ease of Use	r(51) = -.349

5 Discussion

In this section, we provide possible explanations for some of the correlations found and how they lead to design implications. We also discuss limitations of this study.

5.1 Personality and Persuasive Technology Relationship

The number of correlations we found indicates that there is some promise to using personality traits as a method for adapting persuasive strategies to better fit the needs of users. Here we offer possible explanations for some of the correlations we found. Taken together, these findings and implications can help guide future designs of mobile persuasive technology applications for different personalities and give designers a better sense of which designs may work better with specific user groups. Although we attempt to provide explanations, future research is needed for valid explanations of the significant relationships.

Neuroticism describes a tendency toward negative emotionality, which can be described as feeling nervous, sad, tense, and emotional instability [14]. This trait showed the fewest correlations, which could indicate indecisiveness about the different strategies. The two correlations we found were interesting, in that there was a positive correlation toward enjoyment of Negative Reinforcement, which consisted of the transition of a dry, brown field to a lush green one. The decrease in the opinion on the quality of life for Cooperative strategies may indicate that these participants do not prefer working with others to achieve their goals.

Conscientiousness is the tendency toward goal completion, following norms and rules, planned behavior, prioritizing tasks [14]. We believe people with these traits would be most likely to be successful in achieving their health goals, and our study shows that people with higher conscientiousness scores were the most positive in general toward the technologies with five positive correlations. The correlations were all with the two Social strategies of Competitive and Cooperative. Thus, people who are conscientious may be more likely to use socially-based technologies.

Agreeableness is the tendency toward altruism, trust, and modesty as well as compassion and cooperativeness toward others [14]. Interestingly, the only positive correlation to this trait was in the ease of use of the Competitive strategy. We were surprised that we did not see any positive correlations with the Cooperative strategy, although modesty or not wanting to brag or make others feel bad may play into this. We also saw a number of negative correlations with the positive and negative reinforcement strategies. This may indicate that reinforcement systems in persuasive technologies are not as desirable for people who are agreeable.

Extraversion is the tendency for personality traits of sociability, activity, and assertiveness and an engagement with the external world [14]. There were no positive correlations for any of the technologies with regard to extraversion scores and a large number of negative correlations for a number of the different persuasive strategies. This may indicate that persuasive technologies in general are not perceived as desirable by people with high extraversion scores. This could possibly be explained by their tendency to have strong social networks and thus not have as much need for technology to meet their goals, which tends to be more personal in nature.

Openness is the tendency toward art, emotion, unique experiences, and the wholeness and complexity of an individual's life [14]. Our study showed that individuals with higher openness scores were more likely to favor Competitive or

Authoritative technologies. This could be because these are technologies that they have not yet tried, and thus it would be a new experience.

5.2 Limitations of the Current Study

Although we uncovered a number of interesting trends, this study was not without limitations to consider when interpreting these results. First, given that previous researchers have shown that different prototype formats can results in different user feedback, it is important to further study these findings with working prototype or other types of depictions such as videos [22]. Recruiting through Amazon's Mechanical Turk has its own limitations, as described previously. However, these limitations may be balanced by the benefits that AMT offered. The demographic data presented in Table 1 illustrates that using AMT resulted in a fairly good survey distribution for a number of criteria. However, as expected, AMT recruited a larger than average distribution of individuals aged 22-30 and with college and graduate degrees. Finally, we acknowledge that assessing personality through the Big Five model may not necessarily explain all of human personality. It merely represents one form of personality assessment and was used because it allowed us to analyze a large number of personalities at once.

6 Conclusions and Future Work

We investigated the relationship between personality and persuasive technologies, specifically mobile based persuasive technologies that promoted healthy lifestyles. This was the first comprehensive study to investigate the relationship between the Big Five personality traits and different persuasive technology strategies. Although this study showed many interesting and significant findings, we believe there are many areas for future exploration. We will further analyze our dataset by looking at combinations of personality types (*e.g.,* whether there are preferences in technology for people who are high in both Agreeableness and Extraversion), a regression analysis of the findings, and the qualitative statements made about the perceptions of persuasive technologies and general attitudes toward persuasive technologies by personality type. Follow up studies could include comparisons of perceptions of persuasive technology strategies with other similar psychological tests, such as tests for optimism. We plan to use the findings to design mobile-based health applications that can be customized to individual personalities for maximum success across a diverse population. Overall, we believe this study has successfully illustrated the promise of customized persuasion techniques based on personality. We hope the results from this study will be useful to persuasive technology designers, especially those designing for specific populations.

References

1. Arteaga, S.M., Kudeki, M., Woodworth, A.: Combating obesity trends in teenagers through persuasive mobile technology. SIGACCESS (94), 17–25 (2009)
2. Benet-Martinez, V., John, O.P.: Los Cinco Grandes: Across cultures and ethnic groups: Multitrait multimethod analyses of the Big Five in Spanish and English. J. of Personality and Soc. Psych. 75, 729–750 (1998)
3. Chiu, M.-C., et al.: Playful Bottle: a Mobile Social Persuasion System to Motivate Healthy Water Intake. In: Proceedings of Ubicomp 2009, Orlando, Florida, USA (2009)

4. Consolvo, S., Everitt, K., Smith, I., Landay, J.A.: Design Requirements for Technologies that Encourage Physical Activity. In: Proc. of CHI 2006, April 2006, pp. 457–466 (2006)
5. Consolvo, S., et al.: Goal-Setting Considerations for Persuasive Technologies that Encourage Physical Activity. In: Proc. of Persuasive 2009, pp. 1–8 (2009)
6. Consolvo, S., McDonald, D.W., Landay, J.A.: Theory-driven design strategies for technologies that support behavior change in everyday life. In: Proc. of CHI 2009, pp. 405–414 (2009)
7. Fogg, B.J.: Persuasive technology: using computers to change what we think and do. Morgan Kaufmann Publishers, Amsterdam (2003)
8. Froehlich, J., et al.: UbiGreen: investigating a mobile tool for tracking and supporting green transportation habits. In: Proc. of CHI 2009, Boston, MA, USA (2009)
9. Gajos, K.J., Weld, D.S.: SUPPLE: automatically generating user interfaces. In: Proc. of Intelligent User Interfaces 2004, Funchal, Madeira, Portugal (2004)
10. Gajos, K.Z., et al.: Improving the performance of motor-impaired users with automatically-generated, ability-based interfaces. In: Proc. of CHI 2009 (2009)
11. Goldberg, L.R.: The structure of phenotypic personality traits. The American Psychologist 48(1), 26–34 (1993)
12. Grimes, A., Grinter, R.E.: Designing Persuasion: Health Technology for Low-Income African American Communities. In: de Kort, Y.A.W., IJsselsteijn, W.A., Midden, C., Eggen, B., Fogg, B.J. (eds.) PERSUASIVE 2007. LNCS, vol. 4744, pp. 24–35. Springer, Heidelberg (2007)
13. John, O.P., Donahue, E.M., Kentle, R.L.: The Big Five Inventory–Versions 4a and 54, University of California, Berkeley, Institute of Personality and Social Research (1991)
14. John, O.P., Naumann, L.P., Soto, C.J.: Paradigm Shift to the Integrative Big-Five Trait Taxonomy: History, Measurement, and Conceptual Issues. In: Handbook of Personality: Theory and Research, pp. 114–158. Guilford Press, New York (2008)
15. Kittur, A., Chi, E.H., Suh, B.: Crowdsourcing user studies with Mechanical Turk. In: Proc. of CHI 2008, Florence, Italy (2008)
16. van der Lelie, C.: The value of storyboards in the product design process. Personal and Ubiquitous Computing 10(2-3), 159–162 (2006)
17. Lin, J.J., et al.: Fish'n'Steps: Encouraging Physical Activity with an Interactive Computer Game. In: Dourish, P., Friday, A. (eds.) UbiComp 2006. LNCS, vol. 4206, pp. 261–278. Springer, Heidelberg (2006)
18. Lo, J.-L., et al.: Playful tray: Adopting UbiComp and persuasive techniques into play-based occupational therapy for reducing poor eating behavior in young children. In: Krumm, J., Abowd, G.D., Seneviratne, A., Strang, T. (eds.) UbiComp 2007. LNCS, vol. 4717, pp. 38–55. Springer, Heidelberg (2007)
19. Long, J.D., Stevens, K.R.: Clinical Scholarship: Using Technology to Promote Self-Efficacy for Healthy Eating in Adolescents. J. of Nursing Sch. 36(2), 134–139 (2004)
20. Nawyn, J., Intille, S., Larson, K.: Embedding Behavior Modification Strategies into a Consumer Electronic Device: A Case Study. In: Dourish, P., Friday, A. (eds.) UbiComp 2006. LNCS, vol. 4206, pp. 297–314. Springer, Heidelberg (2006)
21. Peng, W.: Design and Evaluation of a Computer Game to Promote a Healthy Diet for Young Adults. Health Communication 24(2), 115–127 (2009)
22. Sellen, K., et al.: The People-Prototype Problem: Understanding the Interaction between Prototype Format and User Group. In: The Proceedings of CHI 2009, pp. 635–638 (2009)
23. Truong, K.N., Hayes, G.R., Abowd, G.D.: Storyboarding: An Empirical Determination of Best Practices and Effective Guidelines. In: Proc. of DIS 2006, pp. 12–21 (2006)
24. Whiteley, J., et al.: State of the Art Reviews: Using the Internet to Promote Physical Activity and Healthy Eating in Youth. Am. J. of Lifestyle Med. 2(2), 159–177 (2008)

Persuasive Features in Six Weight Loss Websites: A Qualitative Evaluation

Tuomas Lehto and Harri Oinas-Kukkonen

University of Oulu, Department of Information Processing Science
Rakentajantie 3, 90570 Oulu, Finland
{Tuomas.Lehto,Harri.Oinas-Kukkonen}@oulu.fi

Abstract. Websites for weight loss have been demonstrating promising results. Still, it is unclear which website components contribute to successful outcomes. The purpose of this paper is to explore the utilization of various persuasive features on six weight loss websites. The websites were selected by using a set of criteria for this qualitative evaluation. The Persuasive Systems Design Model was applied to extract and analyze persuasive system features found in the sites. The results of this study suggest that there is room for improvement in both designing and implementing web-based interventions for weight loss. The evaluated sites provided relatively good primary task support and strong social support. However, there were weaknesses in both dialogue and credibility support. Overall, the evaluation showed that the evaluated weight loss websites may not be very persuasive.

Keywords: PSD model, persuasive, web-based, weight loss, intervention.

1 Introduction

One of the most vibrant areas within health behavior change research has been Web-based software systems promoting weight loss and weight maintenance. Recent research suggests that the Web may be a highly viable channel for delivering weight loss and obesity interventions across diverse populations [1-4]. Barak, Klein and Proudfoot [5] define a web-based intervention as a mainly self-guided online program operated through a website and used by consumers seeking health-related assistance. The intervention program attempts to create positive change and or improve/enhance knowledge, awareness, and understanding via the delivery of reliable, unbiased health-related content and the utilization of interactive functionality.

Web-based weight control applications have the potential to achieve outcomes similar to other lifestyle treatment options [2]. Several randomized trials have demonstrated web-based weight-loss interventions to be efficacious for short-term weight loss [3], [6-10]. However, online programs have not accomplished weight losses of the magnitude typically produced by traditional individual and or group treatment approaches [1], [11]. These findings should be interpreted with caution, however. According to Bennett and Glasgow [1], most randomized controlled trials in

T. Ploug, P. Hasle, H. Oinas-Kukkonen (Eds.): PERSUASIVE 2010, LNCS 6137, pp. 162–173, 2010.

this particular domain have been relatively small and underpowered, suffering from high levels of attrition and occasionally reporting change in only secondary outcomes, e.g., knowledge and self-efficacy, rather than primary outcomes, e.g., behavior change. Tsai and Wadden [12] argue that minimal evidence still exists for recommending the use of commercial Internet-based interventions, whereas Womble and colleagues [13] found in their study that a commercial Internet-based weight loss program produced only minimal weight loss and was not as effective as a traditional manual-based approach. Yet, Harvey-Berino and colleagues [14] reported that participants assigned to an online weight maintenance program sustained similar levels of weight loss over 18 months compared to individuals who continued to meet face-to-face.

The current generation of online weight loss interventions takes advantage of a set of varying software components, such as self-monitoring functionality, food diaries, body mass index calculators, support forums, and coach messaging [1]. Yet, it is unclear which of these features, either in isolation or collectively, are associated with the greatest magnitude of weight loss [1], [2], [11].

Bennett and Glasgow [1] summarize that greater results in weight loss are typically observed with such web-based weight-loss interventions that are highly structured, provide support from a human counselor, utilize tailored materials, and promote a high frequency of website logins. Krukowski and colleagues [11] share this view by concluding that structured interventions comprising behavior therapy components, interactive and dynamic website features, and synchronous communication produce the most significant weight losses.

As noted above, the area of weight-loss applications is still rather unclear. Moreover, the features of the applications, and in particular the persuasive features, are normally not well reported. The purpose of this paper is to explore the utilization of various persuasive features in six web-based weight loss applications. The Persuasive Systems Design Model [15], [16] is applied to extract and analyze persuasive system features from the included web-based weight loss interventions.

2   Related Research

McConnon, Kirk and Ransley [17] highlight the need for process evaluation to help identify the key components of Internet interventions, whether positive, negative, or insignificant. They criticize previous research for focusing primarily on examining the ability of online weight control interventions to promote weight loss, with limited investigations of acceptance, satisfaction, and patterns of use. They suggest that a more comprehensive approach to evaluating the role of computer-based tools, beyond simply demonstrating improved outcomes, is needed.

Krukowski and colleagues [11] underscore the importance of dynamic and interactive website features. They suggest that such Web features which provide participants with visual representations of goal progress, self-monitoring feedback, and social support are predictive of weight loss and maintenance. Different features seem to be important during treatment and maintenance. In their study, progress charts, calculators, and past diaries were included in the factor best predicting weight loss during the baseline to 6 months treatment period. The factor comprising chats and e-mail addresses of peer participants was the best predictor during the maintenance period.

A major challenge in Internet-based weight loss interventions is that participant attrition [18] is generally high (typically more than 25%), and among those participants who are retained, engagement rates usually decline over time [1], [2]. As reducing attrition and increasing website utilization would likely enhance weight loss and management success, designing, implementing, and evaluating features that participants find attractive and captivating should clearly be a priority [11]. This type of knowledge will assist in designing, implementing and evaluating effective interventions that are able to engage and retain large numbers of individuals, potentially enhancing population weight-related health and well-being, and thus of significant public health value [2].

Stevens and colleagues [19] have identified several major lessons from their experience in developing and implementing an interactive website to support the maintenance of weight loss. According to them, it is critical to designate the theoretical underpinnings of the intervention program and the website objectives early in the design process. They point out that website design does not iterate the same way as the development of in-person, counseling-based interventions. Making solid decisions about website objectives and abiding by them during the development process helps eradicate expensive rework.

3   Evaluating Persuasive Systems

Research on persuasive technology has been introduced relatively recently [20]. Briñol and Petty [21] outline persuasion as follows: "In the typical situation in which persuasion is possible, a person or a group of people (i.e., *the recipient*) receives an intervention (e.g., *a persuasive message*) from another individual or group (i.e., *the source*) in a particular setting (i.e., *the context*)." (p. 71)

Persuasive systems may be defined as computerized software or information systems designed to reinforce, change or shape attitudes or behaviors or both without using coercion or deception [15]. Successful persuasion takes place when the target of change (e.g., attitudes, beliefs) is modified in the desired direction [21].

Oinas-Kukkonen and Harjumaa [15], [16] have conceptualized a framework for designing and evaluating persuasive systems, known as the Persuasive Systems Design (PSD) model. The PSD model presents a way to analyze and evaluate the persuasion context and related techniques. Persuasion context analysis includes recognizing the intent (persuader, change type) and the event (use context, user context, and technology context) of persuasion, and recognizing the strategy (message, route) used. In the PSD model, the categories for persuasive system techniques are primary task support, dialogue support, system credibility (the more credible the system is, the more persuasive it is), and social support (the system motivates users by leveraging social influence). Primary task support addresses the target behaviors and employs seven principles, namely reduction, tunneling, tailoring, personalization, self-monitoring, simulation, and rehearsal. Dialogue support addresses the feedback that the system offers in guiding the user to reach the intended behavior and employs praise, rewards, reminders, suggestion, similarity, liking, and social role. System credibility support is a persuasive element, and the PSD model describes seven design principles for supporting it. These are trustworthiness, expertise, surface credibility, real world feel, authority, third party endorsements, and verifiability. The category of social support describes how to design the system so that it motivates users by leveraging social influence. The model operates with the following design principles: social learning, social comparison, normative influence, social facilitation, cooperation, competition, and recognition.

In this study, the PSD framework was applied for identifying the persuasive features that have been incorporated into the web-based weight loss interventions.

4   Research Setting

The research question is: *What kind of persuasive system features, and to what extent, do current web-based weight loss interventions convey?*

Our aim was to gather a short but representative list of current state-of-the-art weight loss websites. The site had to be in English, free of charge (or providing a free trial), require registration, accept international users, and provide extensive interactivity. Web-based weight loss applications were searched for during December 2009–January 2010 from the Internet using public search engines (e.g., Google, Yahoo!, Bing), using the following search terms: weight, loss, control, diet, nutrition, obesity. Even if the search was extensive, the search method cannot be considered as exhaustive. The search phrase "weight loss" yields millions of hits on Google alone. Moreover, going through all possible combinations and variations for search terms is practically impossible and will only lead into highly redundant search results.

Based on the abovementioned criteria, we chose six websites for further evaluation. The sites were:

- Calorie Count (http://www.caloriecount.about.com, later CC)
- CalorieKing (http://www.calorieking.com/, CK)
- Diet.com (http://www.diet.com/, DIET)
- ObesityHelp (http://www.obesityhelp.com/, OH)
- WebMD Healthy Eating & Diet Center (http://www.webmd.com/diet/default.htm, WMD)
- Project Weight Loss (http://www.projectweightloss.com/, PWL)

Four of the sites were free of charge (CC, OH, PWL, WMD), one (CK) offered a free trial for seven days (CK), and one (DIET) charged for premium membership (the free standard membership was evaluated). See table 1 for the types of content the sites provided.

Table 1. Type of content on evaluated weight loss websites

Type of content	CC	CK	DIET	OH	PWL	WMD
Health advice	●	●	●	●	●	●
Nutrition	●	●	●	●	●	●
Diet	●	●	●	○	●	●
Physical activity	●	●	●	○	●	●
Weight loss	●	●	●	●	●	●
Weight maintenance	●	●	●	○	●	○
Obesity	○	○	○	●	○	○

● = yes, ○ = no

The websites included in the study were evaluated based on the persuasive system context and functionality presented in the PSD model. The model does not suggest that all systems should always implement all of the features described in it. However, due to the nature of this study, and as the quality of the implemented features varied tremendously, we found it appropriate to use a scoring system. The authors independently reviewed the sites feature-by-feature. The resulting tables were then compared, discussed and combined. See table 3.

5   Results: Persuasion Context

The persuasion context is composed of the intent, the event, and the strategy [16]. Dey [22] states that context is all about the whole situation relevant to an application and its set of users, and he defines context as any information that can be used to characterize the situation of an entity.

The intent. The *persuaders* behind the websites appeared to be commercial companies. Yet, only two of the sites (CC, WMD) clearly stated the background organization. In fact, it was very hard to determine the underlying motives for persuading users and/or biases other than what was obvious. All of the evaluated sites ultimately aimed at individuals' enhanced health, essentially weight loss, through the utilization of different types of software tools and information. For this reason, self-help, personal goal-setting, and motivation play an important role in the change process in all of these sites. All of the sites failed to explicitly state whether they targeted a change in individuals' behavior only or also in their attitudes (*change type*). However, it is relatively safe to assume that the sites favored behavior change over attitude change. Furthermore, three out of six interventions did not reveal the purpose of the website beyond very general statements. In our view, these shortcomings lower the overall persuasiveness of the website.

The event contains the *use, user* and *technology contexts*. The use context refers to the problem domain dependent features. The user context refers to the individual users' characteristics, including, but not being limited to, users' goals, abilities, and cultural factors. The technology context refers to the features and requirements of the technological platform and/or application.

The use context was described on a very general level in all of the evaluated sites. It would appear that half of the sites failed to recognize different user groups, leading to a questionable one-fits-all approach. In our view, web-based health behavior change interventions without predefined user groups and with at least minimal tailoring for the groups cannot offer much more than educational content with minimal effect on users' behavior. For example, differences in age, gender, culture and lifestyle may play an important role in persuasion. Specific to the users of the evaluated weight loss websites is that they are typically people who are interested in weight loss and/or they are motivated to losing weight personally. None of the sites was targeted at a certain demographic group. See table 2 for an overview of the technology context.

Table 2. Technology context

	CC	CK	DIET	OH	PWL	WMD
Web2.0 functionality	●	●	●	●	●	●
Mobile functionality	●	●	○	○	○	●
Video	●	●	●	●	●	●
Podcasting	●	○	●	○	○	●
Downloadable tools	●	●	○	○	○	●
Social media connectivity	●	○	○	●	●	●

● = yes, ○ = no

Every site provided video clips, and half of the sites offered mobile functionality to the user. Two of the sites provided weight-loss related podcasts. The results from a recent study [23] suggest that the use of behavioral, theory-based podcasting may be an effective way to promote weight loss. Half of the sites offered downloadable tools, and the majority had some type of social media connectivity (e.g., Facebook, Twitter). Bennett and Glasgow [1] argue that the most critical design gap concerns the underuse of Web2.0 features in the current generation of Internet interventions.

The strategy in the PSD model emphasizes two elements, namely the *message* and the *route*. The message refers to the form and/or content selected to deliver the intended transformation in behavior and/or attitude change. The content could be, for instance, statistical data about the health risks of drinking, but the information could be presented to the user in plain text, streaming video, or it could be embedded in a game. The route for persuasion can be direct, indirect, or both. A direct approach provides one or a few solid and convincing arguments, whereas an indirect route is based on a number of facts rather than a single strong argument.

Presumably, the wider the content, the more embedded messages and arguments are likely to be presented to the user. Some of the sites offered very wide content (CC, CK, DIET, WMD) whereas others relied on more compact presentation (OH, PWL). It has to be noted that the total number of embedded arguments may not be necessarily relevant, compared with the manner in which they are presented.

The embedded arguments in all of the sites seem to target appealing to both the emotions and the logic of the users. All of the sites appeared to target the individuals' behavior change through a set of arguments, instead of using one convincingly strong argument only (route, direct vs. indirect persuasion).

6 Results: Persuasive Features

The persuasive features listed of the PSD Model [16] found in the evaluated weight loss websites are presented in table 3.

Table 3. Persuasive features in evaluated websites

Persuasive features	CC	CK	DIET	OH	PWL	WMD
Reduction	●●	●●●	●●	●	●●	●
Tunneling	○	○	○	○	○	○
Tailoring	●●	●●	●	●	●	●
Personalization	●●	●●	●●	●●	●●	●●
Self-monitoring	●●●	●●●	●●●	●●●	●●	●
Simulation	●●	●●●	●	●	●●	●●
Rehearsal	●	●●●	●●	●	●	●
Praise	○	●	●	○	○	○
Rewards	○	●●	●●	○	○	○
Reminders	●	●●	○	○	○	●
Suggestion	●	●●	●	○	●	●
Similarity	●	●	●	●●	●	●
Liking	●	●	●	●	●	●
Social role	●●	○	○	○	○	○
Trustworthiness	●●	●●	●	●●	●●	●●●
Expertise	●●	●●	●●	●●	○	●●●
Surface credibility	●●	●●●	●	●●	●●	●●
Real-world feel	●●	●	●	●	●	●●
Authority	○	○	○	○	○	●●
3rd party endorsements	○	○	○	○	○	●●
Verifiability	○	○	●	○	○	●●
Social learning	●●	●●	●●	●●	●	●
Social comparison	●●●	●●	●●	●●	●	●
Normative influence	●●	●●	●●	●	●	●
Social facilitation	●●●	●●●	●●●	●●	●●	●
Cooperation	○	○	○	○	○	○
Competition	●	●●	●	○	○	○
Recognition	○	●●	●●	●	●	●

●●● = high support, ●● = medium support, ● = low support, ○ = no support

6.1 Primary Task Support

All of the evaluated sites were relatively strong in their primary task support. Self-monitoring functionality (e.g., food/activity/weight logs and trackers) was highly supported in all of the sites. According to Krukowski and colleagues [11], there is some indication that Internet-based programs may facilitate greater self-monitoring than in-person programs due to the ease of self-monitoring through online tools. This may be partially true, but based on our experience, using these tools can initially be quite a laborious task and require a rather high motivation level. After the user is familiar with the tools, and is being provided with an opportunity to save day-to-day patterns (favorite meals, favorite physical activity) into the system, the burden of self-monitoring may decrease slightly.

All of the sites demonstrated functionality that fits within reduction, i.e., the system/application reduces complex behavior into simple tasks helping users to perform the target behavior. This is important because a system that guides users through a process or experience provides opportunities to persuade them along the way. A closely related feature is tunneling [24]. Tunneling may enhance the change process since the user is led through a predetermined sequence of steps and receives the most appropriate content at a proper time. Surprisingly, tunneling was not used in any of the sites.

The level of tailoring, i.e., providing different content for different user groups, was average in two sites and weak in four sites. Bennett and Glasgow [1] urge for future research to determine how and under what circumstances tailored messaging might be used most effectively to stimulate sustained website utilization. According to them, despite tailored approaches being generally accepted and preferred, only a few trials have systematically studied the outcome of different types or the extent of tailoring.

Personalization was relatively good in all of the sites. The quality of web personalization depends on how well the content generated by the personalization agent matches the preferences of the user in a particular domain [25].

Simulation and rehearsal were rather common features. A typical example of simulation was calculating how much calories a specific physical activity burns, or the type and duration of exercise needed to burn the calories from, e.g., a chocolate bar. The rehearsal feature was supported by providing workout plans and exercise ideas to the user. As a highlight, two of the sites (CK, DIET) provided extensive video-based, customizable workout builders.

6.2 Dialogue Support

In comparison to primary task support, the sites demonstrated much weaker support for system-to-user interaction. There was great variety in the feedback the sites offered in guiding the user to reach the intended behavior.

Two of the websites demonstrated praise (e.g., the user is presented with a positive message upon completing a specific task) and also offered virtual rewards, such as medals, and points. Three sites presented suggestions for action to the user. Only one site adopted a social role. This was done by facilitating communication between the user and a nutrition specialist ("Ask Mary, your personal nutrition coach").

Overall, the dialogue support demonstrated throughout the sites was at a below average level. Strategies to improve retention rates and engagement with the web-based intervention (e.g., through email reminders, or via enhanced program features) should be further explored [2]. A persuasive system should remind users of their target behavior during the course of the intervention. A recent systematic review showed that the use of periodic prompts can be effective in behavior change interventions [26]. In the present evaluation, one site provided average support and two sites weak support for reminders.

6.3 Credibility Support

There is a general concern that people are unable to assess the reliability and quality of information presented on websites. Miles, Petrie and Steel [27] examined the first 50 websites found on an Internet search with the search term 'weight loss diets', finding that only three offered good dietary advice, while 26 sites offered the sale of vitamins, minerals, supplements and diet replacements. They concluded that the information available on these websites ranged from solid advice to information that was potentially misleading and dangerous.

In this study, we evaluated the credibility of the selected websites. Obviously, as information systems researchers, we cannot fully evaluate the quality of the advice *per se*, but we can say if the information *appears* trustworthy; showing expertise, authority and verifiability. Combining the elements in the credibility support category gives a good overview of the credibility, reliability and quality of information presented to the potential users.

None of the six sites had any remarkable problems with credibility issues. All of them successfully demonstrated trustworthiness (i.e., the presented information is truthful, fair and unbiased) and expertise (except for PWL). Surface credibility was relatively strong in most of the sites, but at the same time, distracting advertisements and confusing/changing layouts weakened the sites' overall credibility. The real-world feel was weak or at an average level. Only one site referred to an authority, whereas two sites presented third party endorsements. Verifiability of the claims presented to the user was weak or nonexistent in all sites with one exception (WMD).

6.4 Social Support

Most of the evaluated sites offered seemingly strong social support. Several techniques were employed for this purpose, such as journals/diaries/blogs, mailbox, friends/buddies, forums/message boards, groups/clubs, and chat. Harvey-Berino and colleagues [14] claim that the group meetings in the chat forum offer a powerful format to improve overall outcomes for a group-based intervention. Accordingly, synchronous communication could facilitate social support, a component that has been previously found to enhance weight loss in behavioral obesity programs.

The social learning principle means that an individual may be more motivated to perform a target behavior if she can observe others performing the behavior while using the system. This principle was supported in all of the sites. A closely related principle is social comparison; users will be more motivated to perform the target behavior if they can compare their performance with the performance of others. People are also more likely to perform target the behavior if they are able to observe others performing the behavior, or are being observed by others. This principle is called social facilitation. Social comparison and social facilitation were supported widely.

Leveraging competition and cooperation may persuade users to adopt a target attitude or behavior. Features supporting competition were found in half of the sites while none of the sites provided means for cooperation. Normative influence was utilized to some extent in all of the sites.

By offering public recognition for an individual or group, a system can increase the likelihood that the person and/or group will adopt a target behavior. Recognition was utilized in five of the six sites.

Bennett and Glasgow [1] claim that there are no examples of trial designs that would allow for systematic investigation of the relative benefits of various social-networking features.

7 Discussion and Conclusions

This paper provided a qualitative evaluation of the persuasive features in six weight loss websites. The selected sites represent the current state-of-the-art of web-based weight interventions. The results of this study suggest that there is room for improvement in both designing and implementing web-based interventions for weight loss. The evaluation showed that the weight loss websites may not be very persuasive.

Primary task support features were utilized relatively strongly in many of the sites. Tailoring was surprisingly weak, as half of the evaluated sites did not utilize it at all. This finding implies that the interventions may be targeted at too broad an audience. It is reasonable to assume that different approaches might work well for different user groups. In other words, if the user feels the content is not designed for her needs, there is a high possibility that the user will discontinue using the program (i.e., attrition).

The dialogue support (system-to-user) provided by the evaluated sites was not very strong. Half of the websites provided some praise, and some offered some virtual rewards. The use of periodic prompts can be effective in persuasion. Half of the sites used reminders as a persuasion technique and three sites presented suggestions for action to the user.

None of the six sites had any remarkable problems with credibility issues. All of them successfully demonstrated trustworthiness and expertise. However, real-world feel was relatively weak. None of the sites referred to an authority, whereas some of them presented third-party endorsements. Worryingly, the verifiability of the claims put forward was weak or nonexistent for all but one site.

Social support was relatively strong as all of the sites provided online social support to some extent. Several techniques, such as blogs, forums, groups, instant messaging, and chat rooms were employed for this purpose. In our view, providing (expert-moderated) support groups as a part of a web-based intervention is a very important aspect of such interventions. As demonstrated, there are various techniques readily available to facilitate communication between peers. In anonymous online support groups, the participants may overcome the feeling of being stigmatized, and time and location are no longer obstacles for participation. We suggest that web-based interventions and support groups should not be considered as substitutes, but rather as supplements to traditional forms of treatment and peer support.

There are some limitations to this study. First, the evaluated sites represent only a fragment of the available web-based weight loss sites. Second, no outside evaluators were used, and thus the evaluations were at least partially based on the authors' subjective views. Third, the evaluation of the quality of the actual information presented on the sites is critical but beyond the scope of this paper. Finally, the relation between persuasive features and weight loss outcomes was not studied. The results should be regarded as indicatory for future studies.

The use of persuasive technology in the health behavior change arena is still in its infancy. While the field is expanding, it is evident that more research is needed to better determine how the persuasiveness of the systems affects users' intended behavior. Effective face-to-face counseling interventions may not be directly translatable into the Web environment. Designing, implementing and evaluating systems aiming at individual's behavior change requires a thorough understanding of the problem domain, underpinning theories, and the strategies of persuasive systems design. An interdisciplinary team of professionals is often needed. Establishing such teams will be a demanding task for building successful web-based health behavior change interventions.

Current research tends to reveal very little about the underlying persuasive mechanisms that have been built in the systems which target health behavior change. Focusing on the validation of the outcome results only is insufficient; more emphasis should be put on studying what software features and functionalities contribute to the success of the interventions and how they could and/or should be implemented and delivered to diverse populations.

References

1. Bennett, G.G., Glasgow, R.E.: The Delivery of Public Health Interventions Via the Internet: Actualizing their Potential. Annu. Rev. Public Health 30, 273–292 (2009)
2. Neve, M., Morgan, P.J., Jones, P.R., et al.: Effectiveness of Web-Based Interventions in Achieving Weight Loss and Weight Loss Maintenance in Overweight and Obese Adults: A Systematic Review with Meta-Analysis. Obes. Rev. (2009)
3. Saperstein, S.L., Atkinson, N.L., Gold, R.S.: The Impact of Internet use for Weight Loss. Obes. Rev. 8, 459–465 (2007)
4. Weinstein, P.K.: A Review of Weight Loss Programs Delivered Via the Internet. J. Cardiovasc. Nurs. 21, 251–258 (2006)
5. Barak, A., Klein, B., Proudfoot, J.G.: Defining Internet-Supported Therapeutic Interventions. Ann. Behav. Med. 38, 4–17 (2009)
6. Micco, N., Gold, B., Buzzell, P., et al.: Minimal in-Person Support as an Adjunct to Internet Obesity Treatment. Ann. Behav. Med. 33, 49–56 (2007)
7. Rothert, K., Strecher, V.J., Doyle, L.A., et al.: Web-Based Weight Management Programs in an Integrated Health Care Setting: A Randomized, Controlled Trial. Obesity (Silver Spring) 14, 266–272 (2006)
8. Tate, D.F., Jackvony, E.H., Wing, R.R.: A Randomized Trial Comparing Human E-Mail Counseling, Computer-Automated Tailored Counseling, and no Counseling in an Internet Weight Loss Program. Arch. Intern. Med. 166, 1620–1625 (2006)

9. Tate, D.F., Jackvony, E.H., Wing, R.R.: Effects of Internet Behavioral Counseling on Weight Loss in Adults at Risk for Type 2 Diabetes: A Randomized Trial. J. Am. Med. Assoc. 289, 1833–1836 (2003)
10. Tate, D.F., Wing, R.R., Winett, R.A.: Using Internet Technology to Deliver a Behavioral Weight Loss Program. J. Am. Med. Assoc. 285, 1172–1177 (2001)
11. Krukowski, R.A., Harvey-Berino, J., Ashikaga, T., et al.: Internet-Based Weight Control: The Relationship between Web Features and Weight Loss. Telemed. J. E. Health 14, 775–782 (2008)
12. Tsai, A.G., Wadden, T.A.: Systematic Review: An Evaluation of Major Commercial Weight Loss Programs in the United States. Ann. Intern. Med. 142, 56–66 (2005)
13. Womble, L.G., Wadden, T.A., McGuckin, B.G., et al.: A Randomized Controlled Trial of a Commercial Internet Weight Loss Program. Obes. Res. 12, 1011–1018 (2004)
14. Harvey-Berino, J., Pintauro, S., Buzzell, P., et al.: Effect of Internet Support on the Long-Term Maintenance of Weight Loss. Obes. Res. 12, 320–329 (2004)
15. Oinas-Kukkonen, H., Harjumaa, M.: A Systematic Framework for Designing and Evaluating Persuasive Systems. In: Oinas-Kukkonen, H., Hasle, P., Harjumaa, M., Segerståhl, K., Øhrstrøm, P. (eds.) PERSUASIVE 2008. LNCS, vol. 5033, pp. 164–176. Springer, Heidelberg (2008)
16. Oinas-Kukkonen, H., Harjumaa, M.: Persuasive Systems Design: Key Issues, Process Model, and System Features. Communications of the Association for Information Systems 24, 28 (2009)
17. McConnon, A., Kirk, S.F., Ransley, J.K.: Process Evaluation of an Internet-Based Resource for Weight Control: Use and Views of an Obese Sample. J. Nutr. Educ. Behav. 41, 261–267 (2009)
18. Eysenbach, G.: The Law of Attrition. J. Med. Internet Res. 7, e11 (2005)
19. Stevens, V.J., Funk, K.L., Brantley, P.J., et al.: Design and Implementation of an Interactive Website to Support Long-Term Maintenance of Weight Loss. J. Med. Internet Res. 10, e1 (2008)
20. Fogg, B.J.: Persuasive technology: Using computers to change what we think and do. Morgan Kaufmann, San Francisco (2003)
21. Briñol, P., Petty, R.E.: Persuasion: Insights from the Self-Validation Hypothesis. Adv. Exp. Soc. Psychol., 69–118 (2009)
22. Dey, A.K.: Understanding and using Context. Personal and Ubiquitous Computing 5, 4–7 (2001)
23. Turner-McGrievy, G.M., Campbell, M.K., Tate, D.F., et al.: Pounds Off Digitally Study A Randomized Podcasting Weight-Loss Intervention. Am. J. Prev. Med. 37, 263–269 (2009)
24. Danaher, B.G., McKay, H.G., Seeley, J.R.: The Information Architecture of Behavior Change Websites. J. Med. Internet Res. 7, e12 (2005)
25. Tam, K.Y., Ho, S.Y.: Web Personalization as a Persuasion Strategy: An Elaboration Likelihood Model Perspective. Inform. Syst. Res. 16, 271–291 (2005)
26. Fry, J.P., Neff, R.A.: Periodic Prompts and Reminders in Health Promotion and Health Behavior Interventions: Systematic Review. J. Med. Internet Res. 11, e16 (2009)
27. Miles, J., Petrie, C., Steel, M.: Slimming on the Internet. J. R. Soc. Med. 93, 254–257 (2000)

The Dominant Robot: Threatening Robots Cause Psychological Reactance, Especially When They Have Incongruent Goals

M.A.J. Roubroeks[*], J.R.C. Ham, and C.J.H. Midden

Department of Human-Technology Interaction, Eindhoven University of Technology
M.A.J.Roubroeks@tue.nl

Abstract. Persuasive technology can take the form of a social agent that persuades people to change behavior or attitudes. However, like any persuasive technology, persuasive social agents might trigger psychological reactance, which can lead to restoration behavior. The current study investigated whether interacting with a persuasive robot can cause psychological reactance. Additionally, we investigated whether goal congruency plays a role in psychological reactance. Participants programmed a washing machine while a robot gave threatening[1] advice. Confirming expectations, participants experienced more psychological reactance when receiving high-threatening advice compared to low-threatening advice. Moreover, when the robot gave high-threatening advice and expressed an incongruent goal, participants reported the highest level of psychological reactance (on an anger measure). Finally, high-threatening advice led to more restoration, and this relationship was partially mediated by psychological reactance. Overall, results imply that under certain circumstances persuasive technology can trigger opposite effects, especially when people have incongruent goal intentions.

Keywords: Persuasive Robot, Psychological Reactance, Intentionality, Social Influence, Energy Conservation Behavior, Incongruent goals.

1 Introduction

Recently, robots have been developed that are able of showing social behavior (i.e., trigger human-like behavior, e.g., politeness) [12]. However, it remains unclear how these robots should behave and interact with people. For example, what social skills are needed to persuade people to act in a desired way? And what happens when the goals of people are incongruent with the goals of the persuasive robot? Should the robot adapt its persuasive messages in these situations?

Importantly, persuasive messages inherently contain some kind of directive to change a specific attitude or behavior. People could experience these directives as a threat to their autonomy, and consequently will experience some sort of arousal

---

[*] Corresponding author.
[1] In this article "threatening" refers to threat-to-autonomy.

T. Ploug, P. Hasle, H. Oinas-Kukkonen (Eds.): PERSUASIVE 2010, LNCS 6137, pp. 174–184, 2010.
© Springer-Verlag Berlin Heidelberg 2010

termed psychological reactance. In response, people will try to restore their lost sense of autonomy [2; 3]. The current study aims to answer the question whether people also become psychologically reactant when confronted with persuasive technology: a persuasive robot. If so, this persuasive robot could hamper the persuasion processes, which also could structurally damage further relationships with the persuasive technology. Since psychological reactance is a social phenomenon [2; 13]; this would imply that persuasive robots can be viewed as social actors. Furthermore, this would lead to design implications of persuasive robots. For instance, robots should be designed that are adjustable to the person interacting with it. Earlier research already showed that participants became psychologically reactant when confronted with only a picture of a robot [13]. In the current study, we would like to extend these results to an interactive environment, in which participants have to interact with a persuasive robot. Our main research question of this paper focuses on the role of goal congruency on psychological reactance. Imagine that a persuasive robot threatens you to accomplish a goal that is not your own current goal. It could be that people become even more psychologically reactant when the goals of the robot are incongruent with their own goals, because they are forced in a direction that is opposite to their own personal goals. People could get the impression that the robot is working against them, and consequently react opposite to the intended direction; even more than psychological reactance behavior in situations of incongruent goal intentions. In the current study, we investigated what would happen if this robot explicitly states that it has the intention to pursue a particular goal. Therefore, the main question is: "Does it matter whether a high-threatening robot tries to persuade you to reach your own goal, or the opposite of your goal?"

Some studies have assessed the effect of intentions on persuasive messages. A study by [4] investigated the influence of people's prior intentions on their responses to advice messages. A deductive message (i.e., explicit threat-to-autonomy message) resulted in more reactance than an inductive message (i.e., implicit threat-to-autonomy message), when participants had no prior intentions to perform a specific behavior. However, when participants did have prior intentions to perform the specific behavior, there was no difference between a deductive or inductive message [4]. These results could be explained by assuming that participants already made a choice themselves to use sunscreen and therefore did not experience the deductive message as a threat to their autonomy. Support for this conclusion was found in a recent study by [14], who studied the effect of agent similarity on psychological reactance. He found that people experienced less reactance when the agent was very similar to the participant, regardless of threat. On the other hand, when the agent was dissimilar compared with the participant, people experienced more reactance. In other words, when a person had the same goal intentions as the persuader, it seems that it did not matter if high-threatening language was used, whereas different goal intentions led to an increase of psychological reactance [14]. However, according to psychological reactance theory [2], a threat-to-autonomy message will always cause psychological reactance, regardless of people's prior intentions. In the current study, we will investigate this apparent contradiction.

In the current study, we want to address two questions: "Do people become psychologically reactant when their autonomy is threatened by a persuasive robot?", and, if so, "What is the role of goal congruency on psychological reactance?" The current study will assess the influence of a robot's intentionality on psychological reactance. That is, we investigate whether a high-threatening, persuasive robot with an incongruent intentionality to that of the participant will trigger more feelings of psychological reactance, compared to a robot with a congruent intentionality to that of the participant.

In this study, we examined participant's willingness to follow the advice about energy conservation/clean laundry while programming a washing machine. For psychological reactance to occur, participants should experience a threat to their autonomy [2]. Therefore, first, we manipulated the experienced threat to autonomy. The threat-to-autonomy manipulation existed of advice messages given by an agent that were either low-threatening advice messages that contained low-controlling language (e.g., "Could you set the temperature at 40 °C, please?"), or high-threatening advice messages that contained high-controlling language (e.g., "Are you going to set the temperature at 40 °C, or not?!"). To minimize any doubt or incorrect interpretations about the meaning of the message we used concrete language that consisted of specific actions [8]. Furthermore, according to [6], psychological reactance can be measured by measuring the level of anger and the amount of negative thoughts. They claim that these measures serve as the predictors of psychological reactance [6]. Our first hypothesis is in line with prior research about psychological reactance [for an overview see 5]. *H1: Participants who are provided with a high-threatening concrete advice message will experience more psychological reactance (more feelings of anger and more negative thoughts) than participants who are provided with a low-threatening concrete advice message.*

Second, we investigated what would happen if an incongruent intentionality is combined with a high-threatening advice message. To manipulate this, participants were first asked to rate their preference for two goals; energy conservation or a clean laundry. After the rating, the advice-giving agent explicated to have a congruent intentionality (i.e., Like you, I too, prefer energy conservation) or incongruent intentionality (i.e., Different from you, I prefer a clean laundry). To make the manipulation more explicit, the agent also told it was rather good at accomplishing its goal and would give advice on how the participant could accomplish this goal. Our second hypothesis tests whether the fact that the agent has incongruent intentions would add to the amount of psychological reactance that is experienced after receiving a high-threatening message. *H2: Participants, who are exposed to a high-threatening advice message combined with an incongruent intentionality of the agent will experience the most psychological reactance, compared to all other groups.*

Finally, we investigated the restoration people could show after experiencing psychological reactance. If we want to develop persuasive technology to persuade people, it is very important to know the reactions of people in response to psychological reactance. According to the model of psychological reactance [2], a threat to autonomy leads to more restoration and this relationship is mediated by psychological reactance. Our third hypothesis therefore consists of mediation analyses for three measure of restoration. *H3: Participants who are provided with a high-threatening advice message will experience more (a) restoration thoughts during the task, (b) more restoration behavior during the task, and (c) will evaluate the advice-giving agent as more negative, compared to participants who are provided with a low-threatening advice message. In addition, the relationship between threat and* restoration (i.e., restoration thoughts, restoration behavior, negative evaluations) will be mediated by psychological reactance.

The current study can give insights in the effects of intentionality on psychological reactance that can help in the development of persuasive robots. If our hypotheses are confirmed, it is important to adapt advice messages given by persuasive technology in such a way, that psychological reactance and restoration are minimized, especially when a person's intentionality is incongruent with the advice message.

2   Method

2.1   Participants and Design

Seventy-nine participants (46 males, 33 females; age $M = 20.1$, $SD = 2.0$) were recruited at Eindhoven University of Technology, and existed mainly of first-year undergraduates. Participants were randomly assigned to one of four conditions of a 2 (threat: low threat vs. high threat) x 2 (intentionality: congruent intentionality or incongruent intentionality) between-subjects MANOVA. The dependent variables were the negative thoughts score and the anger score [i.e., the predictors of psychological reactance; 6]. All participants were native Dutch speakers. The experiment lasted about 30 minutes, for which participants were paid € 7.50 (approximately $ 11.25 at the time this experiment was conducted).

2.2   Procedure

Participants were invited to participate in a study about technology and interaction. When arriving at the laboratory, participants were seated behind a desk top computer. After some general instructions, the experiment left the room (to minimize possible influences of the experimenter). Participants could begin the experimental task by pressing a "Continue" button. The participants were shown an introduction about programming a virtual washing machine (see Picture 1). Next, participants were introduced to the iCat, called Femke (see Picture 2).

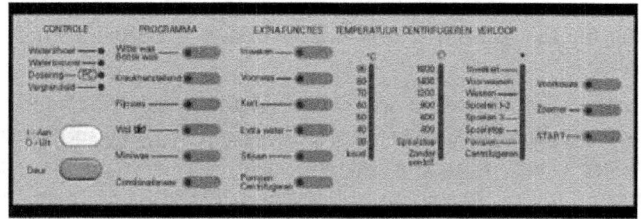

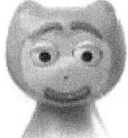

Picture 2: The iCat

Picture 1. Virtual washing machine panel

Before participants began with the practice trial, they were introduced to two goals that people can have during washing their laundry; "A clean laundry", and "Energy conservation". Participants were asked to rank these two goals by their preference of importance of the goal. After stating their preference, participants were told that Femke had also made a preference ranking. In the congruent intentionality condition, participants were told that (depending on their preference ranking) Femke had made the same ranking. Then, participants could push a button and Femke introduced itself. Femke stated its preference ranking again and explicated that this ranking was the same as the participant's ranking. In the incongruent intentionality condition, participants were told that (depending on their preference ranking) Femke had made the opposite ranking. When Femke introduced itself, it stated again its preferences and explicated that this ranking was the opposite as the participant's ranking. After this introduction, participants proceeded to the practice trial. During the washing tasks (including the practice trial), Femke provided the participants with advice about their programming choices. In the low threat condition, participants received advice consisting of low-threatening language (e.g., "You could set the temperature to 40 C°"). In the high threat condition, participants received advice consisting of high-threatening language (e.g., "You have to set the temperature to 40 C°"). Before the 10 trials started, Femke again explicated its preference ranking in comparison with the participant's preference ranking. In addition, the participant was reminded that he/she was not obligated to follow the advice of Femke. After completing the 10 trials, participants were asked to report their demographics, feelings of anger, negative thoughts, perceived threat-to-autonomy, perceived intentionality of Femke, restoration thoughts, and evaluations of Femke. Finally, participants were thanked, paid € 7.50 (approximately $ 11.25 at the time this experiment was conducted), and dismissed.

2.3 Materials

Feelings of anger: This measure is based on the anger questionnaire of [6], and on the STAXI [15]. Statements are presented such as "I felt irritated during the task", "I had the feeling to hit on something during the task", and "I felt angry during the task". The mean score of the feelings of anger questionnaire formed a reliable scale (alpha = .83) and was labeled as "anger score".

Negative thoughts: To obtain negative thoughts a thought-listing task was administered. In this task, participants were asked to report every single thought they had while programming the washing machine. After that, participants were asked to label every thought they reported as either "Negative" (N), "Positive" (P), or "Neutral" (Neu). Additionally, they were asked to report the frequency of every thought. The percentage of the negative thoughts in the thought-listing task was labeled as "negative thoughts score".

Perceived threat-to-autonomy: This measure was based on the perceived threat to autonomy measure used in [6]. Statements were, for example: "I felt free to choose the way I wanted to choose", and "I had the feeling that it was tried to make a decision for me". The mean score of the perceived threat-to-autonomy questionnaire formed a reliable scale (alpha = .85) and was labeled as "threat score".

Perceived intentionality: The intentionality questionnaire assessed whether participants perceived the displayed intentionality of the agent (i.e., Femke) as either cooperative (the same intentions as the participant) or competitive (different intentions as the participant). Statements were for example: "Femke wanted to reach the same goals as I did", and "Femke tried to hinder me in reaching my goals". The mean score of the perceived intentionality questionnaire formed a reliable scale (alpha = .83) and was labeled as "intentionality score".

Negative evaluations of the agent: The agent (i.e., Femke) was evaluated by two items. The statements were: "Femke was an expert at doing the laundry", and "Femke was friendly". The two questions correlated fairly well ($R = .33$, $p < .005$) and were combined to form the "negative evaluations score".

Restoration thoughts: To measure restoration thoughts (i.e., cognitions about restoring the feeling of autonomy) two questions were asked "Often, I had the tendency to do just the opposite of what Femke recommended", and "Often, I deliberately tried to ignore the advices of Femke". The two questions correlated fairly high ($R = .58$, $p < .001$) and were combined to form the "restoration thoughts score".

Restoration behavior: Participant's restoration behavior (i.e., actual behavior to restore the feeling of autonomy) was the behavioral measure in this study. In the washing trials, participants were asked to make programming choices. After each programming choice, participants were provided with advice from the iCat. Then, we checked whether participants adjusted their score after receiving the advice. We calculated a difference score of first washing choice and final washing choice, with taking the advice of the iCat into account.

3 Results

3.1 Manipulation Checks

To check whether our manipulations of threat and intentionality were successful, we conducted two separated one-way ANOVAs. The one-way ANOVA of our threat manipulation on the threat score indicated that participants in the high threat condition experienced a higher level of threat ($M = 3.5$, $SD = .5$), than participants in the low threat condition ($M = 3.0$, $SD = .6$), $F(1, 75) = 16.76$, $p < .001$. This suggests that our threat manipulation was successful. The one-way ANOVA of our intentionality manipulation on the intentionality score indicate that participants in the congruent intentionality condition perceived Femke's (i.e., the iCat) intentionality as more congruent ($M = 3.8$, $SD = .8$) than participants in the incongruent intentionality condition ($M = 2.8$, $SD = .7$), $F(1, 75) = 33.20$, $p < .001$.

3.2 Effects on Psychological Reactance

Our first hypothesis stated that we expected that participants would experience more psychological reactance when they received high-threatening messages compared to low-threatening messages. To test this, we submitted the negative thoughts score and the anger score to a 2 (threat: low threat vs. high threat) x 2 (intentionality: congruent intentionality vs. incongruent intentionality) between-subjects MANOVA. Confirming our first hypothesis, participants in the high threat condition experienced more negative thoughts ($M = 49.7$, $SD = 26.0$) than participants in the low threat condition ($M = 29.3$, $SD = 26.3$), $F(1, 75) = 11.88$, $p = .001$. Also, participants in the high threat condition experienced more feelings of anger ($M = 1.8$, $SD = .6$) than participants in the low threat condition ($M = 1.5$, $SD = .4$), $F(1, 75) = 5.22$, $p = .025$. However, when analyzing the data we discovered two extreme outliers (i.e., on Mahalanobis distance), which had an effect on the anger score. That is, the effect of threat on feelings of anger, after exclusion of the outliers, showed only a marginal difference, $F(1, 73) = 3.00$,

$p = .087$. Because the effects remained the same in all other analyses, we decided to present the data without outliers.

Our second hypothesis stated that participants who interacted with a high-threatening agent that expressed an incongruent intentionality would experience the most psychological reactance compared to all other groups. For psychological reactance to occur, participants have to experience a threat to their autonomy. First, we checked whether an incongruent intentionality alone would be experienced as autonomy-threatening and consequently caused psychological reactance. As expected, no main effects were found for intentionality on the negative thoughts score as well as on the anger score, both Fs < 1, ps > .1, suggesting that intentionality itself did not cause any differences on psychological reactance. That is, the intentionality of the agent did not serve as an autonomy-threatening variable. Second, we checked whether there existed an interaction between threat and intentionality. The interaction effect appeared to be non-significant for both negative thoughts, $F(1, 73) = .25$, $p = .616$, and feelings of anger, $F(1, 73) = 1.83$, $p = .181$. Although the interaction did not reach significance, the means of the anger score are in the predicted direction (see Figure 1).

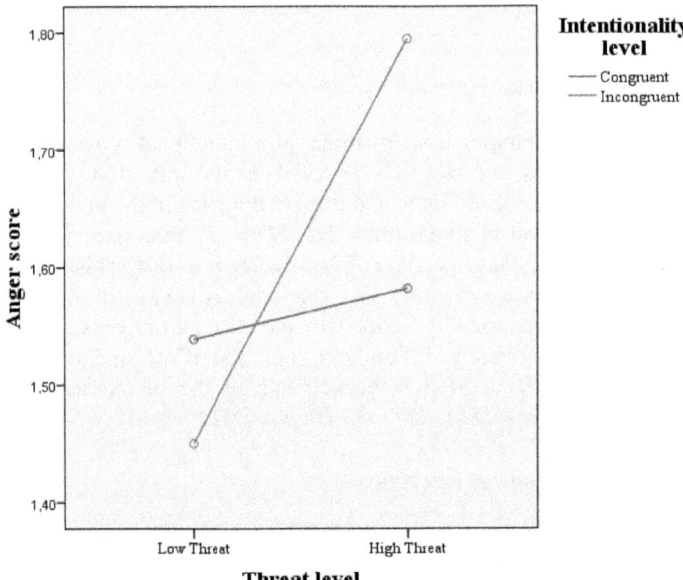

Fig. 1. Feelings of anger by threat level and intentionality level

Closer examination of the mean answers on the anger rating questions suggested that when participants had interacted with an agent that had an incongruent intentionality, they experienced more anger when the agent used high-threatening messages ($M = 1.8$, $SD = .6$) compared to low threatening messages ($M = 1.5$, $SD = .3$), $F(1, 73) = 4.97$, $p = .029$. However, when the agent had a congruent intentionality no differences were observed, $F < 1$, $p > .1$. Also, when participants had interacted with an agent that used low-threat language, results suggest they experienced comparable anger when the agent had congruent or incongruent intentionality, $F < 1$,

$p > .1$. Likewise, when participants had interacted with an agent that used high-threat language, results suggest they experienced comparable anger when the agent had congruent or incongruent intentionality, $F(1, 73) = 1.74, p = .191$. Although the latter effect did not reach significance, the means are in the predicted directions. Indeed, confirming our predictions, a contrast analysis comparing the incongruent intentionality/high threat condition with all other groups, showed that participants who were exposed to a high-threatening agent with an incongruent intentionality experienced the most anger compared to all other groups, $F(1, 73) = 4.55, p = .036$.

In sum, these results suggest partial support for our second hypothesis, indicating that participants in the incongruent intentionality/ high threat condition experienced the most feelings of anger, but showed no differences on negative thoughts.

3.3   Effects on Restoration

Our third hypothesis stated that there exists a relationship between threat and (a) restoration thoughts, (b) restoration behavior, and (c) negative evaluations of the agent. In addition, we hypothesized that the relationship between threat and restoration was mediated by psychological reactance.

First, we checked whether the relationship between threat and restoration thoughts was mediated by psychological reactance. To test this, we performed a mediation analysis as described by [1], with threat as independent variable, psychological reactance (i.e., combined score of the negative thoughts score and the anger score) as the mediator, and restoration thoughts as the dependent variable. Results indicated that the effect of threat on restoration thoughts was significant, $B = .62, SE = .24$, $t(76) = 2.61, p = .011, R^2 = .08$. When including the mediator as a predictor, the effect of threat on restoration thoughts was diminished but remained significant, $B = .54, SE = .26, t(76) = 2.09, p = .04, R^2 = .09$. The effect of psychological reactance on restoration thoughts showed no significant effect, $t(76) < 1, p > .3$. This analysis indicates that psychological reactance did not mediate the relationship between threat and restoration thoughts. It seemed that threat causes both psychological reactance and restoration thoughts.

Second, we checked whether the relationship between threat and restoration behavior was mediated by psychological reactance. Again, we performed a mediation analysis [1], with threat as independent variable, psychological reactance as the mediator, and restoration behavior as the dependent variable. Results showed no effect of threat on restoration behavior, $t < 1.2, p > .1$. Interestingly, when examining the correlation matrix, it can be observed that restoration behavior is significantly related to anger score $(R = .29)$, and to negative thoughts score $(R = .27)$. These results suggest that there is no direct effect of threat on restoration behavior, but do suggest that high levels of psychological reactance are associated with high levels of restoration.

Finally, we checked whether the relationship between threat and negative evaluations of the agent was mediated by psychological reactance. Again, we performed a mediation analysis [1], with threat as independent variable, psychological reactance as the mediator, and negative evaluations of the agent as the dependent variable. Results showed that the effect of threat on negative evaluations was significant, $B = -1.1, SE = .17, t(76) = -6.54, p < .000, R^2 = .36$. When including the mediator as a predictor, the effect of threat on restoration thoughts was slightly diminished but remained highly significant, $B = -.96, SE = .18, t(76) = -5.44, p < .000$,

$R^2 = .4$. Also, the effect of psychological reactance on negative evaluations showed a significant effect, $B = -.01$, $SE = .01$, $t(76) = -2.09$, $p = .04$, $R^2 = .4$. A Sobel test suggests confirmation of this finding, $z = -1.83$, $p = .067$. So, this mediation analysis indicates that threat caused psychological reactance, which in turn caused evaluations of the agent to be more negative.

4   Conclusions and Discussion

The current study investigated whether the intentions of an advice-giving robot have an effect on people's feelings of psychological reactance in response to a threat of autonomy [2]. To examine this, participants were provided with either high-threatening advice messages or low-threatening advice messages. First of all, results present evidence – in line with our expectations – that participants who received high threat-to-autonomy advice messages experienced more psychological reactance (feelings of anger and negative thoughts) than participants who received low threat-to-autonomy advice messages. This finding is in correspondence with previous research that showed that explicit directives resulted in more psychological reactance [6, 8, 9; 10; 11; 13]. Based on these findings we argue that when developing persuasive messages the wording of the message should be carefully planned in order to minimize psychological reactance.

Second, we expected that incongruent goal intentions would add to the effect of psychological reactance caused by a high-threatening message. Results indicated that participants who were exposed to a high-threatening robot with incongruent intentions reported the most feelings of anger compared to all other groups. However, this effect was not found for negative thoughts. Therefore, our second hypothesis was partially supported. A possible explanation for this null effect of the negative thoughts measure could be that the task used to obtain the negative thoughts was not a very valid type of measurement. As can be observed in the raw data, the variance is rather large, which makes it difficult to draw high-quality conclusions. Previous research already showed that it is very hard to measure people's cognitions, because the measures used are often not sensitive enough to elicit cognitive responses [e.g., 16]. Another explanation could be that people may have experienced feelings of psychological reactance, but may not have had the time to construct cognitions about it. Our main conclusion from these findings is that the expression of incongruent intentions can increase the probability of experienced feelings of psychological reactance (or at least anger). A consequence of this could be that users might not want to interact anymore with the persuasive technology in the future.

Finally, we investigated whether psychological reactance mediated the relationship between threat and restoration thoughts during the task. We found that participants reported more restoration thoughts, as a result of a higher threat-to-autonomy message. That is, participants showed a higher tendency to do the opposite of what the advice-giving agent said and a higher tendency to ignore the advice completely. Results indicate that the relationship between threat and restoration thoughts was not mediated by psychological reactance. This suggests that a threatening message can trigger psychological reactance as well as restoration thoughts directly. Next, we investigated whether psychological reactance mediated the relationship between threat and restoration behavior. Although we did not find a relationship between threat and restoration behavior, restoration behavior was significantly correlated with both feelings of anger and negative thoughts. Finally, we investigated whether psychological reactance mediated the relationship between threat and negative evaluations. We found that participants gave more negative evaluations of the robot, as a result of a higher threat-to-autonomy message. That is, they attributed a lower expertise to the high-threatening advice-giving agent, and evaluated it as less friendly than the low-threatening advice-giving agent. For negative evaluations, it seemed that there was a small partial mediation of psychological reactance. That is, the effect of threat diminished when including psychological reactance as a predictor of negative evaluations, but remained highly significant. In short, the current results suggest that participants who experienced a threat to their autonomy became psychologically reactant and consequently evaluated the advice-giving agent more negatively.

Summarizing our findings, we found that participants became more psychologically reactant (reported more feelings of anger and more negative thoughts) when exposed to high-threatening advice provided by a robot. Moreover, this effect increased when the robot explicitly indicated it had incongruent intentions (on the reactance measure of feelings of anger). Finally, although results indicated no behavioral restoration effect, participants did report more restoration thoughts and evaluated the robot more negatively when they received a high threat-to-autonomy advice. This could imply that participants might become reluctant to work with the robot in the future.

Overall, these findings suggest that persuasive technology should consider the formulation of persuasive messages. In correspondence with earlier research [e.g., 4, 7, 8; 13] we advise that in order to minimize psychological reactance, the threats to the user's autonomy should be minimized. Moreover, we argue that it would be wise to always pretest a persuasive message to check for psychological reactance. We argue that the current results are important beyond the effects of language intensity. Of course this study only looked at language intensity (e.g., "could" vs. "have to") as a threat manipulation, but this is only one way to trigger the feeling of threat to people's autonomy. Other studies also showed different ways of a threat manipulation, like choice elimination [3]. As already explained in the introduction, every act of persuasion–thus also every act of persuasive technology–has the possibility of triggering psychological reactance [2, 3]. If you try to change people's behavior (or attitudes), people may feel this as a threat to their autonomy. In other words, the *feeling* of threat to autonomy is enough to cause people to experience psychological reactance and consequently show behavior that is in contrast to the desired behavior. This means that every persuasive technology can suffer from the effect of psychological reactance, which could lead to opposite behavior or even rejection of the persuasive technology. Most importantly, the current research adds to psychological reactance research that it is important to take into account both the intentions of the user, and also the intentions the user attributes to the persuasive technology. That is, we suggest that to improve persuasive effects, persuasive technology can adapt persuasive messages to the user's intentions, especially when the intentions of the user and the intentions of the persuasive technology (or the agent behind it) are in opposite directions. It seems that incongruent goal intentions even can cause a stronger feeling of threat to autonomy that increases the probability of rejecting the persuasive technology. Therefore it is important to design persuasive technology that can adapt to the user's goal intentions. Hereby, we advice to ask the user beforehand for his or her goal intentions and only then start to persuade the user to perform some desired behavior (or change a specific attitude).

Acknowledgements

We would like to thank all the prior and current members of the Persuasive Technology Lab Group and in particular Suzanne Vossen, Ad van Berlo, Eric Postma, and Wilco Moerman for their insights and contributions to this research.

References

1. Baron, R.M., Kenny, D.A.: The Moderator-Mediator Variable Distinction in Social Psychological Research: Conceptual, Strategic and Statistical Considerations. J. of Pers. and Soc. Psycholog. 51, 1173–1182 (1986)
2. Brehm, J.W.: A Theory of Psychological Reactance. Academic Press, New York (1966)
3. Brehm, S.S., Brehm, J.W.: Psychological Reactance: A Theory of Freedom and Control. Academic Press, New York (1981)
4. Buller, D.B., Borland, R., Burgoon, M.: Impact of Behavioral Intention on Effectiveness of Message Features: Evidence From the Family Sun Safety Project. Hum. Commun. Res. 24(3), 433–453 (1998)
5. Burgoon, M., Alvaro, E., Grandpre, J., Voulodakis, M.: Revisiting the Theory of Psychological Reactance: Communicating Threats to Attitudinal Freedom. In: Dillard, J.P. (ed.) The Persuasion Handbook: Theory and Practice. Sage Publications, Thousands Oaks (2002)
6. Dillard, J.P., Shen, L.: On the Nature of Reactance and Its Role in Persuasive Health Communication. Commun. Monogr. 72, 144–168 (2005)
7. Grandpre, J., Alvaro, E.M., Burgoon, M., Miller, C.H., Hall, J.R.: Adolescent Reactance and Anti-Smoking Campaigns: A Theoretical Approach. Health Commun. 15(3), 349–366 (2003)
8. Miller, C.H., Lane, L.T., Deatrick, L.M., Young, A.M., Potts, K.A.: Psychological Reactance and Promotional Health Messages: The Effects of Controlling Language, Lexical Concreteness, and the Restoration of Freedom. Hum. Commun. Res. 33, 219–240 (2007)
9. Quick, B.L., Considine, J.R.: Examining the Use of Forceful Language When Designing Exercise Persuasive Messages for Adults: A Test of Conceptualizing Reactance Arousal as a Two-Step Process. Health Commun. 23, 483–491 (2008)
10. Quick, B.L., Stephenson, M.T.: Further Evidence That Psychological Reactance Can be Modelled as a Combination of Anger and Negative Cognitions. Commun. Res. 34(3), 255–276 (2007)
11. Rains, S.A., Turner, M.M.: Psychological Reactance and Persuasive Health Communication: A Test and Extension of the Intertwined Model. Human Commun. Res. 33, 241–269 (2007)
12. Reeves, B., Nass, C.: The Media Equation: How People Treat Computers, Television, and New Media Like Real People and Places. Cambridge University Press, New York (2002)
13. Roubroeks, M.A.J., Midden, C.J.H., Ham, J.R.C.: Does It Make a Difference Who Tells You What To Do? Exploring the Effects of Social Agency on Psychological Reactance. In: Chatterjee, S., Dev, P. (eds.) Proceedings of the 4th International Conference on Persuasive Technology 2009, Claremont, California, April 26 -29, article No.: 15. ACM, New York (2009)
14. Silvia, P.J.: Deflecting Reactance: The Role of Similarity in Increasing Compliance and Reducing Resistance. Basic and Appl. Soc. Psych. 27(3), 277–284 (2005)
15. Van der Ploeg, H.M., Van Buuren, E.T., Van Brummelen, P.: The Factor Structure of the State-Trait Anger Scale. Psych. Rep. 63, 978 (1988)
16. Wansink, B., Ray, M.L., Batra, R.: Increasing Cognitive Response Sensitivity. J. of Advert. 23(2), 62–74 (1994)

Practical Findings from Applying the PSD Model for Evaluating Software Design Specifications

Teppo Räisänen, Tuomas Lehto, and Harri Oinas-Kukkonen

University of Oulu, Department of Information Processing Science
Rakentajantie 3, 90570 Oulu, Finland
{Teppo.Raisanen,Tuomas.Lehto,Harri.Oinas-Kukkonen}@oulu.fi

Abstract. This paper presents practical findings from applying the PSD model to evaluating the support for persuasive features in software design specifications for a mobile Internet device. On the one hand, our experiences suggest that the PSD model fits relatively well for evaluating design specifications. On the other hand, the model would benefit from more specific heuristics for evaluating each technique to avoid unnecessary subjectivity. Better distinction between the design principles in the social support category would also make the model easier to use. Practitioners who have no theoretical background can apply the PSD model to increase the persuasiveness of the systems they design. The greatest benefit of the PSD model for researchers designing new systems may be achieved when it is applied together with a sound theory, such as the Elaboration Likelihood Model. Using the ELM together with the PSD model, one may increase the chances for attitude change.

Keywords: Persuasive Systems Design Model, specifications, research, practice, guide, analysis.

1 Introduction

As we have gained deeper understanding of the field of persuasive technology, the expectations for persuasive designs have also increased. This is especially evident in competitive markets such as Web 2.0, e-business and the mobile domain. When designing solutions for these kinds of environments, the designers must have a thorough understanding of the various persuasion, motivation and influence strategies to gain competitive advantage.

Oinas-Kukkonen and Harjumaa [1] have conceptualized a framework for designing and evaluating persuasive systems, known as the Persuasive Systems Design (PSD) model. In the PSD model, the categories for persuasive system design principles are: primary task support (supporting the user's primary task), dialogue support (supporting the interaction between the user and the system), system credibility (the more credible the system is, the more persuasive it is), and social support (the system motivates users by leveraging social influence). In addition to this, the model can be utilized to analyze the intent, event and strategy of the persuasion context.

T. Ploug, P. Hasle, H. Oinas-Kukkonen (Eds.): PERSUASIVE 2010, LNCS 6137, pp. 185–192, 2010.

As the PSD model is a meta-level model, it is designed to be used together with suitable theories, such as the Elaboration Likelihood Model [2], the Theory of Reasoned Action [3], the Theory of Planned Behavior [4], Social Cognitive Theory [5], or other behavior or attitude change theories. This paper will describe practical findings from applying the PSD model to evaluating software design specifications.

Section two will discuss persuasive technologies in the light of software requirements engineering. Section three will present the case, and section four the results. Section five will discuss the relationship between the PSD model and the Elaboration Likelihood model (ELM) and how to apply the PSD model in conjunction with the ELM. Finally, section six discusses the findings, and section seven concludes the paper.

2   Requirements Engineering

Requirements engineering is an early part of the software system development process. It is a "branch of software engineering concerned with the real-world goals for, functions of, and constraints on software systems. It is also concerned with the relationship of these factors to precise specifications of software behavior, and to their evolution over time and across software families." [6]. Nuseibeh and Easterbrook [7] have identified the following core requirements engineering activities:

- Eliciting requirements.
- Modeling and analyzing requirements.
- Communicating requirements.
- Agreeing requirements, and
- Evolving requirements.

The first step of requirements engineering is the elicitation of requirements. It aims at identifying all the stakeholders –such as customers, developers and users – as well as the objectives and tasks of the system. Prototyping, brainstorming and focus groups are examples of elicitation techniques. In addition, various elicitation methods provide guidance on how to use the techniques in the elicitation process [7].

Modeling the requirements aims at producing abstract descriptions of the requirements so that they would be amenable to interpretation. For example, in the case of large information systems, data modeling is often used to understand how information is to be manipulated and managed [7]. In the case of behavior-change support systems [8], domain modeling and behavior modeling must be used to gain a deeper understanding of the intent, event and strategy of the targeted behavior change. Various analysis methods should also be used together with modeling techniques to validate and verify the models. Finally, modeling also transfers the requirements into a communicable form. This way they can be presented to the stakeholders.

The core activities of communicating and agreeing on the requirements with different stakeholders aims at establishing a consensus that the requirements and models elicited provide an accurate account of stakeholder requirements [7]. Finally, evolving requirements is about managing the changes to the requirement documents.

The research presented in this paper deals mostly with analyzing models. We utilized the Persuasive Systems Design (PSD) model [1] as a vehicle for the analysis. The next section will present the case.

3 Case Description

In this case, the PSD model was utilized for evaluating the requirements specifications of a mobile Internet device under planning. We received several requirements documents from Company X. The documents related to user interface and user interaction issues. They were rich with life-sized sketches of the proposed solutions. Figure 1 illustrates the pictures and the level of detail found in the set of documents. In addition to the touchpad gestures, the pictures in the specifications also had screenshots of user interface elements to illustrate how the gestures can be used to interact with the elements.

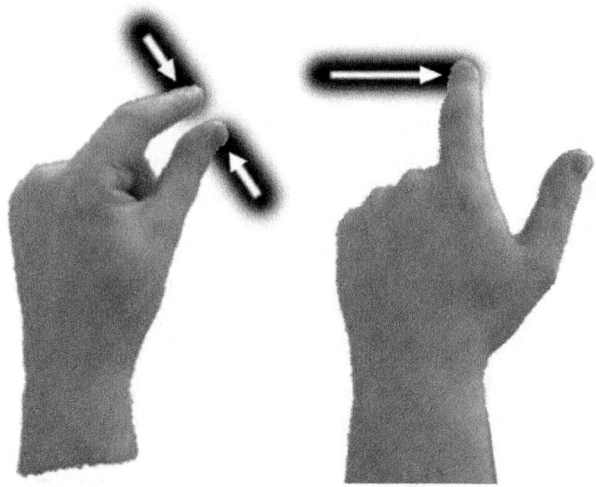

Fig. 1. Example picture from the software design specifications. The pictures demonstrate two touchpad gestures.

The evaluation protocol was as follows. Two researchers independently evaluated the design documents in order to recognize the persuasive features through the PSD model. After this, the findings were discussed and a joint understanding was formed through face-to-face discussion. All persuasive features were graded in terms of how well the planned implementation seemed to support the feature. Company X was then provided with the results and a short list of suggestions on how to improve the persuasiveness and usability of the system. Thus, even if we focused mostly on the analysis of the modeled requirements, we included some elements of requirement communication as well.

4 Results

Software design specifications define the roadmap for the system building process [9]. Evaluation of the specifications aims at ensuring that the requirements are feasible and that no crucial requirements are missing. In addition, the evaluation of the specifications aims at picking up any problems before resources are committed to addressing the requirements [10].

The case demonstrated that the PSD model as such is feasible for evaluating design specifications. In this kind of work, it becomes imperative to clearly identify and define the primary task for the target of the evaluation. With mobile Internet devices, the primary task can vary greatly from browsing the Web to watching videos, social networking and all the way to using the device as a mobile phone. In this case, the device was of general purpose, i.e., it was intended to be used for any of the abovementioned purposes. This made the analysis of persuasiveness regarding the primary task issues somewhat more difficult than with a more precise goal for the device.

The main findings can be summarized as follows:

- The case demonstrated how the various PSD principles work together. For example, the principles of suggestion and reward are interlinked with each other. If the application suggests new ways of doing things for the user, some kind of rewarding feature would naturally supplement it.
- It seems to be that some principles do not work very well together. For example, the abundant use of reduction makes tunneling nearly useless.
- Our experiences confirm the claim put forward by the developers of the PSD model that there is no point in trying to utilize all persuasion techniques in a single case. Rather, a coherent set of the techniques should be recognized and selected. This should be done in such a manner that there would be as much synergy as possible between the different techniques included.

Additional persuasive effects may be achieved through the synergy between different design principles. Many of the principles in the PSD model seem to operate well in pairs or as part of larger sets. Paired principles, such as suggestion–reward, suggestion–personalization, self-monitoring–reminders, similarity–liking, competition–cooperation, and simulation–rehearsal can be effective together. For instance, users could rehearse the target behavior with simulations. Further examples would be a self-monitoring functionality that could be triggered by using reminders, or using suggestion to prompt the user to personalize an application or service.

Yet, harnessing principles with low synergy might result in less persuasive effects than anticipated. Thus, it is indeed a coherent set of persuasive design principles that may be able to provide advantages and the best persuasive results.

An aspect of the PSD model that posed a challenge for us was that some of the social support principles are highly interlinked with each other. The connections between social learning, social comparison, social facilitation, and normative influence are difficult to differentiate from each other. For example, it is difficult to see where social comparison starts and social learning ends. This overlapping makes the utilization of the model for evaluation purposes very challenging. Furthermore, in some cases, the persuasive principles may not be determined based solely on design specifications, as some of the principles (especially in the credibility support and social support categories) might only be observed in the actual system-to-user interaction situations.

The greatest challenge in applying the PSD model was that no explicit evaluation heuristics have been defined for it yet. The model would gain more strength from explicitly defined scales and instructions for evaluating the implementation of each principle. These types of heuristics would substantially reduce the influence of the subjective views of an individual evaluator, and thus would diminish potential bias. Nevertheless, it should be noted that evaluation will always remains subjective. A further challenge is that since the PSD model incorporates a total of 28 design principles, the evaluation of specifications and/or applications may be quite laborious and time consuming.

Beyond the evaluation of persuasive principles, the PSD model can be utilized to recognize the intent (persuader, change type), event (use, user, and technology context) and strategy (message, route) of the persuasion context [11]. In this case, we were not able to extract this information from the software specifications beyond a rather generic level. (It should be noted that we were not part of the design team/organization.) In our view, defining the persuasion context early in the design process is essential and may eliminate costly rework.

5   The Relationship between Theories and the PSD Model

Practitioners with no strong theoretical background can apply the PSD model for their designs and/or evaluations and gain benefits from it, whereas researchers still need a theoretical framework for their own work to gain the full benefit from the PSD model. When applying the PSD model for research purposes for design, it is important to lean on an understanding provided by a persuasion-related theory to be able to select the desirable persuasive features through the PSD model.

For instance, the Elaboration Likelihood Model, or ELM for short, [2] is one of the most widely used theories to explain how attitude change happens. Next, we will describe how the PSD model could be used in conjunction with the ELM to increase the persuasiveness of a designed system. See Fig. 2 and note the arrows.

The figure shows the two parts of the ELM in two separate spirals. These are the central and peripheral routes (the PSD model calls these the direct and indirect routes). The direct route is used when information processing is based upon critical thinking. An example of this could be the decision to stop drinking alcohol. In contrast, the attitude shift through the indirect route is based on rules of thumb. These rules can be, e.g., personalized content [12]. In figure 1, the direct route is the outer spiral formed by persuasive communication, motivation, ability, cognitive processing and direct attitude change. The indirect route is the inner spiral formed by persuasive communication, indirect cues and indirect attitude shift. For clarification purposes, the indirect route is also drawn with dashed arrows. When the ELM is drawn in a spiral, it emphasizes the incremental nature of persuasion (cf. [1]).

Especially important in the ELM are the yes-arrows. The attitude change happens along them. As the direct attitude change is enduring, resistant and predictive of behavior, the outer part of the spiral is crucial. If we want to design the system to help achieve attitude change, the PSD principles should aim at producing this yes-effect (i.e., the principles should support movement along the yes-arrows in the figure). For example, dialogue support should aim at making sure that communication is persuasive (the yes-arrow from "persuasive communication" to "motivated to

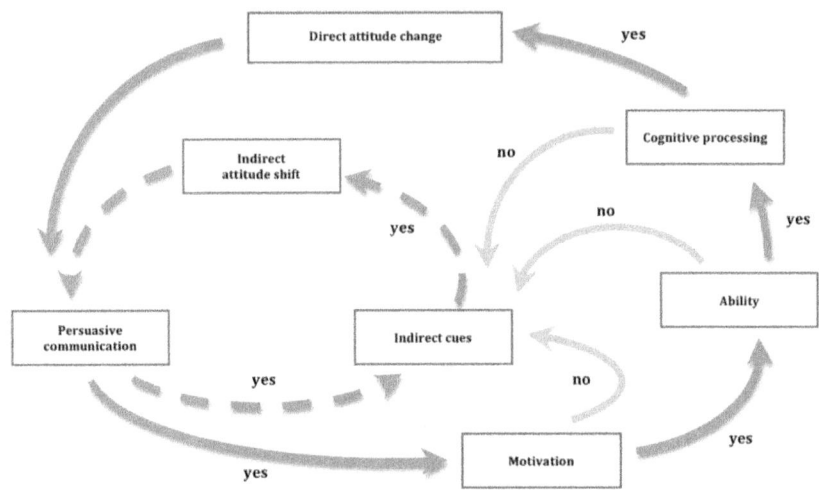

Fig. 2. Two key spirals in the Elaboration Likelihood Model

process"), social support could provide the means to motivate the users to process the message (yes-arrow from motivation to ability), primary task support should strengthen the ability to do this, and credibility support could best match the indirect cue (i.e., it seems to be better suited for an indirect attitude shift rather than change).

Support for the nature of cognitive processing and cognitive structure change seem to be very hard to achieve. In fact, this is the only yes-arrow from the ELM that the PSD model does not directly support. Yet, support for cognitive processing is not only difficult in a persuasion context. Similar problems do exist also in the context of knowledge work [13], where designed solutions can at the same time both support and hamper cognitive performance.

The ELM and the PSD model can be utilized together to achieve attitude change. Similarly, in order to design persuasive systems that aim at producing behavior change, we should apply the PSD model together with behavior change theories and models. For example, the primary task category could be used to make target behavior simpler, thus increasing the chances for behavior change [14]. This would probably lead into gaining further benefits from the PSD model.

6 Discussion

This paper provided a case description of applying the PSD framework to identify the (support for) persuasive features on a mobile Internet device. The main findings of this study were: i) the case demonstrated how the various PSD principles work together, ii) applying the PSD framework as a tool to evaluate the persuasive features of the system (based on software design specifications) is feasible. In addition, our results confirm that trying to utilize all the persuasion techniques in a single case is redundant. Rather, a coherent set (matching the persuasion context) of the techniques should be considered and conveyed. This should be done in such a manner that there would be as much synergy as possible between the different techniques included.

With mobile Internet devices, the primary task can vary greatly from surfing the Web, social networking, playing games and using the device as a mobile phone. This made the analysis of persuasiveness concerning the primary task issues somewhat more difficult than with more defined goals for the device. On the other hand, analyzing dialogue support was rather straightforward, as the dialogue support category deals mostly with system-to-user interaction issues, which were described in detail in the design specifications.

Behavioral modeling is an important part of requirements engineering [7]. With behavioral modeling, we can also identify opportunities for behavior change. In this case, however, the persuasive features were not necessarily directly linked with behavior change *per se*. Most of the persuasive system features (or the support for them) found in the design specifications seemed to enhance the user experience, i.e., boosting the ease of use and usefulness of the device. For instance, reduction (reducing complex behavior into simple tasks) decreases the effort that is required of the users to perform their target behavior.

In this particular context, analyzing persuasive design is a demanding interpretative task. As there are no explicit evaluation heuristics defined for the PSD model yet, there lies a potential bias in the interpretation of the specifications. Nevertheless, in extracting and categorizing persuasive features, we rigorously observed if the specifications clearly included the described variables. Obviously, the specifications did not always follow the very same terminology as found in the PSD model, and thus the analysis was mostly based on interpretive categorization. In spite of its wide coverage, the PSD model still is not an exhaustive list of persuasive features. New persuasion techniques may be identified in the future. The model has been built in such a manner that it may evolve, but even as it stands now, it is an important tool for any persuasive system developer.

7 Conclusions

Based on this case, the PSD model seems to fit relatively well for evaluating software design specifications. Practitioners who have no theoretical background can apply the PSD model to increase the persuasiveness of the systems they design. The greatest benefit of the PSD model for researchers designing new systems may be achieved when it is applied together with a sound theory, such as the Elaboration Likelihood Model. Using the ELM together with the PSD model, one may increase the chances for attitude change. The only part in the ELM that the PSD model does not directly support is the use of the direct route for achieving a positive or negative attitude change.

The level of details of the software design specification plays an important role in the evaluation process. Evaluating highly detailed specification documents enables more reliable and relevant investigation of the persuasive features than evaluating a specification document that is on a very high level of abstraction.

As the evaluation of specifications and/or applications may be quite laborious and time consuming, the PSD model would benefit from explicit heuristics defined for each of its design principles. Also, a clearer distinction between the design principles in the social support category would make them easier to use. Additional persuasive features may be identified from practice.

A potential future research area is supporting cognitive processing and cognitive structural change. Additionally, a very interesting and multidisciplinary line of research is how to design, implement and evaluate (persuasive) behavior change support systems for a multitude of domains such as healthcare and education.

Acknowledgements

We wish to thank the Graduate School on Software Systems and Engineering (SoSE), the National Technology Agency of Finland (Tekes) and the RichWeb project for funding this research.

References

1. Oinas-Kukkonen, H., Harjumaa, M.: Persuasive Systems Design: Key Issues, Process Model, and System Features. Communications of the Association for Information Systems 24, 28 (2009)
2. Petty, R.E., Cacioppo, J.T.: Communication and Persuasion: Central and Peripheral Routes to Attitude Change. Springer, Heidelberg (1986)
3. Fishbein, M., Ajzen, I.: Belief, attitude, intention, and behavior: An introduction to theory and research. Addison-Wesley, Reading (1975)
4. Ajzen, I.: The Theory of Planned Behavior. Organ. Behav. Hum. Decis. Process. 50, 179–211 (1991)
5. Bandura, A.: Social Cognitive Theory of Self-Regulation. Organ. Behav. Hum. Decis. Process. 50, 248–287 (1991)
6. Zave, P.: Classification of Research Efforts in Requirements Engineering. ACM Computing Surveys 29(4), 315–321 (1997)
7. Nuseibeh, B., Easterbrook, S.: Requirements engineering: a roadmap. In: Proceedings of the Conference on The Future of Software Engineering table of contents, Limerick, Ireland, pp. 35–46 (2000)
8. Oinas-Kukkonen, H.: Behavior change support systems: The next frontier for web science. In: The Second Web Science Conference, Raleigh, NC, USA, April 26-27 (2010)
9. Nunamaker Jr., J.F., Chen, M., Purdin, T.D.M.: Systems Development in Information Systems Research. J. Manage. Inf. Syst. 7, 89–106 (1990)
10. Bourque, P., Dupuis, R., Abran, A., et al.: The Guide to the Software Engineering Body of Knowledge. IEEE Software 16, 35–44 (1999)
11. Dey, A.K.: Understanding and using Context. Personal and Ubiquitous Computing 5, 4–7 (2001)
12. Tam, K.Y., Ho, S.Y.: Web Personalization as a Persuasion Strategy: An Elaboration Likelihood Model Perspective. Inform. Syst. Res. 16, 271–291 (2005)
13. Nakakoji, K., Yamamoto, Y., Akaishi, M., et al.: Interaction Design for Scholarly Writing: Hypertext Representations as a Means for Creative Knowledge Work. New Review of Hypermedia and Multimedia 11, 39–67 (2005)
14. Fogg, B.J.: A Behavior Model for Persuasive Design. In: Persuasive 2009, Claremont, California, USA, April 26-29 (2009)

Activity-Based Micro-pricing: Realizing Sustainable Behavior Changes through Economic Incentives

Tetsuo Yamabe[1], Vili Lehdonvirta[2], Hitoshi Ito[1], Hayuru Soma[1],
Hiroaki Kimura[1], and Tatsuo Nakajima[1]

[1] Dept. of Computer Science, Waseda University, Tokyo, Japan
{yamabe,hitoshi_i,hayuring,hiroaki,tatsuo}@dcl.info.waseda.ac.jp
[2] Helsinki Institute for Information Technology, Helsinki, Finland
vili.lehdonvirta@hiit.fi

Abstract. In this paper, we further develop the idea of combining pervasive computing techniques with electronic payment systems to create activity-based micro-incentives. Economic incentives are an effective way to influence consumer behavior, and are used in e.g. marketing and resource coordination. Our approach allows marketers and regulators to induce consumers to perform particular actions in new application domains by attaching micro-prices to a wider range of behaviors. A key challenge is designing incentive mechanisms that result in desired behavior changes. We examine two basic incentive models. Based on the results of preliminary experiments, we discuss how economic incentives can affect consumer attitudes and lead to sustainable behavior changes.

Keywords: Persuasive technology, economic incentives, mobile payment, micropayments, activity-based micro-pricing, virtual currency.

1 Introduction

Economic incentives are a powerful way of shaping consumer behavior towards more commercially efficient and environmentally sustainable patterns. For example, taxation is a common strategy to dealing with the overuse of shared resources. Free resources shared by a number of people, such as a public toilet or the natural environment, tend to be overused in a process called the tragedy of the commons [1]. This happens because each individual derives a personal benefit from using the resource, while any costs are shared between all the users. An example of such behavior is the wasteful use of free plastic shopping bags that are filling landfills. In Japan, plastic bags are usually free, but in Finland shoppers have to pay for them. This provides an economic incentive for individuals to re-use plastic bags or bring own shopping bags to stores.

However, vendors and regulators are currently limited in what behaviors they can set a price on. Only a limited range of consumers' activities can be feasibly observed in a limited number of locations. In the aforementioned example, basically consumers have two options (i.e., purchase a plastic bag or bring one's

T. Ploug, P. Hasle, H. Oinas-Kukkonen (Eds.): PERSUASIVE 2010, LNCS 6137, pp. 193–204, 2010.

own shopping bag) and it is manually checked at the cashier in a store. However, manual observation is efficient only in cases where the consumer does not have too many options and each activity is such that it can be easily observed. Otherwise, the cost of human resources imposes a limit on this approach. If a consumer's activities could be recognized with less cost, the power of economic incentives could be applied in a far greater range of application areas.

Two emerging topics in pervasive computing and HCI research are persuasive applications and electronic payment systems. Pervasive-persuasive applications seek to alter user behavior through the means of a feedback loop between sensor-tracked user behavior and system output [2,3]. In electronic payment systems, pervasive technologies are used to implement and deploy mobile payment solutions that enable small payments in discreet and effortless manners [4,5]. In this paper, we combine these two topics, exploring the possibility of using pervasive computing technologies to create small activity-based economic incentives that discreetly steer consumer behavior towards desired patterns. Some of these applications could be aimed towards preventing overuse of environmental resources, while others would simply enable businesses to charge for their services in a more fine-grained manner, overcoming inefficiencies and stimulating commerce [5,6].

In the following sections, we describe the concept of activity-based billing systems and refer to findings in behavioral economics to discuss how economic incentives affect a consumer's decision making process. We then present an overview of a system architecture for an activity-based billing system that supports two different incentive models. Each model corresponds to a different set of transaction flows, so that services can alter consumer behavior by choosing a different model. Finally, based on lessons learned in the prototyping process, we discuss future directions. In this paper, we particularly focus on the challenge of designing incentives that have a sustainable, long-term influence on behavior [7].

2   Activity-Based Billing System

2.1   Ubiquity of Payments

The rapid growth of mobile computing has transformed mobile devices to a medium of payment. Mobile devices are used to initiate, activate and confirm payment transactions in various kinds of services, collectively known as "mobile payments" [8]. Mobile payments are not simply an extension of normal electronic payments, as they free users from physical constraints (i.e., time and place) and allow flexible decision making that adapts to the mobile use context [9]. While new features have been added to mobile user terminals, our surrounding environments are also increasingly being embedded with ambient intelligence. To support daily tasks and events, living environments are expected to become sensitive to the presence of users. For example, elder people's activities might be monitored with sensors in order to automatically detect emergency situations. Thus, computers, sensors and network connectivity have been installed into buildings, parks, trains and everyday objects [10].

The maturity of mobile payments and the increasingly prevalent ambient intelligence technology suggest the notion of *ubiquitous payments*. As argued in [5,11], sufficiently fine-grained tracking of user activity makes it possible to implement accurate pay-per-use payment models in commercial services. With sufficient context information, vendors can precisely calculate the economic cost of a consumer's action, and bill accordingly. Ubiquitous interaction techniques give consumers real-time information and control over spending. Transactions of small nominal value take place frequently, since payment is associated with the consumer actions. In ubiquitous computing environments, payments become ubiquitous, too. In this section, we introduce the idea of activity-based billing systems. Figure 1 illustrates an example scenario with two types of transaction flows, case A and case B.

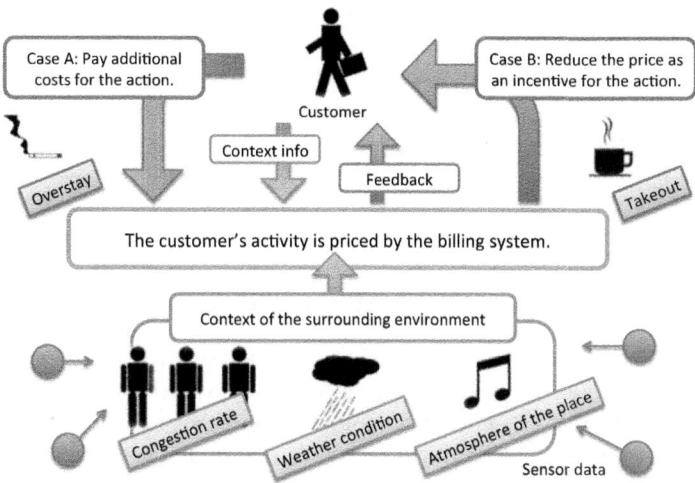

Fig. 1. Overview of the activity-based billing system with two example scenarios

2.2   Pricing Consumer Actions

A common problem for managers of busy cafes and restaurants is that customers linger in the space for a long time after their initial order without placing any additional orders, whilst taking up space from other potential customers. In Tokyo, for example, even dozens of people can be waiting for a seat outside a restaurant at lunchtime. It is difficult to keep track of how long each customer has stayed in the restaurant without making some effort to monitor them. Moreover, it would be troublesome for the staff to collect a fee for the overstay even if such customers could be identified accurately. As a result, limited seats remain occupied and from the manager's point of view, resources used inefficiently.

If the cost of customers' time spent in the cafe could be automatically priced, the situation would be different. Consider a billing system that notifies customers how much they have to pay for spending time in the space: "an additional fee will be charged for further stay: \$0.1 for every 10 minutes", for instance. If the customer continues to stay despite the notification, the system begins to charge the time on their mobile phone. In this way, the manager can charge an additional fee from overstaying customers, which improves the availability of seats while recouping the cost of lost business from occupied seats (case A). On the other hand, it is also possible to give rebates to customers who take actions that are beneficial to the business. For example, coffee price can be reduced if a customer orders coffee to go during lunchtime (case B).

Our key idea in this scenario is coupling economic incentives with specific actions, and implementing the resulting incentive system using ubiquitous computing technologies. Context recognition techniques provide support for tracking consumers' actions. The payment or rebate can be carried out smoothly by mediating it with a mobile payment system. Furthermore, the vendor to determine the current price of a given action can use different pieces of context information. If the overstay charge increases as the cafe becomes increasingly packed, it will motivate customers to move on speedily. The occupancy rate of seats can be manually checked, or automatically detected with pressure sensors embedded in chairs. Methods such as discount coupons and selective taxation are sometimes used for creating economic incentives that steer consumer behavior, but compared to the approach outlined above, they are inflexible and static.

2.3   Psychological Factors and Micro-pricing Models

The prices of these actions will nevertheless be relatively small compared to the price of, for example, a cup of coffee, because the incentives are not a core part of the service. Under the notion of ubiquitous payments, transactions happen anywhere, anytime a consumer takes a relevant action. This leads to an increase in the frequency of transactions, and the price per one action will correspondingly decrease. Thus in the activity-based pricing mechanism design, we must consider how to affect consumers' behavior with stakes of relatively low nominal value.

It is well recognized that consumers' real economic behavior is emotional and sometimes leads to irrational decision making [12,13]. In some cases this lack of economic rationality follows quite predictable patterns. For example, people tend to avoid risk associated with uncertain gains. If there are two choices, such as (a) receive a guaranteed sum of \$10, and (b) receive \$20 with a 50% probability, choice (a) is preferred even though the expected utility is same. While risk-neutral and risk-loving attributes also exist, this preference that most people have is called risk-averse. Risk-averse decision making results from so-called loss aversion bias explained in *prospect theory* [14,15].

The practical implication of this asymmetry for economic incentive systems is that surcharges (losses) and rebates (gains) can be used to create different kinds of incentivizing effects even when their overall economic impact is the same. For example, during busy lunchtime hours, a cafe could charge patrons in the form of a small initial fee and additional time-based surcharges, encouraging short stays. During quieter hours, when the manager wants patrons to linger for as long as possible, the equivalent sum could be charged in the form of a bigger initial fee and tiny time-based rebates. The suitable model can thus be chosen according to desired behavior.

The key challenges in implementing the activity-based billing system are designing an effective context recognition module and suitable billing policies that lead to desired incentivizing effects. In the following sections, we introduce the two basic micro-pricing models built on the earlier discussion on economic incentives, which can be used as the basis of such policies.

UbiPayment Model. As illustrated in Figure 2, the UbiPayment model is used to charge additional costs upon a consumer's specific actions. This transaction flow corresponds to the case A in Figure 1. In the UbiPayment model, the initial cost of a service would be smaller than in the conventional case, because vendors can expect additional revenues from the micro-payments. It also has certain benefits to consumers: they obtain the possibility of leaving out unnecessary options (i.e., actions) that are normally bundled into the price of the service, and reducing costs.

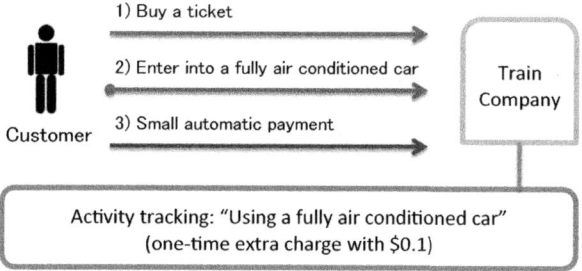

Fig. 2. Transaction flow of the UbiPayment model

UbiRebate Model. In the UbiPayment model, psychological reluctance is an important tool in influencing consumer behavior. However, sometimes it can lead to negative feelings that make customers hesitant to use the service in the first place. We therefore considered how the payment system could reduce this reluctance without changing the total volume of transactions. As illustrated in Figure 3, the idea of the UbiRebate model is to return some amount of money back to the buyer depending on the buyer's actions. The main idea here is eliminating the "paying" process from the automatic payment system. In this approach, the initial payment is set higher than in the UbiPayment model, but rebates are paid for particular activities instead of additional payments.

The concept of this approach comes from psychological aspects of consumption behavior. In general, people resist paying from their wallet, but want to "get" something instead [4]. The UbiRebate model automatically gives micro-rebates that replace the automatic payments for opposite actions. The UbiRebate model enables vendors to implement an automatic billing system that overcomes the consumer reluctance issue. Contrary to the automatic payment case, consumers may feel happy when they get a rebate for their actions, even though the total economic impact would be the same. Moreover, there is no satiation in the pay-as-you-do model, but the amount of maximum payment is ensured in the rebate-as-you-do model. The models consist of simplified transaction flows, and each one represents different incentive design. Thus it is possible to replace, combine, and switch the models according to a vendor's objectives.

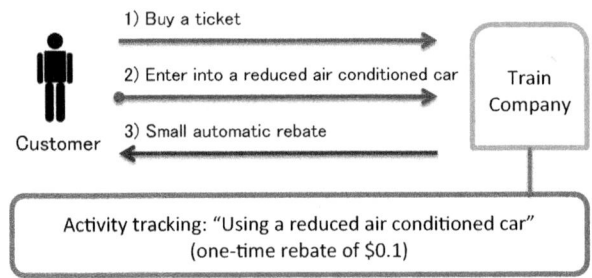

Fig. 3. Transaction flow of the UbiRebate model

3   System Architecture

In this section, we describe the system architecture of the billing system (Figure 4). The system is composed of user side modules and service side modules.

3.1   User Side

Consumers are assumed to have a mobile device for communicating with services and conducting transactions. The transaction management module handles transactions, such as payments and rebates. The module also records all transactions into a database called Log DB, which can be used for error recovery. The service discovery module detects available billing systems within range of the device's wireless connectivity (e.g., Wi-Fi, Bluetooth). The communication module establishes a connection to the detected billing system and encrypts data before transferring it to the service.

3.2   Service Side

The billing system must recognize the consumer's activities within the scope of the service in order to price and bill the behavior, and provide feedback. The context recognition module handles inputs from the consumer's devices as well as sensors that are installed in the environment. Pre-configured sensor analysis algorithms generate context information required by the billing engine. The billing engine gathers the context information and also the consumer's personal information, if necessary. The service's billing rules are pre-configured into a database called the billing policy DB; the engine calculates the applicable payment or rebate amount according to the policies set in the DB.

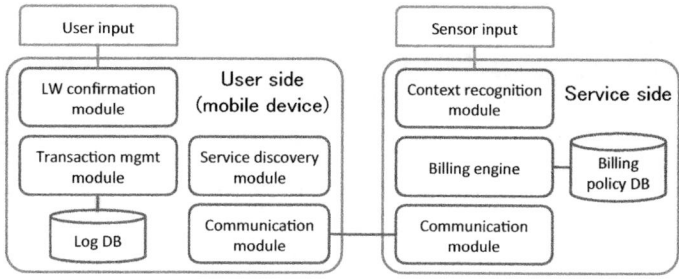

Fig. 4. System architecture of the billing system

4 Evaluation

In the above sections, we explained two basic models of activity-based micro-pricing. In order to evaluate the feasibility of these concepts, we performed an experimental study. In the sections below, we describe the methods, implementation and results of the evaluation.

4.1 Method

In order to observe how consumers might regard activity-based micro-pricing in real settings, we set up an experimental environment in our laboratory. The experimental environment was presented as a Japanese-style comic cafe (*manga kissa*), and several kinds of services were installed as shown in Figure 5. For example, participants could play a game (Nintendo Wii), read comics, browse web sites, and use a toy gadget (Chumby). A display shows a list of possible actions where participants can check which actions are priced and how much they cost. A prototype of the billing system was developed for this study.

A mobile device (iPod Touch) was handed to participants before the study started. 1,000 JPY[1] was virtually charged into the device and participants could freely enjoy the services using the money. The remaining amount is displayed on the mobile device (Figure 5), and the participant can configure feedback settings by flipping the window. Under default settings, the mobile device periodically checks whether any transactions have been conducted or not with a 10 second interval. If remaining amount is changed, sound notification is given to the participant. The participant can change the feedback interval and enable/disable the sound notification. This feature was implemented to provide insights into appropriate feedback design.

In the experiment, we prepared two scenarios: UbiPayment and UbiRebate. Table 1 shows priced actions and corresponding price in the UbiPayment scenario, and Table 2 shows the action list in the UbiRebate scenario. For example, in the UbiPayment scenario, a participant has to pay 100 JPY at the beginning.

---

[1] 1 JPY $\simeq$ 0.01 USD as of 31.3.2010.

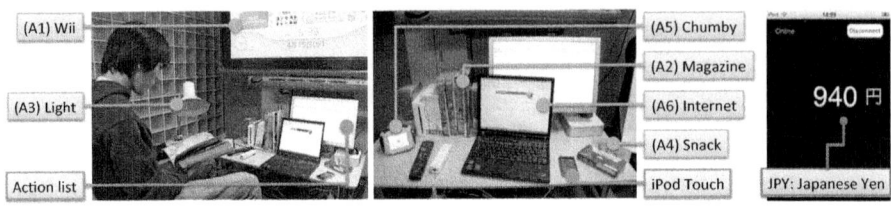

Fig. 5. A comic cafe setup and a mobile user interface for the experimental study

Table 1. Action list in the UbiPayment scenario

ID	Action	Interval	Payment
A0	Initial cost	-	100 JPY
A1	Play Wii	1 min	10 JPY
A2	Read a comic	1 min	5 JPY
A3	Turn on a light	1 min	1 JPY
A4	Have a snack	(per 1 snack)	10 JPY
A5	Play Chumby	1 min	5 JPY
A6	Browse web sites	1 min	5 JPY

Table 2. Action list in the UbiRebate scenario

ID	Action	Interval	Rebate
A0	Initial cost	-	500 JPY
A1	NOT play Wii	1 min	10 JPY
A2	NOT read comics	1 min	5 JPY
A3	NOT turn on a light	1 min	1 JPY
A4	Have a snack	-	- JPY
A5	NOT play Chumby	1 min	5 JPY
A6	NOT browse web sites	1 min	5 JPY

Then, if the participant plays a Wii game, 10 JPY will be automatically withdrawn from their mobile device per minute. In contrast, in the UbiRebate scenario, the participant has to pay a bigger initial cost than in the UbiPayment scenario (500 JPY). However, if the participant does *not* use services, the corresponding amount of money is automatically rebated to their mobile device. For example, if they play a Wii game, the sum of all the actions' prices excluding A1 is rebated each minute.

Participants were instructed to stay in the room for 10 minutes for each scenario. While the study was performed, we monitored the room with a web camera and used the Wizard-of-Oz technique instead of using the context recognition module explained in Figure 4. In the monitor's display, a check list is shown and performed actions can be checked accordingly. Then the amount of payment/rebate is automatically calculated, and the remaining amount is updated on the mobile device's display. Six university students joined this study as participants (male: 5, female:1, age: 22-25). We recorded how they configured the feedback settings in the experiment. We also asked several questions about their impressions regarding activity-based micro-pricing at the end of the test.

4.2   Results

On average, the participants performed approximately 2.5 different types of actions in the UbiPayment scenario, and 2 kinds of actions in the UbiRebate scenario. As shown in Table 3, they felt that the test duration was not long (Q1), and the price of payments/rebates was neither expensive nor inexpensive

(Q2 and Q4). The responses to Q3 and Q5 imply that the UbiRebate model affected the participants' mental state slightly stronger than the UbiPayment model. However, due to the size of the user study, we cannot find significant differences from the results. Moreover, some of the participants pointed out that camera monitoring was one reason for their anxiety, so we cannot assert that loss-aversion effects in the UbiPayment model are the only explanation for the responses to Q3.

Table 3. Questions presented to the participants and the mean responses (5-point Likert scale)

	Question	Point
Q1	What do you think about the duration of the test? (5: too long - 0: too short)	2.5
Q2	What do you think about the size of the payments in the UbiPayment scenario? (5: too expensive - 0: too inexpensive)	3.0
Q3	Did you feel nervous or anxious in the UbiPayment scenario? (5: strongly felt - 0: did not feel)	3.1
Q4	What do you think about the size of the rebates in the UbiRebate scenario? (5: too big - 0: too small)	3.0
Q5	Did you feel happy or satisfied in the UbiRebate scenario? (5: strongly felt - 0: did not feel)	3.3

In the experiments, only two participants customized the time interval of the sound notification. In the questionnaire, they commented that frequent sound interruption was annoying. One of the participant felt that even rebating becomes annoying due to frequent notification. Alternative ideas in their comments are notifications with vibration, notifications without sound, and notification with price limitation. Almost of all participants preferred to decrease notification frequency, and 7.2 minutes was the average interval that they would set if the activity-based micro-pricing got realized. Some of the participants also commented that simple authentication or confirmation is needed in the payment transactions, but it is not necessary in the rebating transactions.

5   Discussion and Future Work

In this paper, we examined the concept of activity-based micro-pricing. Even though economic incentives could potentially be used in a persuasive way to create new business opportunities and resource conservation strategies in many areas, the cost of manual activity recognition prevents their widespread use. We proposed applying ubiquitous computing technologies to implement effective activity recognition, and examined ways of billing consumer activities in a wide variety of situations. In our vision, vendors can effectively charge for users' activities on a per-action basis. At the same time, wider choice is provided to the consumer, who can avoid unnecessary costs that are normally bundled in the price of various services. In order to bring the concept into a concrete shape, we introduced two different models and conducted a small user study. In below sections, we discuss design issues derived from the experiments and identify future directions towards sustainable behavior change.

5.1   Conveying Information for Deeper Understanding of Actions

The activity-based micro-pricing system induces a consumer to perform particular actions by controlling the level of psychological response applied to them (i.e., anxiety in the UbiPayment model and satisfaction in the UbiRebate model). However, a key issue is how to make the behavior changes achieved through such incentives sustainable. For example, if supermarkets start to charge a fee for plastic shopping bags, consumers will stop using them in order to avoid an economic loss, but no real change is achieved in attitudes or knowledge concerning the importance of reducing plastic bag consumption and resource consumption more generally. If the supermarkets start to provide the plastic bags for free again, consumers will go back to their original mode of behavior.

This story can be explained with the *elaboration likelihood model* (ELM) [16]. The ELM postulates that people processes information in two different ways: the central route and the peripheral route. The choice of route affects people's attitude, and the central route that provides high elaboration leads to stronger attitude formulation than the peripheral route. If people processes the messages presented from a persuader (e.g., how plastic bags reduction contributes to protect the environment) in the central route, they understand the meanings of the action consciously; and thus the behavior change will become more sustainable. On the other hand, economic incentives possibly lead people to use peripheral route, since the economic value is intuitive and attractive enough to change their behavior without consciousness.

In the user study, we discovered that the way in which we communicated the pricing system or billing policy to the "customers" of the cafe was probably insufficient. We visualized the billing policy as an action list, but a more detailed explanation (e.g., how each action is defined and recognized by the system) should probably have been available. Moreover, in order to persuade consumers rather than scare them away, the overall idea of activity-based pricing probably needs to be effectively communicated. The presentation method should draw the consumers' attention, and should be lightweight so that consumers can recognize and process the message through the central route. However, the route choice and the cognitive response to the message also changes depending on a consumer's motivation and ability.

5.2   Hybrid Incentive Design for Sustainable Behavior Change

One possible solution to the problem is adding playfulness to the system design. For example, Nakajima *et al.* proposed an "ambient lifestyle feedback system" to effect changes in our daily behavior [17]. They developed several kinds of pervasive applications while considering emotional engagement. For example, if a child does not brush their teeth in the correct manner and frequency, a virtually presented aquarium becomes dirty and its virtual fish fall sick. The virtual aquarium is installed in a bathroom, so pleasant and unpleasant feelings evoked by the application are shared among family members. Thus social pressure provides motivation for each individual to keep the aquarium clean through proper tooth brushing behavior. Providing accumulated feedbacks in the interaction loop allows a user to understand the importance of sustainable behavior change, and emotional engagement contributes to keep their attention to the service.

Affecting a consumer's normative belief is another approach. The *theory of planned behavior* (TPB) defines subjective norm as one of general constructs that guides a person's behavioral intention [18]. The subjective norm represents perceived social pressure, and it composes from normative beliefs that refer to behavioral expectation the person perceives in a social community. As aforementioned, the social pressure is expected to compensate the short comings of an economic incentive based approach. Shiraishi *et al.* developed an application called *EcoIsland*, which is a system persuading individuals to reduce CO_2 emissions [3]. In their work, economic incentives are implemented as EcoPoints, a virtual currency used in EcoIsland. Users can earn EcoPoints by reporting achieved ecological actions, and the points can be used to purchase items to decorate their virtual island in a way that visualizes each family's contributions to CO_2 reduction. In the application window, users can see other families' islands so that they can compete and improve behavior in a playful fashion.

Moreover, this social networking feature decreases dishonest behavior that is otherwise possible due to technical limitations. Since eco-friendly actions are often too complex to detect automatically, it is hard to verify users' self-reported data. The social aspect of EcoIsland allows users to monitor each other, providing peer pressure against cheating. In addition, sometimes economic incentives compel consumers to be under too much mental pressure, and services become to be uncomfortable to use in the end. Requiring too much attention also prevents consumers from enjoying the service. Thus social psychological incentives that appeals to consumers' values and ethics could relax the anxiety and reluctance.

A hybrid incentive approach could cover a wider range of users within an application. Each individual has their own preferences, and multiple types of incentives increase the chances of them developing interest in the application. For example, social psychological incentives work most effectively inside tightly linked groups or communities (e.g., families), while economic incentives operate on the individual consumer level. In a local community, users know each other and they collaborate to maximize their total benefit, instead of taking actions that are detrimental to each other. On the contrary, for bigger groups in which anonymous users are loosely coupled, economic incentives probably work better. This is because users start to make their decisions individually, and economic values become prioritized over other kinds of values. In this sense, the activity-based micro-incentive approach should thus be especially suitable for places and situations involving large numbers of general public. In addition, to avoid the tragedy of the commons with social psychological incentives, it is important to try to bring together a small community and offer a virtual space (e.g., islands in EcoIsland) to smoothen its communication and collaboration.

References

1. Hardin, G.: The tragedy of the commons, vol. 162, pp. 1243–1248 (1968)
2. Oinas-Kukkonen, H., Harjumaa, M.: Towards deeper understanding of persuasion in software and information systems. In: Proc. ACHI 2008, pp. 200–205. IEEE Computer Society, Los Alamitos (2008)
3. Shiraishi, M., Washio, Y., Takayama, C., Lehdonvirta, V., Kimura, H., Nakajima, T.: Using individual, social and economic persuasion techniques to reduce co2 emissions in a family setting. In: Proc. Persuasive 2009, pp. 1–8 (2009)
4. Mainwaring, S., March, W., Maurer, B.: From meiwaku to tokushita!: lessons for digital money design from japan. In: Proc. CHI 2008, pp. 21–24. ACM, New York (2008)
5. Lehdonvirta, V., Soma, H., Ito, H., Yamabe, T., Kimura, H., Nakajima, T.: Ubipay: minimizing transaction costs with smart mobile payments. In: Proc. Mobility Conference 2009. ACM, New York (2009)
6. Accenture Technology Labs: Pay-per-use, http://www.accenture.com/global/services/accenture_technology_labs/r_and_i/payperuseobject.htm
7. Yamabe, T., Lehdonvirta, V., Ito, H., Soma, H., Kimura, H., Nakajima, T.: Applying pervasive technologies to create economic incentives that alter consumer behavior. In: Proc. Ubicomp 2009, pp. 175–184. ACM, New York (2009)
8. Stamatis Karnouskos, F.F.: In: Mobile payment: A journey through existing procedures and standardization initiatives, vol. 6 (2004)
9. Mallat, N., Rossi, M., Tuunainen, V.K., Öörni, A.: An empirical investigation of mobile ticketing service adoption in public transportation. Personal and Ubiquitous Computing 12(1), 57–65 (2008)
10. Kawsar, F., Nakajima, T., Fujinami, K.: Deploy spontaneously: supporting endusers in building and enhancing a smart home. In: Proc. UbiComp 2008, pp. 282–291. ACM, New York (2008)
11. Fitton, D., Sundramoorthy, V., Kortuem, G., Brown, J., Efstratiou, C., Finney, J., Davies, N.: Exploring the design of pay-per-use objects in the construction domain. In: Roggen, D., Lombriser, C., Tröster, G., Kortuem, G., Havinga, P. (eds.) EuroSSC 2008. LNCS, vol. 5279, pp. 192–205. Springer, Heidelberg (2008)
12. Ariely, D.: Predictably Irrational: The Hidden Forces That Shape Our Decisions. Harpercollins (2008)
13. Motterlini, M.: Emotional Economy: In What Do We Waste Money in and Why. Paidos Iberica Ediciones S a (2008)
14. Kahneman, D., Tversky, A.: Prospect theory: An analysis of decision under risk. Econometrica 47(2), 263–291 (1979)
15. Tversky, A., Kahneman, D.: The framing of decisions and the psychology of choice. Science 211(4481), 453–458 (1981)
16. Petty, R.E., Cacioppo, J.T.: Communication and Persuasion: Central and Peripheral Routes to Attitude Change. Springer, New York (1986)
17. Nakajima, T., Lehdonvirta, V., Tokunaga, E., Kimura, H.: Reflecting human behavior to motivate desirable lifestyle. In: Proc. DIS 2008, pp. 405–414. ACM, New York (2008)
18. Ajzen, I.: The theory of planned behavior. Orginizational Behavior and Human Process 50, 179–211 (1991)

Enhancing Human Responses to Climate Change Risks through Simulated Flooding Experiences

Ruud Zaalberg and Cees Midden

Abstract. Delta areas are threatened by global climate change. The general aims of our research were (1) to increase our understanding of climate and flood risk perceptions and the factors that influence these judgments, and (2) to seek for interventions that can contribute to a realistic assessment by laypersons of long-term flooding risks. We argue that awareness of one's own vulnerability to future flooding and insights into the effectiveness of coping strategies is driven by direct flooding experiences. In the current research multimodal sensory stimulation by means of interactive 3D technology is used to simulate direct flooding experiences at the experiential or sensory level, thereby going beyond traditional persuasion attempts using fear-evoking images. Our results suggest that future communication efforts should not only use these new technologies to transfer knowledge about effective coping strategies and flooding risks, but should especially be directed towards residents living in flood prone areas, but who lack direct flooding experiences as their guiding principle.

Keywords: Climate Change, Flooding Experience, Affect, Appraisal, Coping, Persuasive Virtual Environment, Simulation, Presence.

1 Introduction

The rising awareness of the consequences of global climate risks for the local communities, is urging many European governments to warnindividuals and companies about their vulnerability to future flooding. An important question is whether these attempts to inform the general public about the local consequences of global warming truly influence the public opinion about these issues, and will eventually stimulate appropriate adaptive or even mitigating actions against the local consequences of global climate change. A recent opinion poll concluded in 2007 that 75 percent of the Dutch population is concerned about global warming. However, in the end, the effectiveness of information campaigns is solely determined by the extent to which human behavior is influenced.

The current research project was initiated to increase our understanding of climate and flood risk perceptions and to seek for interventions that can contribute to a realistic sense of urgency among laypersons of long-term flooding risks caused by global climate change. The first objective was to assess the significance of direct flooding experiences. The next objective was exploring ways to simulate direct flooding experiences as a means to enhance risk awareness and coping potential for residents who lack direct flooding experiences. A major part of the research consisted of the development of a multi-sensory interactive 3D simulation to mimic direct flooding experiences, evoking coping responses without the dangers present in real life.

T. Ploug, P. Hasle, H. Oinas-Kukkonen (Eds.): PERSUASIVE 2010, LNCS 6137, pp. 205–210, 2010.

2 The Role of Experiences

The first part of the research consisted of a survey study to identify factors capable of motivating individuals to effectively cope with future flooding. Based on a sample of 1,597 households living near the rivers Rhine and Meuse in the Netherlands we compared flood victims struck by high impact floods in 1993 and 1995 with non-victims in locations that were neither flooded nor evacuated in the past, although they were selected in the vicinity of the victim locations (see also Zaalberg, Midden, Meijnders & McCalley, 2009). The findings suggested that subjective experiences not only predict adaptive actions via cognitive appraisals, but form an independent and indispensable part of the mediating process, explaining mean differences in adaptation between flood victims and non-victims. Clearly, both the experiential processing mode based on concrete experiences and the analytical processing mode based on reasoning play a role in decisions how to deal with future risks.

Against this background the idea emerged of achieving behavioral change by simulating real 'disaster experience', thereby going beyond traditional persuasion attempts such as the use of fear evoking images. High-end simulations in a Virtual Environment (VE) could provide participants with a simulated flood experience at the experiential or sensory level. Ideally, flood simulations should make an attempt not only to simulate physical exposure to real flooding, but preferably also to include the emotional component of real flooding experiences.

The next step in our research was to explore the extent to which the immersive quality of different presentation modes influences coping responses to virtual floods. New immersive media technologies such as 3D visualizations (i.e., immersion via media form; Lessiter, Freeman, Keogh, and Davidoff, 2001) might support the persuasive quality of future information campaigns communicating real-world flooding risks. Lab research was conducted to investigate the role of multimodal sensory stimulation by means of interactive 3D technology to simulate real flooding experiences, evoking adequate coping responses. We exposed participants to a simulated dike breach and flooding of their virtual residence positioned in a typical low-lying Dutch polder landscape. The central question was whether multimodal sensory stimulation by means of an interactive 3D simulation facilitated participants coping responses compared to non-interactive 2D simulations. In the next section the theoretical framework will be briefly explained.

2.1 Simulating Real Flooding Experiences: What Should Be Evoked?

Based on the risk analysis literature four interrelated components of disaster experience could be distinguished. First, Dooley, Catalano, Mishra, and Serxner (1992) focused on the *emotional* component of disaster experience, such as being scared. Second, Sattler et al. (2000) assessed also the amount of property damage caused by Hurricane Hugo; i.e., the *material* component of disaster experience. Third, Weinstein's (1989) review referred to physical injuries resulting from disasters; i.e., the *physical* component of disaster experience. Additionally, Zaalberg, Midden, Meijnders and McCalley (2009) assessed the amount of social support residents had received during a threatening flood, i.e., the *social* component of disaster experience.

As our survey results indicated actual flood victims seemed more motivated to take adaptive actions in the future compared to equally threatened non-victims. The psychological processes explaining this influence were that victims' intensified social and emotional experiences increased victims' perceived vulnerability to future flooding, and increased victims' perception of the effectiveness of adaptive actions to deal with these future threats. Three theoretical concepts were identified as intervening processes: cognitive appraisals (Rogers & Prentice-Dunn, 1997), affective appraisals (e.g. Loewenstein et al., 2001), and presence (e.g. Lessiter et al., 2001).

2.2 Research Set-Up and Hypotheses

In a lab experiment we manipulated the extent to which participants were immersed in a VE by using three different presentation modes. One condition consisted of multimodal sensory stimulation by means of an interactive 3D simulation on a 72-inch translucent screen. The remaining conditions consisted of non-interactive 2D simulations. In these conditions participants watched the flood simulation on a 15-inch laptop via film or slides without auditory support. Participants were randomly assigned to one of the three conditions.

In a virtual Dutch polder landscape, participants were exposed to a serious flooding of their virtual residence. The following hypotheses were derived. First, information search and coping intentions are both strengthened in the interactive 3D simulation compared to the non-interactive 2D simulations. Second, presence and affective appraisal are stronger in the interactive 3D simulation compared to the non-interactive 2D simulations. Third, the experimental effects on information search and coping intentions are mediated or explained by presence and affective appraisal. Fourth, the content of the simulation (i.e., the story or media content unfolding in the VE) was kept equal across experimental conditions.

2.3 Method

Participants first watched a 5-minute introduction movie to introduce participants to the cause and consequences of global climate change, and the specific events in the simulation. Participants were then asked to portray themselves as residents living in a low-lying polder landscape at the bottom of the dike and close to a river. Participants were told that they had to go for a walk through the VE once the simulation started. Heavy rainfall was simulated visually and was audio supported with a real-life recording of rain falling on grass and trees. Participants first climbed the stairs towards the top of the dike, where they had the opportunity to watch the river to rise slowly. A clear contrast was visible between the water rising on the outer side and the low-lying polder on the inner side of the dike. After approximately 200 m, participants reached a ditch located behind and at the bottom of a dike. Piping and dike breach were simulated. The fast-flowing water was audio-supported with a recording of real waterfall sounds. Moreover, the sound was localized in such a way that when participants looked around in the VE, the sound source shifted accordingly from one speaker box to the other. The magnitude of the sound decreased when participants moved away from the sound source, which gave the participants an extra sensory 3D cue in the VE, making it even more realistic and persuasive.

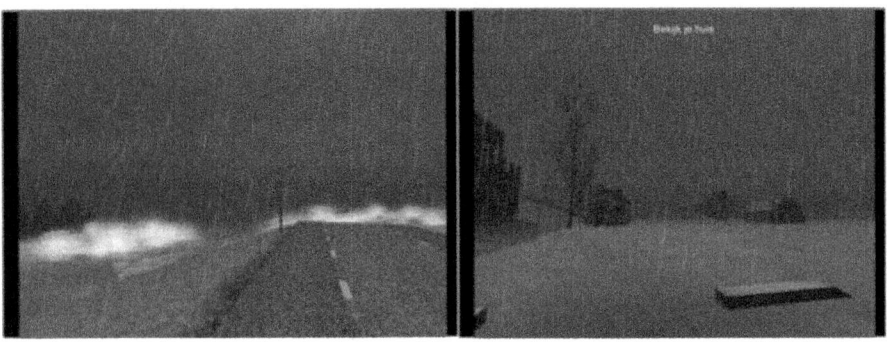

After the dike breached, participants walked back to watch the consequences for their residence. The maximum water level (approximately 300 cm) had flooded the first floor of their residence. At this point the simulation ended. Once seated behind the laptop, participants were asked to imagine a situation in which they would stay in their virtual residence while the dike was about to breach. A post-simulation task gave the participants the opportunity to search for information related to different coping responses to protect their health and belongings in the threatening situation of an imminent dike breach. Participants also answered questions about their coping intentions, cognitive appraisals, affective appraisals, and presence.

For participants in the film and slide conditions the simulation was shown on the 15-inch laptop in full-color without supportive audio recordings. The film simulation lasted for 288 seconds. The slide show consisted of 26 slides of 11 seconds each. Information search was measured using a so-called information board holding pieces of information that users can choose to read. Coping intentions were assessed with seven items, ranging from likelihood is very low (0) to likelihood is very high (4). Preventive evacuation (e.g., evacuation of family members) and preventive actions (e.g., the use of water pumps) were distinguished. A single item about buying flood insurance to protect one's belongings in the real world was added to this list.

Cognitive appraisals, such as perceived vulnerability and perceived consequences, were assessed by means of rating scales in relation to 3 hypothetical flood outcomes.

Affective appraisals were assessed with four rating scales, ranging from not at all (0) to very much (4). For example, the extent to which participants expected to feel anxious about their imaginary belongings being damaged.

Presence during the simulation was assessed with the Igroup Presence Questionnaire (IPQ; e.g. Schubert et al., 2001).

2.4 Results

A series of multiple regression analyses were used to test the effects of presentation mode on information search and coping intentions (Hypothesis 1). Also the indirect, mediated effects via affective appraisals and presence were tested (Hypothesis 2 & 3).

Controlled for age differences in information processing, reading time related to preventive evacuation was longer for participants in the 3D condition (M_a= 46.7 s) compared to participants reading time in the film and slides conditions (M= 35.1 s;

contrast effect hierarchical modeling: $R^2 = .26$, $p < .01$). No (mediating) effects were found for reading time related to preventive actions.

Controlled for differences in the perceived water level at the end of the simulation, participants in the 3D condition were more willing to evacuate from the virtual polder landscape compared to participants in the slides condition, but not to participants in the film condition (($M_{adj} = 3.6$) compared to participants in the slides condition ($M_{adj} = 3.3$), but not to participants in the film condition ($M_{adj} = 3.6$; contrast effect hierarchical modeling $R^2 = .23$, $p < .01$) . This significant contrast was reduced when we controlled for subjective time perception (indicator of presence). Participants in the 3D condition were more willing to evacuate from the virtual polder landscape than participants in the slides condition, because they experienced a greater sense of presence during the simulation (M=2.5 vs. M=1.6; hierarchical modeling $R^2 = .36$, $p < .01$)). Participants' motivation to take *preventive* actions in the 3D condition was similar to participants' motivation in the film and slides conditions ($M_{adj} = 2.0$ vs. $M_{adj} = 1.8/1.8$; $R^2_2 = .01$, ns).

Controlled for differences in the perceived water level at the end of the simulation, participants in the 3D condition were more willing to buy flood insurance compared to participants in the film condition, but no more willing than participants in the slides condition (M=1.6 vs. M=0.7 vs. M=1.0; R2=.16, $p < .05$). This contrast effect reduced when we controlled for spatial presence.(β= -.38 vs. -.29; R2=.24, $p < .01$).suggesting that participants in the 3D condition were more willing to buy flood insurance than participants in the film condition, because they experienced a greater sense of presence during the simulation.

In contrast to our predictions, affective appraisals were not influenced by presentation mode. As predicted, no effects for presentation mode were found for cognitive appraisals. In sum, both affective and cognitive appraisals did not act as mediating processes in the relationship between presentation mode versus information search and coping intentions.

3 Conclusions and Discussion

Multimodal sensory stimulation by means of interactive 3D technology was used to simulate real flooding experiences. An interactive 3D simulation increased not only the motivation to evacuate from the threatened virtual polder, but also increased the motivation to buy flood insurance in the real world. Human intentions changed in response to simulated flooding provided that humans felt 'physically' present in the VE. We believe this to be an essential feature of future information campaigns when aiming at changing people's perceptions and coping responses in response to real-world flooding risks. Awareness of one's own vulnerability to future flooding due to climate change, and insights into the effectiveness of coping actions to deal with these new risks are driven by direct flooding experiences. Future research should test the effects of technology-induced emotions in a VE on threat and coping appraisals as intervening variables predicting flood protection intentions. Future communication efforts should not only use these new technologies to transfer knowledge on effective coping strategies and flooding risks, but should especially be directed towards the millions of residents living in flood-prone areas and who lack direct flooding experience as their guiding principle.

The present research delivers practical insights for developing intervention instruments to motivate the large numbers of residents who live in flood-prone areas in the Netherlands, to protect themselves effectively in case of an imminent flood.

References

Intergovernmental Panel on Climate Change, Climate change 2007: Synthesis report (Fourth Assessment Report), Valencia, Spain (November 2007)

Lessiter, J., Freeman, J., Keogh, E., Davidoff, J.: A cross-media presence questionnaire: The ITC-Sense of Presence Inventory. Presence 10, 282–297 (2001)

Loewenstein, G.F., Weber, E.U., Hsee, C.K., Welch, N.: Risk as feelings. Psychological Bulletin 127, 267–286 (2001)

Rogers, R.W., Prentice-Dunn, S.: Protection motivation theory. In: Gochman, D.S. (ed.) Handbook of health behavior research 1: Personal and social determinants, pp. 113–132. Plenum Press, New York (1997)

Sattler, D.N., Kaiser, C.F., Hittner, J.B.: Disaster preparedness: Relationships among prior experience, personal characteristics, and distress. Journal of Applied Social Psychology 30, 1396–1420 (2000)

Schubert, T., Friedmann, F., Regenbrecht, H.: The experience of presence: Factor analytic insights. Presence: Teleoperators and Virtual Environments 10, 266–281 (2001)

Zaalberg, R., Midden, C.J.H., Meijnders, A.L., McCalley, L.T.: Prevention, adaptation, and threat denial: Flooding experiences in the Netherlands. Risk Analysis 29, 1759–1778 (2009)

Pitfalls in Persuasion: How Do Users Experience Persuasive Techniques in a Web Service?

Katarina Segerståhl[1], Tanja Kotro[2], and Kaisa Väänänen-Vainio-Mattila[3]

[1] University of Oulu, Department of Information Processing Science,
P.O. Box 3000, FI-90014 Oulu, Finland
katarina.segerstahl@oulu.fi
[2] National Consumer Research Center, P.O. Box 5, FI-00531 Helsinki, Finland
tanja.kotro@ncrc.fi
[3] Tampere University of Technology, Unit of Human Centered Technology
P.O. Box 589, FI-33101 Tampere, Finland
kaisa.vaananen-vainio-mattila@tut.fi

Abstract. Persuasive technologies are designed by utilizing a variety of interactive techniques that are believed to promote target behaviors. This paper describes a field study in which the aim was to discover possible pitfalls of persuasion, i.e., situations in which persuasive techniques do not function as expected. The study investigated persuasive functionality of a web service targeting weight loss. A qualitative online questionnaire was distributed through the web service and a total of 291 responses were extracted for interpretative analysis. The Persuasive Systems Design model (PSD) was used for supporting systematic analysis of persuasive functionality. Pitfalls were identified through situations that evoked negative user experiences. The primary pitfalls discovered were associated with manual logging of eating and exercise behaviors, appropriateness of suggestions and source credibility issues related to social facilitation. These pitfalls, when recognized, can be addressed in design by applying functional and facilitative persuasive techniques in meaningful combinations.

Keywords: User experience, web service, qualitative field study, web-based health promotion, Persuasive Systems Design Model.

1 Introduction

Persuasion is a social influence mechanism or a form of interaction that aims at changing the way people think or behave. When the persuading agent is, instead of a person a software system, it is called persuasive technology [2]. Oinas-Kukkonen and Harjumaa [8,9] have further defined persuasive technology as "computerized software or information systems designed to reinforce, change or shape attitudes or behaviors or both without using coercion or deception". Persuasive technologies have been applied for example in the domains of health and wellness promotion and increasing environmental awareness [4,13,11,1]. Persuasion is a tricky and sensitive process and there are certain strategies and techniques that can be applied to improve the chances for success [2]. However, there is little research on how these strategies – when implemented as software functionalities – work in interactive situations.

T. Ploug, P. Hasle, H. Oinas-Kukkonen (Eds.): PERSUASIVE 2010, LNCS 6137, pp. 211–222, 2010.

This study was carried out in order to identify and analyze possible pitfalls of persuasive functionalities as identified based on reported user experiences. Our research question was: *What are the pitfalls of persuasion; when and why persuasive techniques evoke negative user experiences?*

We conducted a qualitative field study where we collected data from users of a persuasive web service targeting weight loss. In the next section we will discuss the conceptual background of our study, then we will describe our method and the web service under investigation. After this we will present our findings and continue with analysis focusing on pitfalls associated with persuasive functionality. Finally, we will discuss our findings in light of practical implications.

2 Background

While many empirical studies on persuasive technologies are successful in constructing persuasive applications and evaluating their effect, few provide an in-depth understanding of the mechanisms by which persuasive technologies influence. Reviews on the effectiveness of digital interventions show that even though they can in some cases promote positive behavioral outcomes, they are in many cases still inefficient and sustainability of their impact has not been verified. [7,10] A more detailed understanding of computer-mediated persuasion needs to be obtained in order to design effective applications. A study by Harjumaa et al [4] shows that persuasive techniques are often applied in combinations when incorporated as actual software functionalities. Their effects are interdependent and closely tied to the context of persuasion. We take this understanding further by investigating how different techniques are experienced by users and what kinds of pitfalls are associated with them. We also analyze further the functional relationships between persuasive techniques.

In this study, we used the *Persuasive Systems Design model* (PSD) [9] to identify and analyze persuasive techniques that were applied via distinct software functionalities. The model will be briefly introduced in the next section on methodology. We investigated the effect of techniques by focusing on reported user experiences. Quite understandably, and as claimed in prior work, positive user experience is an essential antecedent of effective computerized persuasion [12]. *User experience* is a concept that defines the user's reactions and feelings, which arise from interactions with a system in certain situations or use contexts [3]. The aim of interaction design is to support positive user experience by providing features or qualities in the system supporting both pragmatic (goal-oriented) and hedonic (pleasure-oriented) experiences [5]. With persuasive systems, this aim should be integrated with the aim of promoting behavior change.

3 Method and Approach

We conducted a qualitative case study with a web service promoting weight loss. Data was collected from real users of the service with an online questionnaire and analyzed using interpretative methods. This study investigated the Pudottajat web service (www.pudottajat.fi), designed to support weight loss by promoting healthy nutrition and exercise. The service is free of charge and incorporates a variety of persuasive functionalities. Primary content in the service is based on informative tidbits about ways to loose weight and improve everyday behaviors as well as research-based articles about the benefits of target behaviors. The service also contains a recipe database to support a healthy, low-calorie diet. It includes calculators and tests as well as tools for food and exercise journaling. The service facilitates social interaction and support by hosting blogs and discussion forums and through functionality that enables comparing one's progress with others.

Data was collected with an online questionnaire that was distributed through the website's news-section and the weekly newsletter subscribed to by registered users. The questionnaire was designed to collect basic information such as users' age and gender and how long they have been using the service and how frequently they use it. An open-ended question was used for collecting brief narratives about users' goals regarding weight loss/management. Information about usage contexts and users' experiences with the service and its functionality were collected with the following open-ended questions: *"Describe the situation in which you last used the service:"*; *"What was your experience of that situation?"* The following questions were posed to collect data specifically on the problematic user experiences that might correlate with "pitfalls" in persuasion: *"Which features in the service do not work in your case? Why?"*; *"What annoys you about the service? Why?"*

A total of 435 users responded to the questionnaire over the three weeks that it was online. After removing duplicates and extracting responses in which open-ended fields were filled in, we ended up with a total of 291 informants. Majority of informants were women (95%). Most of them had used the service for 3-6 (27%) or 6-12 (28%) months. However, there were also some, who had just started using the service within the past couple of months (29%) and some, who had used it for over a year (16%). 24% reported using the service monthly, 56% used it weekly, while 11% used it on a daily basis and 9% less than monthly. We found that 46% of respondents were actively involved in the process of behavior change, stating that they are currently making choices that will take them closer to their goal. 22% of participants reported that they are determined to achieve their goal, but not in the near future. 33% stated that they would achieve their goal in the near future. 15% reported having relapsed in an earlier attempt to reach their goal. Only 6% reported having reached their goal and having maintained it for over 3 months.

To support the analysis procedure, we used the Persuasive Systems Design Model (PSD) that provides a conceptual framework for identifying and analyzing persuasive techniques within software functionality [9]. The PSD encourages understanding the context of persuasion in investigating persuasive functionalities. The context of persuasion includes understanding the *intent, situation* and the *strategy* of persuasion. The model also provides a scheme including a total of 28 persuasive techniques. These techniques are grouped under four categories based on whether they support the primary task, i.e., the desired target behavior (primary task support) for example by breaking down the behavior to smaller steps; the dialogue between the user and the system (dialogue support) for example by incorporating verbal feedback; or facilitation of social influences (social support), such as providing means to interact or compete with peers. The PSD scheme was used for coding techniques associated with use situations and user experiences reported by informants. (See [9] for more details about the PSD model.)

Data was extracted to a spreadsheet that supported assigning persuasive techniques (based on the PSD) for each distinct user response. Responses were also color-coded based on their experiential valence. Based on the analysis we discovered persuasive techniques that were in this case specifically vulnerable, i.e. could be recognized as "pitfalls" in persuasion. These were identified through situations that were coded as evoking moderate or strong negative experiences.

4   Findings

In this section, we present our findings with respect to pitfalls that were referred to most frequently in users' statements. These pitfalls we recognized are associated with three core techniques in computer-mediated persuasion, as defined in the PSD model [9]: *self-monitoring*, *suggestion* and *social facilitation*.

4.1   Self-monitoring

The goal behind self-monitoring is to offer the user system functionality that helps logging and keeping track of the user's performance or status and make behavioral patterns and their outcomes visible. This is believed to increase users' awareness of their behaviors and support them in achieving their personal goals. [2,9].

In Pudottajat.fi self-monitoring is supported with a food and training diary. The user can manually log, on a daily basis, his/her intake of calories (amount and type of food consumed), as well as the calories burned by exercising (estimates of calories burned). The user calculates the calorie estimates, by using external calorie counters referred to in the service. The service provides links to sites where calories of certain foods can be calculated. The user also independently estimates his/her training amount and calories burned. The service graphs the user's progress over time in achieving their predefined weigh-loss goals.

Many users mentioned the food and exercise diary as one of the most important features of the system. This implies that users' expectations regarding this functionality were high. However, several users commented that the food and exercise diary (coupled with manual calorie counting) did not support their goals as expected.

In the data, there were frequent user statements of unsatisfying user experiences with self-monitoring. Several users stated that the calorie counter is too complicated to use, requires filling in too much small details, or demands too regular recording of information. *"One must search calories (food and training) from different sites and after that, calculate total sums. I do not have time for this, nor do I want to do it. This is why I have started to mainly use another service."* (#262) *"I feel that the diaries are complicated to fill in here. I write on paper what I eat."* (#234).

Many users also commented that using the calorie counter takes too much time or attention, or they seemed reluctant to make changes in their behavior. *"Weigh-loss diary does not work. It's too tedious to count the daily calorie intake and I don't remember to write down what I have consumed. It takes too much time."* (#345) The lack of time was also reflected against the user's life situation. For example, small kids, daily rhythm or eating lunch at work were mentioned as reasons for not using the logging functionality: *"Training and calorie counters [do not work for me]. In my work I have to eat certain foods, and I don't have time to follow a certain training program"* (#185). Some users also blamed themselves for not using the food diary: *"I guess I'm just too lazy to keep the food diary..."* (#190) Counting calories was also mentioned as being boring, and thus alternative ways to control calorie intake were used: *"Counting calories is so boring. I just don't count them but instead I use the recommended food portions and eat often enough."* (#76).

Effective self-monitoring was in this case problematic mainly because the user could not (or it was experienced too tedious to) find information of the exact calorie amounts. *"Exact information of calorie amounts cannot be found but everything has to be found through extra effort. As a mother of small children, counting and marking down food calories is too much, because I have to have time for household chores. I simply don't have time to look for calorie amounts for each oat flake or food I have prepared."* (#68).

For some users, the whole idea of counting calories was new and was felt foreign: *"Counting calories [is irritating]. I have never needed to do that. It's a weird situation for me"* (#438) One user commented the counter reaction of seeing one's development, if one fails: *"I'm afraid that counters are the reason why I might be turned away from the service in case of a relapse. I don't want to see when and what kind of relapses I have had. It's really dismotivating to see negative development."* (#45).

In summary, self-monitoring with the food and exercise diary was experienced as being too complex: requires too frequent (and accurate) usage; requires fetching information (calorie amounts) from various sources; requires too much input and complex calculations (takes time and is cognitively demanding); is tedious and boring. Many users also described contextual hindrances for using the service feature: busy family life, eating at work, of being too "lazy" for such accurate recording of one's activity.

4.2 Suggestion

The principle of suggestion means that systems should offer fitting suggestions to have more persuasive power. This means, as Oinas-Kukkonen and Harjumaa [9] put it, that "systems should suggest users to carry out behaviors during the system use process" and applications for healthier eating habits can "suggest that children eat fruits instead of candy at snack time".

There are three main functions in the Pudottajat service related to the principle of suggestion. These are low-calorie recipes ("Calorie Kitchen"), including suggestions for cooking healthier food, and research related articles on loosing weight. Suggestions are also delivered in the form of tips for exercise, such as how to avoid loosing one's interest in regular exercising.

Based on our data, most of the suggestions in the Pudottajat service fit the main intent of the service, which is to support the user in loosing weight. Yet, some of the suggestive advertisements[1] appearing in the service where experienced by the users as

---

[1] Even though advertisements were not meant as suggestive system functionality, they were interpreted as suggestive by the respondents and were a salient part of the user experience.

unfitting regarding the intent of the service. For example, one of the respondents reported that s/he's annoyed with *"Advertisements that say you don't have to do anything in order to loose weight. I wonder why they even accept these kinds of advertisements???"* (#234). Advertisements linked to the system have suggestive elements in them. These are in this case experienced as intrusive. It is important that suggestions are linked to the expertise of the service provider, not to a compromised third party. Also some users experienced some service based suggestions to be misleading from the perspective of the aim to loose weight: *"with the daily amount of calories the calorie counter suggests I would gain A LOT of weight"* (#435).

What we found interesting was that in this case, most of the problems related to the unfitting suggestions refer to the imbalance between suggestions offered by the system and the actual context of using the service. For example, when the system suggests healthy food recipes, the user might ignore them simply because of the lack of resources to cook one's own food that may originate from everyday practices of work. Other causes for this imbalance may result from personal choice or otherwise restricted food diet. Everyday practices of work means for example eating out: *"I work in a kitchen and I eat the food that is prepared there"* (#175). Personal choice often means personal food diet by choice *"I am a vegetarian, therefore meat-related issues do not suit me"* (#191). *"Recipes do not work for me, since I aim at a zero-tolerance towards white wheat"* (#277). Recipes as suggestions might also not fit because of physical restrictions such as high blood sugar. *"Everything is not suitable for everybody, as these instructions suggest. For example, I have high blood pressure."* (#188).

We found that suggestions may have more persuasive power when they offer multiple solutions to the user's current need of information and need to change one's habits. *"Counting calories [doesn't suit me]. I just don't care to think about that kind of stuff. It would be much better if I could fill in my own estimate of daily eating."* (#462).

Also, a suggestion is experienced as useful if it is linked to current time of the year, for example tidbits that were linked to avoiding unhealthy food during the festive season were experienced motivating and useful: *"Up-to-date advice support good choices. Christmas goodies frighten already."* (#188) Therefore suggestions do not work if they are not up-to-date: for example seasonal suggestions that are not removed from the system (for example tips to avoid gaining weight during Christmas in summer time). *"In the middle of summer there can be an article in the main page about avoiding gaining weight during Christmas"* (#230).

Most of the unfitting tips for exercise are either linked to the physical restrictions (chronic or temporary diseases) of the user or regional differences: *"Exercise [doesn't suit for me] since I have many obstacles because of injuries."* (#134), *"Instructions for exercise, where one needs to use the knees (other knee is a prosthetic knee)."* (#403) *"First of all, I cannot exercise at the gym, or do any kind of endurance training, and I have to satisfy with less [exercise] in a positive spirit."* (#297). Regional differences mean that users of a web based service live in very different areas where local services are not in line with the web service content. For example, if suggestions require the use of urban fitness facilities, they might not fit users who live in the countryside: *"Exercise guidance does not fit for the countryside"* (#242).

4.3 Social Facilitation

The system includes functionality such as blogs and discussion forums to leverage social facilitation and peer-support. These functionalities apply namely the principles of social learning or social facilitation, which are fairly similar. Social learning means that "a person will be more motivated to perform a target behavior is s/he can use a system to observe others performing the behavior", whereas social facilitation proposes that "system users will have a greater motivation to perform the target behavior if they discern via the system that other's are performing the behavior along with them." [9].

We found that social support, if delivered via blogs and discussion forums is very sensitive to pitfalls. A number of respondents reacted to them as being "uninformative" or "lay-opinions" and thus not credible. *"People's conversations are based on opinions and they don't have scientific background. They can't be trusted"*. [#]; *"I don't usually bother to follow conversations. There is often not much substance there."* (#107); *"Users' own stories [are annoying]. The web is full of people's own experiences and I don't want to read those."* (#212); *"Conversations are not the nicest as they don't contain or provide "factual" information"* (#217); *"It's disappointing to realize that when you follow an interesting topic, it turns out that it's actually discussion about someone's unique experience"* (#162); *"I want to read about things that have actually been studied, I'm not that much interested in others' stories, even though I do browse them occasionally for random tips..."* (#227).

Many would also avoid discussion forums and blogs due to their time-consuming nature. Blogs and discussions were therefore perceived as rather a form of consuming time than relevant in terms of actual target behaviors: *"Discussions [do not work for me], I don't really have the time or the motivation to follow them"* (#240); *"Discussions as such are ok, but as I have limited time, I don't need others' experiences as much as I need factual information..."* (103#).

Regarding peer-support, users often felt as if other users of the service would not share the same goals with them or they had difficulty finding other users similar to them. This issue with similarity resulted to inflation of peer-support and indicates that it is only effective, when the person can relate to the community: *"I am not interested in peer groups. If I was substantially more overweight, I think the groups would be more helpful"* (#296). This contrast to peers would in some cases also raise irritation and clearly negatively toned reactions: *"Other people's weight losses [are annoying] and generally I don't bother to read discussion forums!"* (#146).

5 Analysis and Discussion

In this section we will discuss the role of persuasive techniques and principles (identified with the PSD model) and the role of other aspects, such as convenience of use and emotional preconditions that influenced users' experiences of persuasive functionality. This analysis will contribute to persuasive systems design by distinguishing functional and facilitative principles in persuasion and by emphasizing the importance of experiential system qualities such as enjoyability and fluency of interactions.

5.1 Functional and Facilitative Principles

Our findings suggest that there are different *types* of principles in computer-mediated persuasion. Some of the principles are clearly "functional", some are more "facilitative" by nature. In the following, we will elaborate this argument further by analyzing the functional techniques of self-monitoring, suggestion and social facilitation and explaining how these principles benefit from other more facilitative principles in order to work in a desired manner.

Self-monitoring. In our study, positive user experience associated with self-monitoring was clearly hindered by the complexity of continuously filling in calorie and training diaries. Self-monitoring can be seen as consisting of two iterative phases; *reporting* (logging information) and *interpretation* (cognitive processing of this information). In this case reporting was considered as the main hindrance to effective self-monitoring. The way reporting was carried out with the service (manually and requiring fetching external information) was excessively burdensome. The main practical challenge with self-monitoring in the studied service was the need for users to find the exact calorie amounts via external calorie calculators. Some users expressed strong frustration in having to do this tedious task. This can be seen as a usability problem, as the task required too many steps and cognitive effort from the users. As a consequence, the overall positive user experience of self-monitoring was hindered and thus this persuasive technique failed.

Self-monitoring, and in this case specifically the logging, could be facilitated by *tunneling*, i.e. guiding the user through a process e.g. by offering calorie information or estimates directly within the same service. Another potential solution would be to support self-reporting with mobile solutions that could be used in automating the logging process. However, the question remains: how easy and invisible does logging actually have to be in order to engage users over long term? Logging could also be supported with *reduction*, i.e., reducing this complex behavior into simpler steps. This could be implemented with auto fill suggestions to diaries based on previous user behavior and providing users with templates that they can use for logging. Users also mentioned that self-monitoring took too much time or effort. They sometimes blamed themselves for being "lazy" or expressed that filling in calorie details was "boring". Giving the user *virtual rewards* for logging could possibly compensate this situation. Users could be gradually rewarded when they have filled in the diary to a certain extent. According to Hassenzahl and Tractinsky's [5] model of hedonic product qualities, such, game-like features could support a more positive user experience. Delightful user experience could be further advanced by supporting users' curiosity by offering them simulations of how weigh loss may progress with various amounts of calorie intake and training.

In summary, self-monitoring and in particular self-reporting was experienced as *burdensome* and this hindered its effective use. In the case of self-monitoring the role of facilitating principles is mainly in promoting a more positive user experience and micro-persuasion, i.e., using other persuasive techniques to make it easier and more tempting to use persuasive functionalities which are beneficial for primary behavior change. Also, employing mobile data collection technologies may be considered to support a more fluent reporting process. A mobile version of the service could also be used to support the interpretation phase of the reported data, and thus provide means for the whole self-monitoring experience.

Suggestion. Based on our findings, it can be noted that the principle of suggestion benefits significantly from two other, facilitative principles. According to our analysis, most of the examples suffered from lack of *tailoring* the suggestion to the use contexts. The suggestions fit the intent of the service but they do not often fit the use context of the service because of personal and local differences of service users. Tailoring is needed to fit suggestions with the interactive situation and users' differing contexts. This means that the actual use context and routines of everyday life should be recognized and suggestions, at their best, are tailored to match these. Also personal differences, such as one's physical condition and constraints should be realized when tailoring suggestions. Also, if suggestions are not up-dated or they do not fit into the context of the calendar year, they are not effective and can be experienced as irritating, as was found in our empirical examples.

Coherence of information provided by the service was found to be crucial. Therefore, all the material in the services should aim at the same conclusion (in this case loosing weight by actively eating healthier and exercising) if suggestions are to have persuasive effects. Advertisements cannot therefore suggest "miracle diets" but they should be built on the expertise on loosing weight.

Social facilitation. Social facilitation in this case did not turn out as powerful as might have been expected. The reason why users felt that discussions and blogs would not be useful for them and they could not relate to the other users partially resulted from lack of *tailoring*. If socially constructed content was tailored in the sense, that it was prioritized and presented to users based on their profiles, goals and interests, they may more easily find others with similar agendas in the service. For example, by connecting users based on their goals may increase the likelihood of discussion and blog content to be relevant for the user.

Many users commented that they're not interested in discussions and blogs because they're based on others' individual opinions and thus are not to be trusted. There were also users, who would just not be interested in other peoples' endeavors or stories and some even expressed them to be irritating. It appears that social facilitation is closely coupled with expertise and credibility issues. Users don't consider socially constructed content as credible, when they do not know whether the source is trustworthy. In social situations, an individual's reputation is something that strengthens the impact of their message. Thus, incorporating reputation-based functionality, such as collaborative filtering of people's suggestions and stories may be helpful in promoting social facilitation.

Another issue was that discussion and blog functionality was perceived as difficult to navigate and use. Quite understandably this may become a significant hindrance to effective persuasive interactions. It was also reported that many of the blogs and discussions were outdated and thus not current and fitting with the users' temporal context a similar issue to what was observed with suggestions. Blogs and discussion forums in this case suffered from insufficient *tailoring* and *trustworthiness* or expert sourcing, as well as lack of *currentness*.

In sum, our analysis suggests that functional principles often need facilitative principles, such as tailoring to work appropriately. *Facilitating principles define, how a functional principle can be applied.* Based on the analysis, we suggest that in addition to recognizing the different characteristics of persuasive principles, it is crucial to understand how they function when coupled. Another important issue is in supporting positive user experience. Hedonic elements in persuasive systems may facilitate commitment and engaging interactions – which in turn may support persuasion. In addition, general usability issues and experiential aspects of interactions appeared as highly relevant in determining the effectiveness of persuasive functionalities. These issues should not be tackled in isolation when studying and designing persuasive functionality, but considered as essential to effective behavior change.

5.2 Overcoming Pitfalls

Our study shows that there are situations in which persuasive functionalities may be perceived as negative or even discouraging. Reactions can be justified either rationally or emotionally. For example, a suboptimal user experience with discussion forums could result from the perception that forums do not contain enough factual information (rational justification) or from annoyment with others' individual stories (emotional justification). These situations are a challenge for persuasive design, and it is therefore important to recognize what causes them.

In our analysis of self-monitoring, suggestion and social facilitation, we identified three distinct types of situations that evoked frustration with service functionality that could not directly be explained with the PSD. First, frustration was experienced when the content of the service was outdated and not regularly renewed. To reduce experienced frustration, the service should contain material that is linked to the time of the year and that is renewed continuously: otherwise the service is experienced as being passive. In persuasion, the service needs to be dynamic and adapt to the behavior change process. New content provision is experienced as stimulating. We refer to this as content *currentness* and suggest it as an important characteristic or technique to consider in persuasive design.

Second, frustration and negative experience occur when incorporating persuasive interactions (such as facilitating self-monitoring) requires a high degree of cognitive effort from the user. Negative experiences arouse from the experienced lack of time and willingness to devote to the service when using it was experienced as burdensome. It is important to ensure that using the persuasive system does not induce excess burden on users. To reduce the negative experience of a time-consuming service, the concrete tasks required from the user should be simple and easy to use. Therefore we suggest that cognitive effort associated with tasks central to the persuasive process (such as self-reporting) should be minimized and can be reduced with micropersuasive techniques, such as *reduction*, or with mobile support for more automated logging which in this case may contribute to better usability or fluency of interactions.

Third, frustration appeared when the users became aware of negative patterns in their behavior or relapses in their progress, and the system in a way reminded them of this. A system needs to adapt to changing situations and the true state of things but the fact that the persuasive system reminded users about negative development was sometimes experienced as pinpointing failure. This could be approached by a way of hiding unpleasant information from the users automatically or at the user's request. Also, the system could provide *encouragement* or consolation to the users, for them to feel motivated to continue using the service.

We suggest that applying functional principles together with facilitative principles may notably improve the chances of successful computer-mediated persuasion. Even though most users were on the path to healthier behaviors, few reported having achieved their goals. The service was perceived as very useful by 16% of participants and quite useful by 52%, which is quite an encouraging result despite the problems that may be associated with its use. Perhaps addressing the pitfalls in persuasion may help in supporting the remaining 32%, who were either undecided or did not think the service was useful for them. Despite our findings it is important to note that Pudottajat is one of the most popular web services for supporting weight loss in Finland. The core of its success is in its accessibility (being free of charge), broad information content with health, exercise and nutrition advice and newsletters. These were reported by users as the most useful and motivating qualities of the service.

Yet, the greatest challenge appears when a user perceives that s/he does not possess the initial will power or self-discipline to carry out with the behavior change process. Users need help in stepping on the path to the behavior change and the ways to encourage users during various phases of this path need more attention in the future.

6 Conclusions

Positive user experience is a key target in the design of interactive systems. It is also an essential prerequisite of successful persuasion. User experience is generated throughout users' interactions with a system in the contexts of use, and thus the persuasive techniques must be based on the understanding of those use situations. This study illustrates how negative user experiences can be used for identifying situations where persuasive techniques do not function as intended. In this case techniques that were especially vulnerable to pitfalls include *self-monitoring, suggestion* and *social facilitation.* Pitfalls are often associated with excessive cognitive effort that a persuasive functionality may require, contextual and temporal misfit of the functionality or emotional counter-reactions to persuasion often resulting from the high demand for accuracy and credibility of content. We identified the complementary roles of *functional* and *facilitative* principles in persuasion. Facilitative principles, such as tailoring and simulation can be applied in avoiding pitfalls that are easily encountered with functional principles of self-monitoring, suggestion and social facilitation. In addition, the role of, e.g, currentness and fluency of use as facilitating techniques should be considered. Further research is needed in order to establish the functional relationships between functional and facilitative principles in other cases.

Acknowledgments. We express our gratitude to the Pudottajat web service and Mari Kataja for collaboration, Santtu Pakarinen for research assistance and anonymous reviewers for commenting the manuscript. We also thank the RichWeb project and OASIS research group of the University of Oulu, the unit of Human-Centered Technology (IHTE) of Tampere University of Technology and the National Consumer Research Center of Finland for supporting the study.

References

1. Consolvo, S., McDonald, D., Toscos, T., Chen, M., Froelich, J., Harrison, B., Klasnja, P., La Marca, A., LeGrand, L., Libby, R., Smith, I., Landay, J.: Activity Sensing in the Wild: A Field Trial of UbiFit Garden. In: Proceedings of the Conference on Human Factors and Computing Systems, CHI 2008 (2008)
2. Fogg, B.J.: Persuasive Technology. Using Computer to Change What We Think and Do. Morgan Kaufmann Publishers, San Francisco (2003)
3. Forlizzi, J., Battarbee, K.: Understanding experience in interactive systems. In: Proceedings of DIS 2004, pp. 261–268. ACM, New York (2004)
4. Harjumaa, M., Segerståhl, K., Oinas-Kukkonen, H.: Understanding Persuasive Software Functionality in Practice: a Field Trial of Polar FT60. In: Proceedings of the Fourth International Conference on Persuasive Technology (Persuasive 2009), Claremont, California, US, April 27-29. ACM International Conference Proceeding Series, vol. 350 (2009)
5. Hassenzahl, M., Tractinsky, N.: User Experience - A Research Agenda. Behavior and Information Technology 25(2), 91–97 (2006)
6. Bång, M., Gustafsson, A., Katzeff, C.: Promoting new patterns in household energy consumption with pervasive learning games. In: de Kort, Y.A.W., IJsselsteijn, W.A., Midden, C., Eggen, B., Fogg, B.J. (eds.) PERSUASIVE 2007. LNCS, vol. 4744, pp. 55–63. Springer, Heidelberg (2007)
7. Norman, G.J., Zabinski, M., Adams, M.A., Rosenberg, D.E., Yaroch, A.L., Atienza, A.A.: A Review of eHealth Interventions for Physical Activity and Dietary Behavior Change. American Journal of Preventive Medicine 33(4), 336–345 (2007)
8. Oinas-Kukkonen, H., Harjumaa, M.: A Systematic Framework for Designing and Evaluating Persuasive Systems. In: Oinas-Kukkonen, H., Hasle, P., Harjumaa, M., Segerståhl, K., Øhrstrøm, P. (eds.) PERSUASIVE 2008. LNCS, vol. 5033, pp. 164–176. Springer, Heidelberg (2008)
9. Oinas-Kukkonen, H., Harjumaa, M.: Persuasive Systems Design: Key Issues, Process Model, and System Features. Communications of the Association for Information Systems 24(28), 485–500 (2009)
10. Portnoy, D., Scott-Sheldon, L.A.J., Johnson, B.T., Carey, M.P.: Computer-delivered interventions for health promotion and behavioral risk reduction: A meta-analysis of 75 randomized controlled trials, 1988-2007. Preventive Medicine 47, 3–16 (2008)
11. Consolvo, S., Dillahunt, T., Froehlich, T.J., Harrison, B., Klasnja, P., Landay, J.A., Mankoff, J.: Ubigreen project,
http://dub.washington.edu/projects/ubigreen/
12. Segerståhl, K., Oinas-Kukkonen, H.: Distributed User Experience in Persuasive Technology Environments. In: de Kort, Y.A.W., IJsselsteijn, W.A., Midden, C., Eggen, B., Fogg, B.J. (eds.) PERSUASIVE 2007. LNCS, vol. 4744, pp. 80–91. Springer, Heidelberg (2007)
13. Shiraishi, M., Washio, Y., Takayama, C., Lehdonvirta, V., Kimura, H., Nakajima, T.: In: Proceedings of the Fourth International Conference on Persuasive Technology. ACM International Conference Proceedings Series, vol. 350 (2009)

Using Persuasive Design Principles in Motivational Feeling towards Children Dental Anxiety (CDA)

Sobihatun Nur-Abdul Salam[1,*], Wan Ahmad Jaafar-Wan Yahaya[2], and Azillah-Mohd Ali[3]

[1] Information Technology Building, College of Art and Sciences, Universiti Utara Malaysia,
06010 Sintok, Kedah, Malaysia
[2] Centre of Instructional Technology and Multimedia, Universiti Sains Malaysia,
11800 Pulau Pinang, Malaysia
[3] Department of Pediatric Dentistry, Hospital Sultanah Bahiyah,
05460 Alor Setar, Kedah, Malaysia
sobihatun@uum.edu.my, wajwy@usm.my, azillah@gmail.com

Abstract. This paper is focusing the potential use of persuasive design principles in motivating children's dental anxiety. The main intention of the paper is to emphasize an attempt of how persuasive design principle can be designed into educational material using CD ROM based multimedia learning environment to overcome the CDA. Firstly, we describe a problem domain which discuss about the universal feeling of CDA and secondly the current practices in handling those negative feelings. Thirdly, the conceptual background of PMLE and how the principle has been applied in designing the information interfaces and presentation of a persuasive multimedia learning environment (PMLE) are described. Fourthly, an experimental design was used to validate the effects of prototype which assessed children dental anxiety level before and after the demonstration and utilization of a PMLE. Primary school children age between seven and nine years old are selected as respondents. Fifthly, the result of the study has revealed the feedback from children regarding baseline test and children dental anxiety test. It shows how by using persuasive design principles as an overall strategy in designing PMLE was able to motivate children feelings towards dental anxiety and could let the children behave in a good manner for dental visit in the future.

Keywords: children dental anxiety (CDA), persuasive technology principles, multimedia design principles, persuasive multimedia learning environment (PMLE).

1   Introduction: Universal Feeling towards Children Dental Anxiety (CDA)

Dental anxiety is a universal feeling and widespread problem among children. This study defines anxiety as unpleasant emotional feeling with physiological symptoms

---

* Corresponding author.

T. Ploug, P. Hasle, H. Oinas-Kukkonen (Eds.): PERSUASIVE 2010, LNCS 6137, pp. 223–237, 2010.
© Springer-Verlag Berlin Heidelberg 2010

and effects on negative implication such as uncooperative behaviour. Besides, dental anxiety is categorized as a type of generalized anxiety disorder (GAD) which is characterized by excessive worrying about a variety of dental events, including those in the past, present, and future. The majority of the psychological field believes anxiety is learned. Learners, particularly children learned dental anxiety from four major factors which are direct conditioning such as experience of pain, vicarious learning such as learning negative experience from their mother, latent inhibition, and dentist behavior. Berge (2007) highlights that in children; it is often the main reason of behavioral management problems, of interference with regular treatment and of subsequent referrals to dental pediatrics practitioner.

The other problem is that individuals, especially children, have feelings of pain denial. Chapman and Kirby (1999) reported that the children were experiencing pain during the treatment, but the dentists ignored them and carried on. This unpleasant experience at the dentist may make children to be less willing to attend to the treatment again. Reappraisal of threat may solely be due to greater cognitive ability producing at different assessment of situations. Children also insist that no-one has told them any horror stories; it seems to be that greater maturity brings an increased awareness of the potential threat and re-appraisal of the situation (Chapman and Kirby, 1999). Wells (2003) also agreed that the dental anxiety problem is also specific to an individual, such as negative cognition concerning previous treatment and poor self-monitoring capabilities. Subsequently, Carson and Freeman (1997) stated that a child's subjective perception of a dental visit is decisive in the acquisition of dental fear.

2   Current Practice of Handling CDA

There are many techniques identified for the treatment of anxiety (Newton, 2003; Berge et al. 1999; Berge et al. 2002; Lyndsay et al. 2004; Chapman and Kirby., 1999; Naini, et al. 1999; Carson and Freeman., 1997). Treatment for dental anxiety can be pharmacological or psychological, or a combination of both. Table 2.8 describes the treatment options of dental anxiety.

Psychological treatments incorporates communicative management which comprises specific techniques of tell-show-do, voice control, non-verbal communication, positive reinforcement, effective relaxation techniques and distraction (AAPD, 2006; Colgate, 2005; Chapman and Kirby, 1999 and Naini, et al., 1999).

Pharmacological agents may be used as a complement to behavioural techniques to assist in the management of anxiety in some paediatric dental patients. These agents are usually sedative in action and do not, in themselves, eliminate anxiety but merely enhance patient acceptance by reducing arousal and modifying anticipation of danger (Folayan, et al., 2002). The agents used are varied and diverse and include nitrous oxide, benzodiazepines, and narcotics. In pharmacological treatments, general anaesthesia is also used (AAPD, 2006 and Naini, et al., 1999).

These treatments have been shown to be beneficial for patients, but there are some major limitations. The major problem with these programme is that they are often costly to conduct and resource intensive because of the various methods that are utilized. In the Tell-Show-Do approach for example, this treatment require trained staff to coordinate and conduct the treatment programme as well as a suitable venue, materials and equipment to demonstrate the concept. The items may also be costly to purchase and maintain. Therefore, we concern to approach a persuasive multimedia learning environment (PMLE) in manipulating some of the psychological treatment with using the power of persuasive technology principles and multimedia design principles to overcome above issues.

3   PMLE: Persuasive Multimedia Learning Environment

The use of multimedia in learning programs has grown exponentially in recent years. Numerous researchers such as Clark (2007), Kashi (2007), Shank (2005), Mayer (2001), McGloughlin (2001), and Stemler (1997) have found that multimedia offers many benefits that are able to facilitate learning. Some of the benefits include meaningful learning, self-paced interaction and better retention, better understanding of the content, cost effectiveness, intuitive interface, gets the learner's attention and helps the learner to integrate information into her or his knowledge base.

Multimedia also has the advantage as a persuasive technology. According to McCracken and Wolfe (2004), multimedia can engage the human senses to inform, persuade or entertain. Fogg (2003) has coined a word 'captology' that is about understanding how what is known about motivation and persuasion that can be applied to computer and consumer devices. The objective is to change behaviours and attitudes in predictable ways.

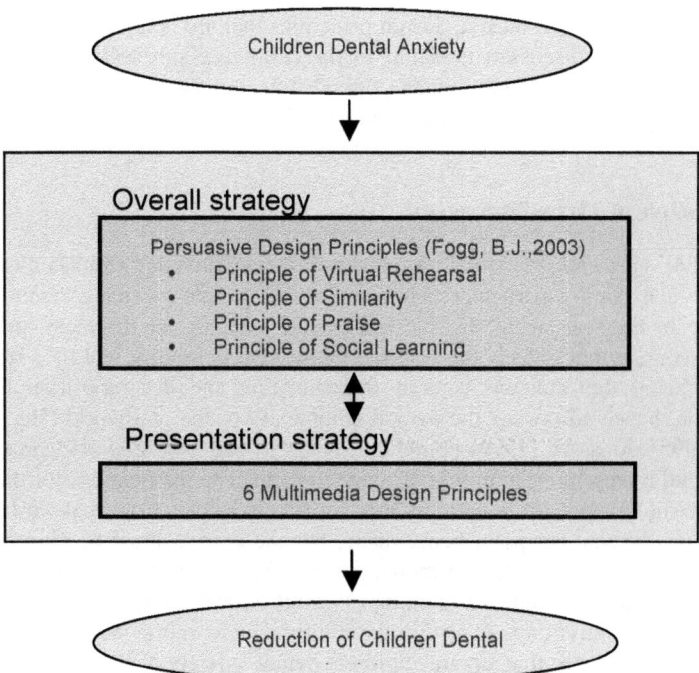

Fig. 1. Theoretical Design Framework of the PMLE

With this element of captology integrated in a multimedia learning environment, we have designed and developed a prototype namely a Persuasive Multimedia Learning Environment (PMLE) for children aged seven to nine year old who have problems associated with dental anxiety. The PMLE is an interactive educational CD-based courseware which also can be used by parents, dental practitioner, teacher to educate and motivate the children in gaining confidence when attending dental visit. The overall instructional theoretical design framework that guides the design of the PMLE has taken such an approach by combining the persuasive technology principles (Fogg, 2003) multimedia design principles. Persuasive technology principles are described as the overall strategic plan which concerned with the selection, sequence, and organization of the subject-matter that are to be presented. While, multimedia design principles are concerned with presentation strategies with the details of each individual presentation to the learner (Chen, 2001). Fig. 1 illustrates the overall instructional theoretical design framework that incorporates both the persuasive technology principles and multimedia design principles.

4   Persuasive Design Principles as Motivational Feeling Driving Factors

Persuasive design comprises studies on carefully planned information activities, where the goals are related to some kind of change in the behaviour of the receivers (Fogg, 2003). Therefore, a persuasive design approach is needed to pursue the desired goals. There are four persuasive design principles that are being applied in this study. The principles are discussed in detail in the following sub section. There are four persuasive principles that have been applied into this study. They are principle of virtual rehearsal, principle of similarity, principle of praise and principle of social learning.

4.1   Principle of Virtual Rehearsal

Fogg's (2003) principle of virtual rehearsal provide a motivating simulated environment in which rehearsing a particular behaviour enable people to change their attitude or behaviour in the real world. In this multimedia learning environment, providing an authentic context that reflects the way the knowledge is used in real-life, preserves the full context of the situation without fragmentation and decomposition that invites exploration, hence allows for the natural complexity of the real world (Herrington and Oliver, 1995). Jonassen (1999) points out that with authentic context learners will get engaged and represent meaningful challenge to them. The implications for the design of interactive multimedia are not simply that suitable examples from real-world situations are used to illustrate the point being made, but the context must be all-embracing, in order to provide the purpose and motivation for the use of the program, as well as to provide a sustained and complex learning environment that can be explored at length.

The simulated environment within the multimedia learning environment attempted to replicate situations that create children dental anxiety feeling. There are three simulated environment situations which are in the house, in the dental waiting room and in the dental treatment room. The main character called "Gg" described the experience of a child being informed about dental check up a day before dental appointment at home, experience of the child being attended to dental clinic in a waiting room and experience of the child undergoing dental treatment.   This multimedia learning environment provides a safe 'place' to explore good behaviours of attending dental appointment with new perspectives. Unlike real environments, persuasive multimedia learning environment is controllable whereby users can start or stop the experience at any time, and when they return for additional multimedia learning experience, they can pick up where they had left it off. For example, Fig. 2 shows the main screen of the multimedia learning environment.

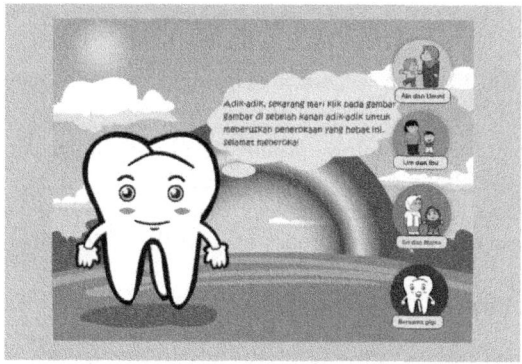

Fig. 2. A snap-shot screen of PMLE main screen

This persuasive multimedia learning environment (PMLE) attempted to persuade children to reduce their dental anxiety through creating situations that motivate them to achieve a target behaviour as shown in the prototype. It also allowed users to practise a target behaviour by imitating how the animated children characters behave in the multimedia learning environment. This prototype also facilitated role-playing by playing the role of children's mothers, nurses, dentist and the children themselves. The role-playing was attempted to let the anxious children adopting another persons behaviour in a good new perspective so that the role-playing can influence the children to behave positively when attending dental appointment.

4.2 Principle of Similarity

In this PMLE, researcher has made the prototype more persuasive by making them similar to the target audience which is the children at the age of seven to nine years old. It conveyed similarity through the use of children language, narration done by children, use of children cartoon characters in a cartoon simulated environment with two dimension animations, and fun games designed for children. For example, in Fig. 3 illustrates the dental setting situation involving children attending a dental treatment so that the children felt that they were experiencing the situations while observing other children of a similar age going through the same process. This is in line with the principle of similarity which stated that people are more readily

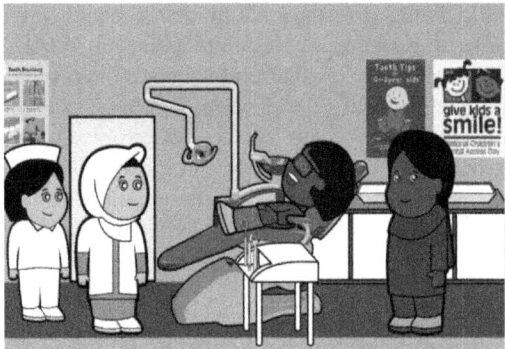

Fig. 3. A snap-shot screen of the simulated dental setting

persuaded by computing technology products that are similar to themselves in some ways. The more the children can identify with the cartoon characters in a cartoon simulated multimedia learning environment, the more likely they will be persuaded to change their anxiety feelings and attitudes in ways the PMLE suggested.

4.3 Principle of Praise

This principle stated that by offering praise, via words, images, symbols, or sounds, computing technology can lead users to be more open to persuasion. In this multimedia learning environment, praises were provided through sounds and visuals to influence children in reducing their dental anxiety feeling. For example, at the end of games section as illustrated in Fig. 4, the children will receive feedback when they answer the question provided correctly. The computer gives feed back in the praise condition like "*Tahniah* / Congratulations!". This prototype also offers praise via voice over character such as a praise from a mother to a child who is well-behaved in the waiting room. The video clip included in the prototype demonstrated a dentist treating a child patient in a welcoming situation with praise and friendly gestures. By applying this principle, researcher hopes that the children who faced dental anxiety will feel better about themselves, are in a better mood and found the interaction engaging.

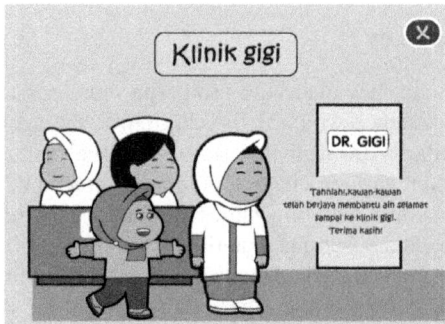

Fig. 4. A snap-shot screen of the ending of games section

4.4 Principle of Social Learning

A person will be more motivated to perform a target behaviour if she or he can use computing technology to observe others performing the behaviour and being rewarded. The important aspect in this principle is the power of modelling.

In this PMLE, a modelling of success personal experience by a boy at the age of seven having a dental check up procedure at a dental clinic has been filmed-up in a short video clip provided in the application. Children, who explored the prototype, will see the boy undergoing a treatment such as a drilling procedure without adverse consequences like crying in which drilling can be threatening to most anxious children. This is in line with the principle which believes that people tend to observe and learn most when behaviour is modeled by others who are similar to themselves. Furthermore, success personal experiences raise a person's expectation of future success. The repeated personal success will lead to the development of strong self-efficacy.

In this persuasive multimedia learning environment, the dentist will treat the boy using a psychological approach which is "tell-show-do" technique. Using this technique, the aim is to allow the patient to feel more in control of the frightening situation. In this study, the boy as a patient was told what he could expect to feel during a procedure. He was also given an idea of how long a procedure would be take place. Furthermore, information on any procedure had been given in concise lay terms. Then, dentist showed the boy or gave a rehearsal for the procedure that he would undergo. After the boy felt confident, then the dentist did the real treatment to the patient. It is hoped in this study that the children will persuade themselves that if others can do it, they should be able to achieve at least some improvements in performance of attending dental appointment. The snap-shot screen of the short video clip is depicted in Fig. 5 below.

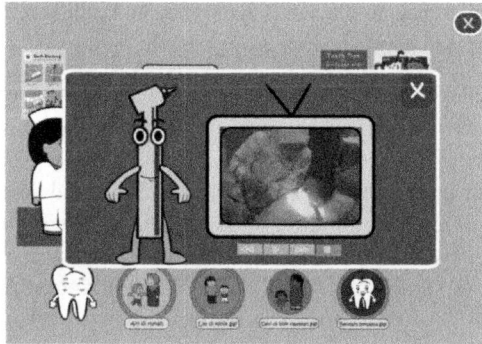

Fig. 5. A snap-shot screen of a short video clip in PMLE

5 Multimedia Design Principles as a Presentable Elements

There are six multimedia design principles that have been applied into this study. They are principle of multimedia design, principle of spatial contiguity, principle of temporal, principle of coherence, principle of modality and principle of redundancy.

Principle of Multimedia Design
Mayer's (2001) first principle of multimedia design stated that learning could be enhanced when pictures were added to words rather than words alone. In this persuasive multimedia learning environment, appropriate words or labels are provided in the images shown in the prototype. As example shown in Fig. 2, all icons are viewed with a simple and meaningful word that represents what is an icon all about and this short words is called the "tool tip ". This was an example of adding text to illustrate in helping learners understand the presented material.

Principle of Spatial Contiguity
The images in the cartoon environment and the corresponding description of instruction in each simulated situation were presented near to each other on the screen. These were all in line with the spatial contiguity principle where presenting words and pictures near to each other encouraged learners to build mental connections between them.

Principle of Temporal
The principle of temporal states that users learn better when corresponding words and pictures are presented simultaneously rather than successively. In this persuasive multimedia learning environment, corresponding portions of narration and animation were presented at the same time. Therefore, the children are more likely to be able to hold mental representations of both in working memory at the same time, and the children are more likely to be able to build mental connections between verbal (narration) and visual (animation) representations.

Principle of Coherence
The coherence principle says that users learn better when extraneous words, pictures, and sounds are excluded rather than included. Thus, PMLE avoided seemingly interesting words, pictures, and sounds that were not relevant to the main message, and the presentation was kept as concise as possible.

Principle of Modality
Based on the modality principle, children will find to learn better when words in a message were presented as spoken text rather than printed text. Hence this persuasive multimedia learning environment provided instruction and feedback in the form of narration during children's exploration of the simulated environment. This principle is applied into the presentation mode two of the prototype which comprises the combination of texts, graphics, audio, video, and narrated animation without on-screen text.

Principle of Redundancy
As stressed in Mayer (2002), the redundancy principle recommended that multimedia learning environment should avoid redundant on-screen text presented at the same time as on-screen graphics. This principle is applied into learning mode two of the prototype which comprises the combination of texts, graphics, audio, video, and narrated animation with on-screen text.

6   Experimenting a Persuasive Multimedia Learning Environment (PMLE)

An experimental research design was used to evaluate the prototype, which assessed children dental anxiety before and after the exploration of a persuasive multimedia learning environment. This design involved two treatment groups, they were presentation mode 1 group and presentation mode 2 group. Relating to this study, presentation mode 1 (PM1) was a learning mode which comprised of combination of narrated animation with on-screen text. Whereas, presentation mode 2 (PM2) comprises of combination of and narrated animation without on-screen text. This study excluded control group because there is no standard benchmark established by Ministry of Health in Malaysia.

This study involved random assignments of the intact groups to treatment with specific criteria, rather than assignment of individuals. The sample of this study must be a group of students that have a feeling on dental anxiety. Therefore, to make sure whether the two groups were equivalent, the baseline test in the phase 1 (see Fig. 6) for both treatments of presentation modes was used to measure the dental anxiety understanding among children. The measurement instrument used was Smiley Faces Programme which was given and analyzed in term of homogeneity of dental anxiety level. The baseline test for both treatments of presentation mode was used as a basis understanding of children who used to have dental anxiety feelings.

The two treatment groups were given a baseline test and a dental anxiety test. Both treatment groups performed a different set of a persuasive multimedia learning environment which was intended to develop their understanding of dentistry, particularly dental treatment. Fig. 6 illustrates the research design in this study. This research design involved four phases. Phase one was the baseline test, phase two was exploration and the use of presentation modes, phase three was the dental anxiety test and the phase four was the motivation test.

Treatment	Phase 1	Phase 2	Phase 3	Phase 4
Group 1	$O_1=$ Baseline test (using SFP instrument)	$Y_1=$ Presentation Mode 1 (PM1)	$O_2=$ Dental anxiety test (using SFP instrument)	Motivation test (using PMMS)
Group 2	$O_3=$ Baseline test (using SFP instrument)	$Y_2=$ Presentation Mode 2 (PM2)	$O_4=$ Dental anxiety test (using SFP instrument)	Motivation test (using PMMS)

Fig. 6. Research design

6.1   Sample Characteristics

The selection of the sample was randomly done by using random sampling technique. The location of study was a selected primary school which has dental treatment facility. The sample size was 240 children aged from seven to nine from primary schools which were selected from one state in Malaysia. Children who were going to have a test on PM1 and PM2 were randomly selected.

Two to three intact classes were chosen from each of five different primary schools. A total of 267 Year 1 to 3 primary school students participated in this experiment. However, out of these students, 27 of them were not taken in the analyses due to the out of the range from the target limit of respondents which was 240. Hence, only 240 participants of children who had dental anxiety feeling were taken into consideration in the analyses.

6.2   Instrument: Smiley Faces Program (SFP)

According to Buchanan (2005), the SFP is a dental anxiety measurement for children which consist of five dimensions of children dental anxiety. The SFP instrument is attached in Appendix A. All five dimensions are the major causal factors of children dental anxiety. Fig. 7 illustrates the children dental anxiety dimensions in the SFP.

SFP: Children dental anxiety dimension
1. Going to the dentist tomorrow
2. Sitting in the waiting room
3. About to have a tooth drilled
4. About to have tooth taken out
5. About to have an injection

Fig. 7. Dental anxiety dimensions in SFP

The measurement scale for SFP used a set of five faces representing the feeling of children's responses towards the dimensions of dental anxiety. The five dimensions included in the SFP score ranged from 1 to 5 equivalent to mean score ranged from 1 to 5. Hence, the minimum score possible was 1 and the maximum was 5 which higher scores indicated higher anxiety. Therefore, the tolerance rate for this study was at range 1 to 3 mean scores.

The reliability of SFP was measured by cronbach alpha and the value was 0.8. This instrument has no effect for age or gender among children. However, this study looked at the effect on the age and gender among children with dental anxiety after using the prototype. The SFP was employed in phase one and three. The result of SFP in phase one was used to indicate scores for children's dental anxiety dimension and in phase three to show scores for children dental anxiety.

7   Results and Discussion

Data analysis of the study is using statistical software, Statistical Package for Social Science (SPSS) version 14.0 (Carver and Nash, 2006). The findings to the research questions (RQ) for the evaluation aspects of this study are discussed as follows.

7.1 Is There a Difference in Children Dental Anxiety Scores between the Two Presentation Modes (RQ1)?

Overall, both text version and non-text version presentation modes had significant positive effects in minimizing children dental anxiety. This was evidenced by the statistical results that both text version and non-text version presentation modes obtained significantly higher mean score for the baseline test which means the children used to have the dental anxiety feeling. In relation to CDA scores, both text version and non-text version presentation modes obtained significantly lower mean score for the CDA test which means the children were successful in reducing their dental anxiety level.

In testing RQ1, Paired samples test was used. This paired samples t-test analysis indicated that there was a mean difference between Baseline test and Children dental Anxiety (CDA) test for both treatments as depicted in Table 1. In non text version, the mean score on the CDA test (M=2.6338) was lower than the mean score on the Baseline test (M=4.0745). In relation to text version, the mean score on the CDA test (M=2.6338) was lower than the mean score on the Baseline test (M=4.0745). This means that there was a reduction in the children dental anxiety level after having both of the non-text version and text version treatments. The reduction scores based on the mean scores difference between Baseline test and CDA test using PMLE as a treatment is illustrated in Fig. 8. In addition, text version presentation mode was slightly higher than non-text version presentation mode in reducing children dental anxiety.

Table 1. Paired Samples t-Test Statistics

Treatment			Mean	N	Std. Deviation	Std. Error Mean
Non-text version	Pair		4.1225	120	.60146	.05491
Baseline			2.5904	120	1.10511	.10088
1	CDA					
Text version	Pair		4.4258	120	.50385	.04600
Baseline			2.7628	120	1.14876	.10487
1	CDA					

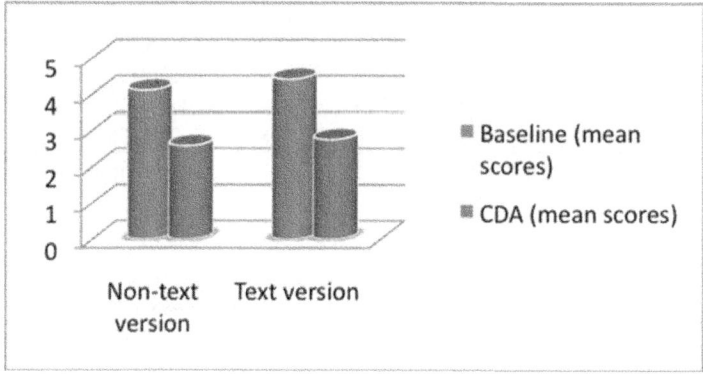

Fig. 8. Mean scores difference between Baseline and CDA for both presentation modes

7.2   Is There a Difference in Score of Each Child Dental Anxiety Dimension between the Two Presentation Modes (RQ2)?

The learners who were exposed to the text version and the non-text version presentation modes obtained significant reduction in each child dental anxiety dimension. In non-text version, the mean scores of the CDA test for each dental anxiety dimension was lower than the mean score of the Baseline test for each dental anxiety dimension. In relation to text version, the mean scores of the CDA test for each dental anxiety dimension was also lower than the mean scores of the Baseline test for each dental anxiety dimension.

Table 2. Paired-samples t- test statistic of difference in mean scores of each children dental anxiety dimension between the two presentation modes

Treatment			Mean	N	Std. Deviation	Std. Error Mean
Non-Text Version	Pair 1	P1a	3.5417	120	1.48322	.13540
		P2a	2.2000	120	1.45867	.13316
	Pair 2	P1b	4.0167	120	.96130	.08775
		P2b	2.8500	120	1.44740	.13213
	Pair 3	P1c	4.1833	120	.95251	.08695
		P2c	2.6500	120	1.48748	.13579
	Pair 4	P1d	4.4333	120	.89568	.08716
		P2d	2.7250	120	1.60860	.14684
	Pair 5		4.4407	118	.66077	.06083
		P1e	2.5339	118	1.55075	.14276
		P2e				
Text version	Pair 1		4.0583	120	1.03140	.09415
		P1a	2.2500	120	1.38570	.12650
			4.4083	120	.66731	.06092
		P2a	2.7750	120	1.44631	.13203
	Pair 2		4.5083	120	.50203	.04583
		P1b	2.7750	120	1.56780	.14312
			4.6723	119	.56911	.05217
		P2b	3.1345	119	1.59939	.14662
	Pair 3	P1c	4.4746	118	.72456	.06670
		P2c	2.9153	118	1.71756	.15811
	Pair 4	P1d				
		P2d				
	Pair 5	P1e				
		P2e				

In testing RQ2, Paired samples t- test was used. This paired samples t-test analysis indicates that there was a mean difference in scores of each child dental anxiety dimension between the two presentation modes as depicted in Table 2. In non-text version, the mean scores on the CDA test for each dental anxiety dimension was lower than the mean score on the Baseline test for each dental anxiety dimension. For example, the mean score on p2a (M=2.2000) was lower than the mean score p1a (M=3.5417). In relation to text version as depicted from Table 5.9, the mean scores on the CDA test for each dental anxiety dimension was also lower than the mean scores on the Baseline test for each dental anxiety dimension. For example, the mean baseline score on p2a (M=2.2500) was lower than the mean CDA score on p1a (M=4.0583). This means that there was a reduction in a children dental anxiety level after having both treatments of the non text version and text version presentation modes. The reduction scores based from the mean scores difference in scores of each children dental anxiety dimension between the two presentation modes using PMLE as a treatment are illustrated in Fig. 9.

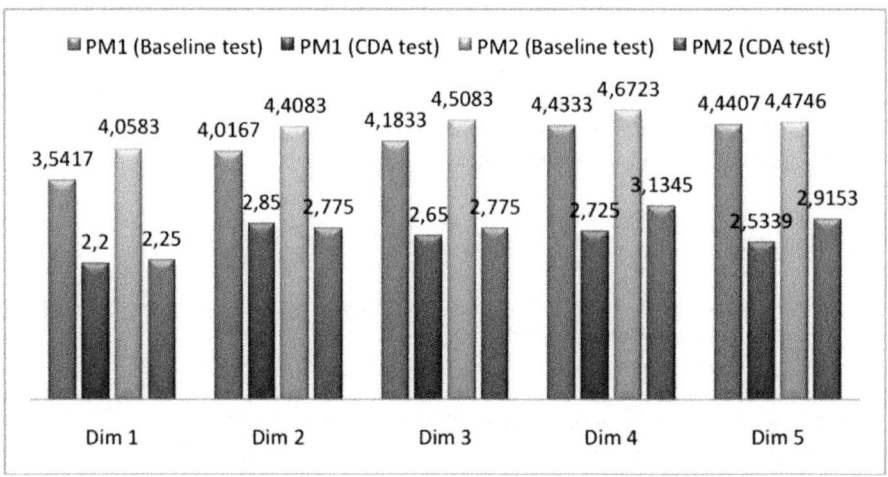

Fig. 9. Mean score differences between each children dental anxiety dimension for both presentation modes

7.3 Is There a Difference in Perceived Children's Motivation Scores between the Two Presentation Modes (RQ3)?

The statistical results showed that the learners who were exposed to the text version and the non-text version presentation modes obtained significantly higher in perceived children's motivation scores. In testing RQ3., One-sample t-test was used. The following section is the result from RQ3 test. This test analysis indicates that there are 92 learners involved in the non text version treatment and 105 learners involved in the text version treatment as depicted in Table 3.

This one-sample t-test analysis indicates that there is a mean difference in perceived children motivation scores between the two presentation modes as depicted from Table 3.

Table 3. Group Statistics

Treatment		N	Mean	Std. Deviation	Std. Error Mean
minPMMS	non-text version	92	4.5363	.82958	.08649
	text version	105	4.5786	.53926	.05263

8   Conclusion

Overall, both text version and non-text version presentation modes had significantly positive effects reducing   children dental anxiety. This was evidenced by the statistical results that both text version and non-text version presentation modes obtained significantly higher mean score for the baseline test which means that the children used to have the dental anxiety feeling. In relation to the children dental anxiety scores (CDA), both text version and non-text version presentation modes obtained significantly lower mean score for the CDA test which means that the children were successful in reducing their dental anxiety. This result proves that persuasive technology principles have been successfully used in motivational feeling of dental anxiety. PMLE is perhaps an alternative solution in reducing children dental anxiety, particularly in Malaysian context.

References

[1] AAPD, American Academy of Paediatric Dentistry. Guideline on behaviour guidance for the paediatric dental patient (2006),
    http://www.aapd.org/media/Policies_Guidelines/
    G_BehavGuide.pdf
[2] Berge, T.M.: Dental fear in children: Clinical consequences (2007),
    http://www.kinderzahn.ch/Dental%20fear%20in%20children_
    Consequences.pdf
[3] Berge, M.T., Veerkamp, J.S.J., Hoogstraten, J.: The etiology of childhood dental fear: the role of dental and conditioning experiences. Journal of Anxiety Disorders 16, 321–329 (2002)
[4] Berge, M.T., Veerkamp, J.S., Hoogstraten, J., Prins, P.J.: Treating Fearful Dental Patients. British Dental Journal 187, 408–412 (1999)
[5] Buchanan, H.: Development of a computerized dental anxiety scale for children: Validation and reliability. British Dental Journal 199, 359–362 (2005)
[6] Carson, P., Freeman, R.: Assessing child dental anxiety: The validity of clinical observations. International Journal of Paediatric Dentistry 7, 171–176 (1997)
[7] Carver, R.H., Nash, J.G.: Doing Data Analysis with SPSS Version 14. Thomson (2006)
[8] Chapman, H.R., Kirby, N.C.: Dental fear in children: A proposed model. British Dental Journal 187(8) (1999),
    http://www.nature.com/bdj/journal/v187/n8/full/4800293a.html
[9] Chen, C.J.: The Design, Development and Evaluation of a Virtual Reality (VR)-based Learning Environment: It's Efficacy in Novice Car Driver Instruction. PhD Thesis, Universiti Sains Malaysia (2005)

[10] Clark, R.: Leveraging multimedia for learning: use instructional methods proven to align with natural learning processes (2007),
http://www.adobe.com/products/captivate/pdfs/
captivate_leveraging_multimedia.pdf

[11] Fogg, B.J.: Persuasive technology: Using computers to change what we think and do. Morgan Kaufmann Publishers, San Francisco (2003)

[12] Folayan, M.O., Faponle, A., Laminkara, A.: A review of the pharmacological approach to the management of dental anxiety in children. International Journal of Paediatric Dentistry 12, 347–354 (2002)

[13] Gardner, H.: Changing minds: The art and science of changing our own and other people's minds. Harvard Business School Publishing, USA (2006)

[14] Herrington, J., Oliver, R.: Critical Characteristics of Situated Learning: Implications for the Instructional Design of Multimedia (1995),
http://www.ascilite.org.au/conferences/melbourne95/smtu/
papers/herrington.pdf

[15] Jonassen, D.: Designing Constructivist Learning Environment. In: Reigeluth, C. (ed.) Instructional Design Theories and Models: A new Paradigm of Instructional Theories, vol. II, pp. 215–239. Lawrence Erlbaum Associates, Mahwah (1999)

[16] Kashi, J.: The multimedia lawyer (2007),
http://www.abanet.org/lpm/lpt/articles/tch02071.shtml

[17] Lyndsay, C., Lauren, D.: Strategies for Combating Dental Anxiety. Journal of Dental Education 68(11), 1172 (2004)

[18] Mayer, R.E.: Multimedia learning. Cambridge University Press, Cambridge (2001)

[19] McCracken, D.D., Wolfe, R.J.: User-Centered Web Site Development: A Human-Computer Interaction Approach. Prentice Hall, Englewood Cliffs (2004)

[20] McGloughlin, S.: Multimedia: Concepts and Practice. Prentice Hall, Englewood Cliffs (2001)

[21] Naini, F.B., Mellor, A.C., Getz, T.: Treatment of dental fears: Pharmacology or Psychology? Dental update 26, 270–276 (1999)

[22] Newton, J.T.: Is childhood dental anxiety a result of irregular attendance? British Dental Journal 194(9), 495 (2003),
http://www.nature.com/bdj/journal/v194/n9/full/4810068a.html

[23] Shank, P.: The value of multimedia in learning: How do you create a truly effective multimedia learning experience? (2005),
https://www.adobe.com/uk/designcenter/thinktank/valuemedia/

[24] Stemler, L.K.: Educational characteristics of multimedia: a literature review. Journal of Educational Multimedia and Hypermedia 6(3/4), 339–359 (1997)

[25] Toscos, T., Faber, A., An, S., Gandhi, M.P.: Chick clique: Persuasive technology to motivate teenage girls to exercise (2006),
http://www.cs.indiana.edu/surg/Projects/ChickClique/
chickCliquePaper_final.pdf

Facilitation of Goal-Setting and Follow-Up in an Internet Intervention for Health and Wellness

Kirsikka Kaipainen[1], Elina Mattila[1], Marja-Liisa Kinnunen[2], and Ilkka Korhonen[1]

[1] VTT Technical Research Center of Finland, P.O. Box 1300, FI-33101 Tampere, Finland
[2] University of Jyväskylä, Department of Psychology, P.O. Box 35,
FI-40014 University of Jyväskylä, Finland
{Kirsikka.Kaipainen,Elina.M.Mattila,Ilkka.Korhonen}@vtt.fi,
Marja-Liisa.Kinnunen@jyu.fi

Abstract. Chronic work-related stress and insufficient recovery from workload can gradually lead to problems with mental and physical health. Resources in healthcare are limited especially for preventive treatment, but low-cost support can be provided by Internet-based behavior change interventions. This paper describes the design of an Internet intervention which supports working-age people in managing and preventing stress-related health and wellness problems. The intervention is designed for early prevention and aims to motivate individuals to take responsibility for their own well-being. It allows them to choose the approach to take to address personally significant issues, while guiding them through the process. The first iteration of the intervention was evaluated with three user groups and subsequently improved based on the user experiences to be more persuasive, motivating and better suited for independent use. Goal setting and follow-up were especially enhanced, tunneled structure improved, and the threshold of use lowered.

Keywords: Internet intervention, computer-aided cognitive behavioral therapy, behavior change, goal-setting, stress, well-being.

1 Introduction

Stress and work exhaustion are taking their toll on the mental well-being of working age population in Western countries. It is estimated that one in four people suffers from mental health problems at some point in their lives [1], and it is likely that the number is increasing. Prolonged stress, coupled with insufficient recovery from workload, can elevate the risk of cardiovascular diseases [2,3] and expose to mental disorders such as depression. High job strain has been shown to predict subsequent work disability pension [4], and work-related mental health problems are the leading cause of sick leave and disability in OECD countries [5]. Depression is expected to be the disorder with the highest disease burden in high-income countries by the year 2030 [6]. Since there are insufficient resources in healthcare to treat these problems before they escalate [1,7], there is a need for novel treatment methods which can be used independently or with minimal professional support and be taken into use when the symptoms are still mild.

T. Ploug, P. Hasle, H. Oinas-Kukkonen (Eds.): PERSUASIVE 2010, LNCS 6137, pp. 238–249, 2010.
© Springer-Verlag Berlin Heidelberg 2010

Internet interventions offer a partial solution to the scarcity of healthcare resources. Access to web-based resources is mostly independent of time and place [7]. Moreover, the possibility of self-management can empower individuals to better master their own well-being. Digital intervention methods may lower the barrier to seek help by assuring anonymity for those who, in fear of stigma, do not wish to attend face-to-face therapy [7]. Internet interventions are gaining acceptance as an alternate treatment to face-to-face therapy; for example, in the United Kingdom, some web-based systems are recommended for treatment of depression and anxiety [8].

Computerized and Internet-based interventions for mental and physical health problems are becoming commonplace and are subject to extensive research [7]. Several Internet interventions have been shown to have positive effects in the treatment of various problems, including depression, anxiety, stress, insomnia, and weight management [9], and the effectiveness of Internet-based therapy in general is comparable to face-to-face interventions [10]. Out of the possible therapeutic approaches employed online, cognitive-behavioral therapy (CBT) has been the most effective [10]. However, many studies report high attrition rates [9] and it is unclear whether this is caused by the intervention design, characteristics of participants, or some other factors. There is a lack of reports describing the detailed development of interventions and their methods, making it difficult to assess particular design decisions. Moreover, persuasive design strategies seem to have been systematically utilized in relatively few interventions [11], although propositions on design practices have been made [12]. Persuasive strategies [13] should be utilized in interventions to a large extent to make them appealing and to motivate attitude and behavior changes.

This paper describes the iterative design of an Internet intervention *GoodLife* (*Hyväksi*, in Finnish) for self-management of mental and physical well-being with focus on stress and recovery. The intervention was developed as a part of a larger concept which involved technologies such as mobile phone applications and measurement devices for daily self-monitoring and assessment, and a brief group intervention comprised of three two-hour face-to-face sessions held by a psychologist [14]. The psychological methods used in the face-to-face and web-based interventions were based on CBT [15] and acceptance and commitment therapy (ACT) [16]. The concept was evaluated with three user groups and improved based on the user experiences and feedback. The focus of this paper is on reporting the lessons learned and presenting the improved design of the web-based *GoodLife* intervention.

2 Design of Internet Interventions

Current Internet-based therapeutic interventions imitate psychological face-to-face therapies in terms of their content, methods and structure [17]. Structured face-to-face therapies, such as CBT, usually progress linearly in sessions, possibly with homework assignments performed between sessions [15]. The therapist and client form a *therapeutic alliance*, the sense of working together towards a shared goal, which is considered to be a key component in the success of therapy [15,18]. The therapist also facilitates the process by guiding the client fluently through a sequence of tasks required in the therapy, and tailors the content to the particular client's needs. Internet-based therapeutic interventions attempt to create positive cognitive and behavioral changes by delivering similar treatment models through Internet and using multimedia and interactive features to provide feedback and enhance motivation [17].

Web-based interventions are usually designed to be highly structured and modularized [17]. This is achieved by tunneling, i.e. designing the program to consist of subsequent sessions which are revealed upon completion of earlier sessions. This leads the user through a change process in a predetermined order, providing appropriate information at right times [12]. Most existing interventions have focused on a single problem or behavior type [7]. In contrast, an intervention which targets several related problems may benefit the most from a hybrid design consisting of multiple tunnels [19]. For instance, eCouch (http://www.ecouch.anu.edu.au) uses a model which incorporates three modules for related disorders.

Therapeutic alliance may be difficult to achieve in self-guided or minimally supported interventions. Supportive guidance and feedback should be provided to aid users in the change process and to hold their interest. Persuasive technology research indicates that building social cues into a system increases motivation, acceptance and adherence [13,20]. These cues can be e.g. positive feedback and tailoring of responses. Interactivity is widely considered to increase user interest and engagement [17]. Although purely information-directed websites can have an effect in promoting health and well-being [21], interactive designs in general show higher adherence [13] and larger effect sizes in health promotion interventions [22,23]. Interactivity can be enriched by tailoring of content and feedback, and by reminder emails or text messages, which provide suggestions within the context of users' daily lives.

Effective components in behavior change interventions have been thus far analyzed relatively little [24]. Research indicates that goal-setting and self-monitoring may be key techniques in interventions designed to promote healthy habits [24]. Goal-setting is considered an effective strategy for changing behavior in general [25]. Forming goals in the form of implementation intentions, which means defining concrete actions to take when specific situations are encountered, has been shown to be an effective method in facilitating goal achievement [26].

Tailoring is another recommendable strategy; tailoring of information and content to users' personal needs have outperformed non-tailored messages across several behaviors [27]. Tailoring criteria can include information needs, risk factors, health behaviors, and stages of change. The identified message tailoring tactics consist of personalization of information, feedback by individual recommendations, and adaptation of content based on individual responses [28]. Provision of comparisons with the user's social group, such as people of the same age or background, increases understandability of feedback and motivation to initiate behavior changes [13].

3   The First Iteration of the *GoodLife* Website

The *GoodLife* website was originally developed as a part of a service concept which combined brief face-to-face psychological group interventions with technology tools to support behavior change [14]. The purpose of the concept was to provide early intervention for stress-related problems with low-barrier and cost-efficient methods for self-management of health and wellness on various areas of well-being.

The first version of the *GoodLife* website was primarily designed to be used with professional support during and between the group meetings. Technology tools – website, mobile applications, and personal devices – were used to facilitate behavior change in daily life as well as to support self-management and maintenance of changes after the end of the face-to-face intervention.

3.1 Initial Design

The idea behind the concept was to empower individuals to make the decisions and take responsibility for their own health and well-being. Thus, the intervention allowed the individuals to choose the issues that they considered to be personally most important to their well-being, as well as motivating and convenient to address at that moment. The role of the *GoodLife* website was to provide users relevant information and tools, facilitate analysis of personal problems and setting of relevant goals, and provide means for follow-up and maintenance of lifestyle changes. The website was divided into five modules, each focusing on one theme of well-being (*stress, exercise, sleep, mood,* and *good life*), to enable the user to choose the personally most relevant starting point. The layout of the website is depicted in Fig. 1.

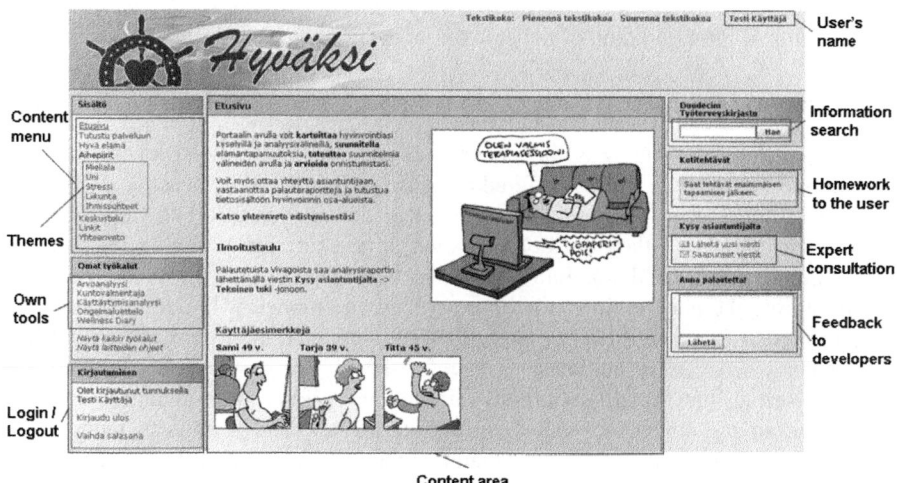

Fig. 1. The layout of the first iteration of the *GoodLife* website

Each module consisted of educational material and four phases: assessment, planning of changes, action, and follow-up. Each phase contained appropriate tools, e.g. assessment phases had questionnaires and in-depth analysis methods, whereas action phases provided tools for execution of plans, such as self-observation diaries and relaxation exercises. The phase division was inspired by the stages of change in the Transtheoretical Model [29]. The general methods of CBT and ACT were tailored for each problem area with customized information and examples.

To gain an overview of their situation, the users could access a summary view which contained color-coded information of their latest questionnaire results, analyses and other entries. The home page was tailored to display the users' active goals right after login. In addition, the website included a discussion board for peer support and a private messaging utility for expert consultation.

3.2 Evaluations

The *GoodLife* website was evaluated alongside with the other technologies and the group intervention with three middle-aged user groups during 2009. Group 1 included 12 men of 32-59 years of age (mean age 48), Group 2 had 23 participants (12/11 female/male) of 37-62 years of age (mean age 54), and Group 3 was composed of 20 women of 27-57 years of age (mean age 45). They were recruited through a newspaper advertisement looking for people suffering from burnout symptoms and/or sleep problems (Groups 1 and 3) and through an email invitation to a well-being program (Group 2). They were familiar with computers and the Internet; majority of them used the Internet on a daily basis and virtually everyone on a weekly basis.

The participants used the intervention website for 8-14 weeks, received the group intervention, and had mobile phone applications and measurement devices in their use at the same time. Questionnaires and website usage log information were used to gather information about the user experiences and usage of the technologies. In the following section, we briefly summarize the findings regarding the *GoodLife* website. The results of the evaluation of the entire concept are reported elsewhere.

3.3 Lessons Learned

The *GoodLife* website was in general considered useful. However, the users commonly felt that the website offered too little guidance and it was easy to get lost in it. For example, many participants commented that it took effort to find personally relevant material and they did not know where to begin after logging in. Thus, one clear improvement need was tailoring of the front page to users' personal needs and restructuring the intervention to be more guided and tunneled. In addition, several of the methods offered in different modules were similar in their core, which produced redundancy between the modules.

Goal-setting functionality was fairly limited and offered little guidance. It did not stand out among other tools and the program did not prompt users to monitor their progress, since self-monitoring was mainly achieved by personal devices and mobile applications. Reminders of the goals and their target dates were missing from the implementation. Considering the effectiveness of goal-setting in behavior change, it should be designed as a central and well-guided function.

Importance of social support was emphasized in the feedback – discussion forum was also one of the most regularly visited website sections, although the number of users was too small to carry out active conversations in long term. The possibility to consult a professional was also appreciated. Opportunity for social contact with others who have similar problems seems to be important in self-management of well-being.

One common theme in the attitudes of the users was reluctance to use Internet-based services after a workday. The usage logs also showed that the visits to the website declined after the first weeks of the evaluation periods. One reason for this could be that some users may have got all they needed from the website on one or two visits; after all, they had more readily available self-observation devices at hand. However, there was certainly a lot of room to make the website more engaging and motivational, starting from visual aspects such as lessening the amount of text and adding graphics. The substantial time commitment required from users due to the length of the programs and sessions has also been noted elsewhere to result in lessened motivation [30]. For early intervention, lighter and less time-consuming design might result in higher adherence and interest.

To summarize, the web-based intervention did not appear to be optimal for independent use. This is understandable, as it was originally developed to be a part of a larger concept. Still, the usability of the website had several shortcomings and persuasive strategies should have been used to a greater extent in the design. Especially further tailoring of content to make it more personally relevant, and more strictly tunneled structure to lead the user through the process, would most likely have reduced the unnecessary cognitive load. However, the inclusion of several different problem areas related to stress into the same intervention seemed to be a good approach, since the problems the users had were diverse. Motivation and adherence to continued use are challenges in Internet interventions in general [9]. One step further in the design could be to increase "fun" elements in the intervention to make it more appealing and engaging. The main evaluation findings, their underlying issues, and our solutions for them are summarized in Table 1.

Table 1. The main weaknesses in the first iteration and their solutions

Finding	Underlying issue	Solutions
It was hard for users to find personally relevant material	Lack of guidance	Clearer and guided structure Better tunneling and tailoring Emphasis on personal motivation in goal-setting and planning
Importance of goal-setting was not emphasized	Inadequate goal-setting and follow-up functions	Goal-setting as a central function Reminders of goals Prompted follow-up Rewarding of achieved goals
Users got lost in the website	Redundancy of content in different modules Lack of guidance	One main tunnel with tailored content to cover all themes Clearer and guided structure
Users' reluctance to spend a lot of time using a computer	Intervention lacked engaging and motivating features	Lessening text, adding graphics Lightened structure Reminders of goals

4   Improved Design of the *GoodLife* Website

The goal in redesigning the *GoodLife* website was to make the web-based intervention suitable for independent use by making it easier and more effortless to use, enhancing persuasive elements to increase users' motivation, and further stressing the importance of personal choice (see Table 1). We follow the philosophy of libertarian paternalism [31] and hypothesize that by suggesting recommendable options, but allowing freedom to choose, users will be likely to plan such behavioral changes they are most motivated and able to carry out. Their perceived self-efficacy [32] and positive intention toward change are thus likely to be the highest. Hence, we focused on facilitation of setting and follow-up of personally relevant goals.

4.1   Website Structure

The website is structured into one main tunnel for the users to follow to lower the threshold of initiating the intervention and to better guide the process. The designed structure of the intervention is depicted in Fig. 2. After the users log in, they receive instructions according to the phase they are in the tunnel. The main phases are learning about personal well-being risks, setting personally relevant goals, and monitoring progress. In the end, the success of goal achievement is evaluated. The system keeps track of the users' actions and displays their history on their home page. To allow the freedom of choice, all content and tools, along with some extra content, are also accessible through the main navigation menu. In addition, the main tunnel includes a few side-tracks at specified points for those who wish to have more elaborate methods for considering their situation.

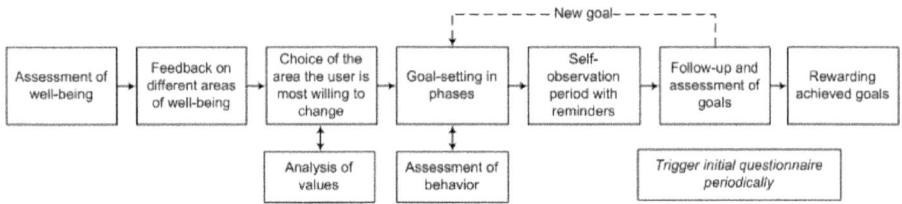

Fig. 2. The tunneled structure of the *GoodLife* website

4.2   Functions

Assessment of well-being. On the first login, the user is instructed to fill in an initial questionnaire which covers eight areas of well-being which are relevant in terms of recovery from stress: *stress, recovery, sleep, mood, exercise, time management, relationships* and *substance use*. The questionnaire is relatively short, with three to five questions per theme, to ensure that it is quick to complete.

Feedback to the questionnaire consists of visual, numerical and textual components. Scores are calculated for each area and visualized by traffic lights related to risk level in each area. Traffic lights were chosen as representations since the meaning of different-colored lights is conceptually familiar to the target group. As data from many users accumulates to the system, feedback given on personal risks related to well-being could be enhanced by displaying comparisons with reference groups. The feedback display is followed by a view where the users can choose the area they are most willing to change. The traffic lights are intended to guide, but not dictate the choices, and thus the user is free to choose any area – even one with the lowest risk score.

In the situation in which the users cannot or do not want to choose any of the eight predetermined areas, they have two options. They can move directly forward to general goal-setting, but pay the price of not having tailored instructions for specified problem areas. They can also choose to analyze their well-being in a more elaborative way with a method called analysis of values. The purpose of the method is to aid people to identify the significant things in his/her life, i.e. values, and to assess how well they have succeeded in living according to their values. After the analysis has been completed, its results are imported to the choice display in addition to the results of the initial well-being assessment questionnaire. The users can then choose one of their values as a basis for goal-setting.

Goal-setting. Goal-setting is done in phases with instructions and example scenarios on how to formulate a goal and a plan. The instructions are tailored to the specific problem areas. Good goals have several characteristics: they are specific, timely, appropriately challenging, personally relevant, and measurable [25]. The goal-setting phases are described in Fig. 3. In each phase, suggestions and default options are offered to the user. For example, in setting of a target date, the program calculates the length of time between the current date and the user-selected target date and gives feedback based on the distance of the target date. If the time period between the two dates is long, the program suggests setting of subgoals and offers defaults for their possible target dates.

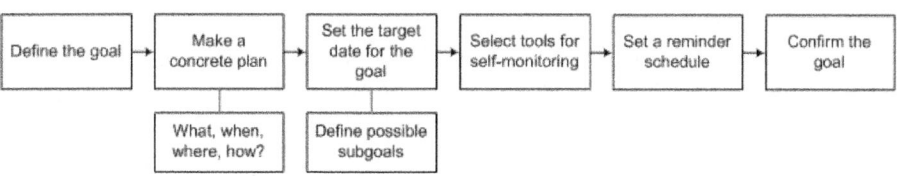

Fig. 3. Phases of goal-setting

A goal is something the user wants to achieve; a plan contains the concrete steps required for goal achievement. Plans are advised to be set in the form of implementation intentions ("If situation Y is encountered, then I will initiate goal-directed behavior X!") [26]. This helps people to make implementation intentions by clarifying and concretizing when, where, and how they intend to achieve their goals.

For those users who might have difficulties in determining appropriate goals for themselves, an analysis method for further assessment of the problematic behavior is provided. With mind-map like display and graphical feedback, the method guides the user to identify the significant factors influencing his/her well-being.

Self-observation period. Continued use of an intervention may be essential for successful behavior change at least for certain problem behaviors [9]. For instance, adding reminders to an Internet-based depression intervention resulted in significant, positive effects, whereas a previous program with no reminders found no program effect [33]. To ensure that the users do not forget their goals and plans, the *GoodLife* program sends them email or SMS reminders on predetermined intervals. The reminders include information on the user's active goals and their target dates.

The *GoodLife* website provides a general self-observation tool for monitoring long-term progress, since effective goals require progress feedback [25]. The users rank their success in pursuing the goal on a scale from 0 to 10, and observe their progress as a graph or a listing of entries. However, this tool is not meant for daily self-observation, since Internet access may not be readily available in most situations calling for self-observations. It would be best to make an entry right after the action has happened to avoid recall bias and to ensure more faithful representation of what truly happened. Thus, users are encouraged to monitor their progress towards goals by other means, such as mobile phone applications or even paper diaries, but the website tool can be used to monitor daily or weekly progress as well.

Follow-up and evaluation of goals. When the user-set target date for a goal arrives, the user is instructed to assess the success of goal achievement on a simple visual rating scale of five smiley faces, ranging from unhappy to happy expression. The achievement is determined by the users' satisfaction regarding their progress towards the goal, not the exact achievement of the goal. This distinction is based on the finding that setting challenging goals leads to better performance, even though it is more difficult to actually achieve the goal [25]. Hence, it would be demoralizing to evaluate the success of a behavior change strictly by assessing the fulfillment of a challenging goal. We assume that if the users are fairly satisfied with the progress they have made, they have in essence achieved the goal.

The goals which the users are satisfied with are rewarded with virtual coins, which are accumulated into a reward chest on the home page. Each coin has a symbol representing the problem area the fulfilled goal was related to. This way the gradual progress toward better well-being is visualized and the users are reminded of their past achievements whenever they log in to the service. Rewarding is also one way to make the intervention slightly more game-like and possibly increase the positive reaction toward it.

Relapse prevention. It is very likely that the users do not always reach their goals or return to do the follow-up when the target date has arrived. Internet interventions should be designed to account for such occasions [12]. In case the user rates a goal as a failure, he/she is provided tools for analysis of possible barriers and problems which hindered the achievement of a goal. The user can also take the failed goal as a basis for setting a new goal and modify it e.g. to a more realistic one. In addition, the program recognizes if the user has neglected to make progress-tracking entries on the schedule, and modifies the content of the reminders to include information about possible ways to analyze difficulties in behavior change.

Long-term follow-up. The summary view enables the users to see their past actions at a glance. To facilitate the long-term follow-up of well-being, the initial questionnaire assessing the variety of factors is offered to the user to refill after a certain period of time has passed.

Social support. A discussion forum for peer support and a private messaging service for expert consultation are integrated into the system.

5   Conclusions

We developed an Internet intervention called *GoodLife* for self-management of health and wellness and evaluated it with three user groups. Based on the evaluation feedback, the design of the intervention was improved to better facilitate goal-setting and follow-up, which were identified as essential factors for behavior change. Persuasive strategies were further applied in the design to increase motivating and engaging features. The intervention structure was lightened to lower the threshold of use, to make finding relevant content easier and faster, and to reduce the users' overall cognitive burden. We assume that when problems are still relatively mild, people need only a simple tool to manage their life and to keep their long-term goals in mind.

In the context of early intervention, people rarely wish to devote a considerable amount of time in working through their possible problems, especially if they are busy and stressed in their daily lives. The improved website attempts to address this issue by having a clear tunnel for the user to follow, still accommodating various problem areas. The concerns of users can potentially range from mild troubles with time management or a wish to lose some weight, to insomnia or depressive symptoms. The delivery of this kind of a service is probably best suited through employers to their employees or from service providers to their customers as a benefit; it might be less likely that the target user group would seek out the intervention by themselves.

Even though the improved design attempts to increase motivation and ease of use, there are still various possibilities to further enhance the persuasive power and appeal of the intervention. For example, to increase user involvement, interactivity could be further increased [12]. Feeling of interactivity could be improved by combining data from different sources, e.g. users' questionnaire scores and self-observation entries, to provide more informative and tailored feedback and instructions. This requires careful design and testing of all possible combinations to ensure that they do not result in misleading advice. However, this would provide significant added value to the users.

It is proposed that digital interventions should offer instant help in situations which cause peaks in the users' relapse proneness [12]. Internet interventions by themselves are not well equipped to provide such assistance. Mobile applications and personal devices have more potential in this sense, and a good self-management system would most likely incorporate and integrate various technologies. Internet interventions are best suited for deeper contemplation and education, whereas personal devices can better facilitate self-monitoring and in-time relapse prevention. Future work can utilize the advantages of both approaches by integrating data from web-based and mobile systems and providing easy mobile access to web resources.

Acknowledgments

This research was partially conducted in the P4Well project, supported by the Finnish Funding Agency for Technology and Innovation (Tekes). The authors wish to acknowledge the companies and research partners in the project consortium: Mawell Ltd., Varma, Firstbeat Technologies Ltd., Suunto Ltd., Mehiläinen Ltd., Solaris, JTO

School of Management, University of Jyväskylä, and VTT Technical Research Centre of Finland. The authors also thank Duodecim Medical Publications Ltd.

This work is partially supported by the PREVE project. PREVE – Prevention of Diseases project (www.preve-eu.org) is partially funded by the European Commission under the 7th Framework Programme (cordis.europa.eu/fp7/ict/ and ec.europa.eu/information_society/index_en.htm)

References

1. Report from the WHO European Ministerial Conference: Mental Health: Facing the Challenges, Building Solutions. WHO (2005)
2. Chandola, T., Britton, A., Brunner, E., Hemingway, H., Malik, M., Kumani, M., Badrick, E., Kivimäki, M., Marmot, M.: Work Stress and Coronary Heart Disease: What are the Mechanisms? European Heart Journal 29, 640–648 (2008)
3. Rosmond, R.: Role of Stress in the Pathogenesis of the Metabolic Syndrome. Psychoneuroendocrinology 30, 1–10 (2005)
4. Laine, S., Gimeno, D., Virtanen, M., Oksanen, T., Vahtera, J., Elovainio, M., Koskinen, A., Pentti, J., Kivimäki, M.: Job Strain as a Predictor of Disability Pension: The Finnish Public Sector Study. Journal of Epidemiology and Community Health 63(1), 24–30 (2009)
5. OECD: Policy Brief: Mental Health in OECD Countries (2008)
6. Lopez, A.D., Mathers, C.D.: Measuring the Global Burden of Disease and Epidemiological Transitions: 2002-2030. Annals of Tropical Medicine & Parasitology 100(5-6), 481–499 (2006)
7. Marks, I.M., Cavanagh, K., Gega, L.: Hands-on Help: Computer-aided Psychotherapy. Psychology Press, San Diego (2007)
8. National Institute for Health and Clinical Excellence: Computerized Cognitive Behavioural Therapy for Depression and Anxiety. Review of Technology Appraisal 51. NICE (2006)
9. Strecher, V.: Internet Methods for Delivering Behavioral and Health-Related Interventions (eHealth). Annual Review of Clinical Psychology 3, 53–76 (2007)
10. Barak, A., Hen, L., Boniel-Nissim, M., Shapira, N.: A Comprehensive Review and a Meta-Analysis of the Effectiveness of Internet-Based Psychotherapeutic Interventions. Journal of Technology in Human Services 26(2/4), 109–160 (2008)
11. Zhu, W.: Promoting Physical Activity Through Internet: A Persuasive Technology View. In: de Kort, Y.A.W., IJsselsteijn, W.A., Midden, C., Eggen, B., Fogg, B.J. (eds.) PERSUASIVE 2007. LNCS, vol. 4744, pp. 12–17. Springer, Heidelberg (2007)
12. Kraft, P., Drozd, F., Olsen, E.: Digital Therapy: Addressing Willpower as Part of the Cognitive-Affective Processing System in the Service of Habit Change. In: Oinas-Kukkonen, H., Hasle, P., Harjumaa, M., Segerståhl, K., Øhrstrøm, P. (eds.) PERSUASIVE 2008. LNCS, vol. 5033, pp. 177–188. Springer, Heidelberg (2008)
13. Fogg, B.J.: Persuasive Technology: Using Computers to Change What We Think and Do. Morgan Kaufmann, San Francisco (2003)
14. Happonen, A.P., Mattila, E., Kinnunen, M.-L., Ikonen, V., Myllymäki, T., Kaipainen, K., Rusko, H., Lappalainen, R., Korhonen, I.: P4Well Concept to Empower Self-Management of Psychophysiological Wellbeing and Load Recovery. In: Proceedings of the 3rd International ICST Conference on Pervasive Computing Technologies for Healthcare, London, UK, April 1-3 (2009)

15. Dobson, K.S. (ed.): Handbook of Cognitive-Behavioural Therapies. Guilford Press, New York (2001)
16. Hayes, S.C., Luoma, J.B., Bond, F.W., Masuda, A., Lillis, J.: Acceptance and Commitment Therapy: Model, Processes and Outcomes. Behavior Research and Therapy 44, 1–25 (2006)
17. Barak, A., Klein, B., Proudfoot, J.: Defining Internet-Supported Therapeutic Interventions. Annals of Behavioral Medicine 38(1), 4–17 (2009)
18. Silverman, D.K.: What Works in Psychotherapy and How Do We Know? What Evidence-Based Practice Has to Offer. Psychoanalytic Psychology 22(2), 306–312 (2005)
19. Danaher, B.G., McKay, H.G., Seeley, J.R.: The Information Architecture of Behavior Change Websites. Journal of Medical Internet Research 7(2), e12 (2005)
20. Bickmore, T., Gruber, A., Picard, R.: Establishing the Computer-Patient Working Alliance in Automated Health Behavior Change Interventions. Patient Education and Counseling 59(1), 21–30 (2005)
21. Christensen, H., Griffiths, K.M., Jorm, A.F.: Delivering Interventions for Depression by Using the Internet: Randomized Controlled Trial. British Medical Journal 328, 265–269 (2004)
22. Hurling, R., Fairley, B.W., Dias, M.B.: Internet-Based Intervention Systems: Are More Interactive Designs Better? Psychology & Health 21, 757–772 (2006)
23. Duffett-Leger, L., Lumsden, J.: Interactive Online Health Promotion Interventions: A "Health Check". In: Proceedings of the 2008 International Symposium on Technology & Society (ISTAS 2008), Fredericton, New Brunswick, June 26-28 (2008)
24. Michie, S., Abraham, C., Whittington, C., McAteer, J., Gupta, S.: Effective Techniques in Healthy Eating and Physical Activity Interventions: A Meta-Regression. Health Psychology 28(6), 690–701 (2009)
25. Locke, E.A., Latham, G.P.: Building a Practically Useful Theory of Goal Setting and Task Motivation: A 35-year Odyssey. American Psychologist 57(9), 705–717 (2002)
26. Gollwitzer, P.M., Sheeran, P.: Implementation Intentions and Goal Achievement: A Meta-analysis of Effects and Processes. Advances in Experimental Social Psychology 38, 69–119 (2006)
27. Noar, S.M., Benac, C.N., Harris, M.S.: Does Tailoring Matter? Meta-Analytic Review of Tailored Print Health Behavior Change Interventions. Psychological Bulletin 133(4), 673–693 (2007)
28. Lustria, M.A., Cortese, J., Noar, S.M., Glueckauf, R.L.: Computer-Tailored Health Interventions Delivered Over the Web: Review and Analysis of Key Components. Patient Education and Counseling 74, 156–173 (2009)
29. Prochaska, J.O., Norcross, J.C.: Stages of Change. Psychotherapy 38(4), 443–448 (2001)
30. Amstadter, A.B., Broman-Fulks, J., Zinzow, H., Ruggiero, K.J., Cercone, J.: Internet Based Interventions for Traumatic Stress-Related Mental Health Problems: A Review and Suggestion for Future Research. Clin. Psych. Rev. 29(5), 410–420 (2009)
31. Thaler, R.H., Sunstein, C.R.: Nudge: Improving Decisions about Health, Wealth, and Happiness. Yale University Press, New Haven (2008)
32. Bandura, A.: Health Promotion by Social Cognitive Means. Health Education & Behavior 31(2), 143–164 (2004)
33. Clarke, G., Eubanks, D., Reid, E., Kelleher, C., O'Connor, E., et al.: Overcoming Depression on the Internet (ODIN) (2): A Randomized Trial of a Self-Help Depression Skills Program with Reminders. Journal of Medical Internet Research 7(2), e16 (2005)

Persuasive Dialogue Based on a Narrative Theory: An ECA Implementation

Marc Cavazza[1], Cameron Smith[1], Daniel Charlton[1], Nigel Crook[2],
Johan Boye[2], Stephen Pulman[2], Karo Moilanen[2], David Pizzi[1],
Raul Santos de la Camara[3], and Markku Turunen[4]

[1] School of Computing, Teesside University, Middlesbrough, United Kingdom
[2] Oxford University Computing Laboratory, Wolfson Building, Oxford, United Kingdom
[3] Telefonica I+D, C/ Emilio Vargas 6, 28043 Madrid, Spain
[4] Department of Computer Sciences, 33014 University of Tampere, Finland
{m.o.cavazza,c.g.smith,d.charlton,d.pizzi}@tees.ac.uk,
{nigel.crook,stephen.pulman,karo.moilanen}@comlab.ox.ac.uk,
johan.boye@speechact.se, e.rsai@tid.es, mturunen@cs.uta.fi

Abstract. Embodied Conversational Agents (ECA) are poised to constitute a specific category within persuasive systems, in particular through their ability to support affective dialogue. One possible approach consists in using ECA as virtual coaches or personal assistants and to make persuasion part of a dialogue game implementing specific argumentation or negotiation features. In this paper, we explore an alternative framework, which emerges from the long-term development of ECA as "Companions" supporting free conversation with the user, rather than task-oriented dialogue. Our system aims at influencing user attitudes as part of free conversation, albeit on a limited set of topics. We describe the implementation of a Companion ECA to which the user reports on his working day, and which can assess the user's emotional attitude towards daily events in the office, trying to influence such attitude using affective strategies derived from a narrative model. This discussion is illustrated through examples from a first fully-implemented prototype.

Keywords: Affective Dialogue Systems, Persuasive Dialogue, Embodied Conversational Agents, Attitude Persuasive Systems.

1 Introduction: ECA and Affective Dialogue

Recent developments in Embodied Conversational Agents (ECA), which support better expressiveness and more sophisticated dialogue, make them good candidates to constitute a specific class of persuasive systems. This is even more the case since recent progress in ECA implementations of Affective Dialogue Systems [1] [2]. The persuasive potential of an ECA derives from its believability and the ability to incorporate affective aspects in its dialogue strategy, whether it analyses the user's emotional state or is able to express specific emotions itself as part of its communication strategy. In particular, the fact that contemporary ECA rely on increasingly sophisticated dialogue systems creates a framework to support persuasive strategies based on communication and argumentation techniques.

T. Ploug, P. Hasle, H. Oinas-Kukkonen (Eds.): PERSUASIVE 2010, LNCS 6137, pp. 250–261, 2010.
© Springer-Verlag Berlin Heidelberg 2010

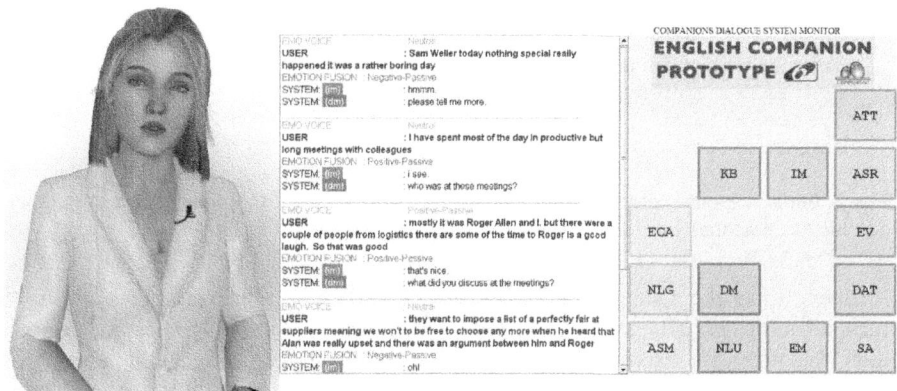

Fig. 1. Overview of the system interface featuring the ECA and including a real-time transcript of the whole dialogue, including output from the emotional speech recogniser. In this example, the dialogue is clearly led by the user (user utterances are displayed in a black font).

In this paper, we describe the implementation of a Companion ECA whose aim is to influence user attitude towards her daily life and in particular relations at work. Our system presents itself as an ECA with whom the user engages in free conversation about her working day, expecting to receive a sympathetic hearing of her difficulties.

We have termed this application the "How Was Your Day?" (henceforth HWYD) scenario. The ECA platform is a fully-implemented, end-to-end spoken Affective Dialogue System designed to support free conversation albeit on a quite limited set of topics. This departs from the dominant philosophy of dialogue systems in which user input tends to be shorter and where user and system dialogue turns regularly follow each other. From a language technology perspective it uses Information Extraction (IE) techniques to recognise key events described by the user. IE techniques are known for their robustness and are hence well-adapted to process lengthy utterances potentially containing speech recognition errors. The system is able to recognise over 40 event templates, which form the basis for its persuasive strategy, as the system will respond to the user's attitude from the perspective of current events. A dialogue manager controls the overall conversation, prompting the user for additional information where necessary, although the dialogue itself remains largely user-led, as illustrated in Figure 1. Affective aspects are also thoroughly integrated in the process: the system records the emotional state of the user using emotional speech recognition and stores them with the event description; the persuasive component is based on an appraisal of the user's emotional reaction and controls the ECA's expression; the ECA supports communicative acts described in an FML-like language [3] [4], which controls both animation and affective Text-To-Speech.

In a typical session, the ECA listens sympathetically to the user's account of her work difficulties, whilst also reacting to apparent discrepancies between her perceived mood and the affective content of the recognised events.

In the following example from a real conversation, the user announces a company restructuring, but in a rather cheerful tone:

```
(EmoVoice: Positive_Active)
<User1>: I have just learnt that my department is going to be
merged with the Barcelona one
<System2>: You sound a bit too ecstatic!
<System3>: I'm  doubtful   that   your   workload   could   be
maintained.
```

Fig. 2. Initial response corresponding to a warning strategy: the ECA aims to correct the user's attitude to a potentially serious event

Every time the Companion has gathered sufficient information it will try to respond more globally to the situation at hand. In the following separate example, after the user has expressed various concerns, the Companion summarises these negative elements picked from throughout the conversation[1]:

```
<System4:> who was at the meeting?
(EmoVoice: Negative-Active)
<User5>: only my team they gave me a set of PowerPoint slides
from the meeting I spent the rest of the day leading the
slides but my computer crashed several times because of the
updates
<System6>: it's forgivable how you must be feeling!
<System7>: it is always sad when you get more work because of
the technical problems.
<System8>: the  technical   problems   are   something   I   rather
hate.
<System9>: it's right to be down about such a bad situation.
<System10>: unfortunately missing the deadline is looking
likely if the technical problems persist.
<System11>: I   can   sympathise   with   the   situation   but
unfortunately the technical problems are out of your control.
```

Fig. 3. Example dialogue corresponding to a sympathetic strategy: the ECA, after empathising with the user's attitude, responds sympathetically to the negative consequences of the situation

These long utterances, or 'tirades', are the main mechanism through which the ECA attempts to influence the user. Whilst they form a natural part of a conversation, they actually constitute a short narrative whose elements are responses to the user's situation and the preoccupations expressed in his/her recollection of the working day. Tørning and Oinas-Kukkonen [5], in their classification of persuasive techniques, have identified 'suggestion' as one of the techniques supported by dialogue, and our approach is compatible with that framework.

The HWYD Companion is a fully-implemented multimodal affective dialogue system, which regularly supports meaningful dialogues exceeding 20 minutes in duration [6]. In the next sections, after discussing relevant previous work we introduce the theory behind these influencing statements, its formalisation and implementation

---

[1] We are using actual system transcripts, hence the inclusion of speech recognition errors such as, in the current example, 'leading' instead of 'reading'.

using AI planning techniques to support text generation, and finally how the quality of the ECA can be evaluated from the perspective of affective dialogue.

2 Previous and Related Work

In their classification of persuasive systems, [5] have distinguished those aiming at influencing user behaviour from those influencing user attitudes. This is an important distinction for our work, as our HWYD Companion agent is designed primarily to influence attitudes, unlike our early *Health and Fitness Companion* prototype [7], which was more similar in its philosophy to [8]. Inherent within human to human conversation is the communication, to varying degrees, of the emotional state of the participants. In developing ECA this brings about the dual challenges of understanding the emotional state of the user and correctly applying this information within the agent's responses. Cavalluzzi et al [2] describe an ECA designed to give advice to the user, adapting the advice-giving policy based on the attitude of the user.

Within the context of an agent giving advice on healthy eating, Cavalluzzi et al employ strategies based on the Transtheoretical Model (from [9]) that outlines five "Stages of Change" in a user's behaviour. From each stage a corresponding set of actions is derived to transition the user onto the next stage. Bickmore and Sidner [8] also employ the Transtheoretical Model combined with Motivational Interviewing, a client-centred counselling technique, in an agent designed to promote physical activity. Grasso et al [10] use a multi-layer approach with their nutrition adviser, *Daphne*. A high-level 'strategist' layer uses a combination of the Transtheoretical Model and the complementary Health Belief Model with a mid-level 'tactician' layer employing an informal argumentation theory (namely the New Rhetoric theory) and a low-level 'orator' level composed of linguistic knowledge. Across each of these advice-giving agents the common factor in the selection of the particular dialogue strategy is an understanding of where, in terms of the emotional landscape, the user is currently and where the agent wishes the user to be.

On the other hand, the emphasis of the work presented here is, firstly, on influencing users' attitudes towards a given situation rather than triggering change in a specific behaviour and, secondly, to blend influences within free conversation with the ECA rather than support them within task-oriented (or purposeful) dialogue.

3 A Narrative Model of Influence

Models of influence tend to rely on a combination of communication and behavioural strategies. The situation is somewhat more complex for persuasive systems which target attitude change, in particular when they rely on a significant affective component. One notable difficulty of affective dialogue is the seamless integration of communication and persuasion strategies: in other words, how to embed influence within the flow of natural dialogue rather than turn the dialogue itself into a negotiation session. To that effect, we have turned ourselves towards narrative models of influence. Tørning [11] has emphasised the role of rhetorics in persuasive systems and relations between narrative and rhetorics are well-known: these have included the adoption of rhetorical concepts by narratology [12] [13] and even the use of rhetorical structures to display information as a narrative [14]. Our interest in narrative does not stem so much from their obvious ability to elicit emotion but how this feature can be blended within their linguistic communication component. This is a point where traditional narratology [12] and some contemporary work on interactive narrative [15] [16] do converge. We have adapted Bremond's narrative theory of influence, which posits that one character can be influenced by another on the basis of his expected outcome for key narrative actions. For instance, a character expecting a loss is more readily influenced by another character mentioning how the prospect of that loss can be reduced.

Bremond's theory comprises two aspects: one relates influence to communicative acts to suggest when to expect advice, warning, or even commination. The other one identifies prototypical examples in narratives of such situations and proposes an ontology of influencing roles: this part is however difficult to generalise beyond the analysis of prototypical narratives. We have thus adapted it by relying on a default structure of events which allow for the better identification of helpers/antagonists, resources, conditions for event completion... as described in forthcoming sections.

Yet, the power of Bremond's model rests with its ability to recursively describe influences within a uniform framework (e.g. causal chains such as "a helper stopping a deterioration process") and to map these onto a set of simple communicative acts. This principle has been implemented in the Companion's appraisal strategy, which identifies the different roles of an event in terms of their influence. This can be extended beyond the strict (default) definition of an event: for instance, an event describing the promotion of the user to a higher position can be extended to include various antagonists such as competitors (persons applying for the same job) or opponents/facilitators (those involved in the decision process).

This makes it possible to define an influencing strategy from the event structures and the communicative acts most appropriate to convey that influence. Following Bremond, the key elements are the event's expected outcome and whether it would improve or deteriorate the user's situation. The next section describes how we have made these principles computational by defining influence strategies using planning techniques, whose operators seek inspiration in Bremond's influence rules.

4   Affective Strategies: Advice, Warning and Comforting Tirades

The ECA's affective strategy targets the user attitude towards his/her situation in the workplace and aims to positively influence that attitude. However, it is not meant to make this attitude the central topic of the conversation and to turn the whole dialogue into a coaching session. Rather, it inserts elements of affective dialogue within the normal flow of the conversation while that conversation remains driven by the user. This may consist of reinforcing positive situations, reassuring or sympathising in negative situations and to challenge user expectations that run counter to the ECA's expectation. To achieve maximum impact the ECA replies are organised as an influencing strategy adopting a narrative structure. This structure organises generic affective statements (empathy, etc.), comments on what may affect the event outcome, discussion of the implications of the outcome itself and finally the global philosophy of the situation. The module controlling the generation of the influencing strategy, which ultimately is translated into a short textual narrative, is referred to as the Affective Strategy Module (ASM).

The first step for the ASM consists of an appraisal process analysing the user's situation and how appropriate to that situation her emotional reaction is. The starting point of the appraisal process is an instantiated event template which also contains the emotional state recorded during the utterances reporting that event.

Table 1. Representative selection of operators with associated categorisation and communicative acts

Operator	Operator Category	Operator Sub-Category	Comm. Act
Empathise	Spontaneous Emotional Reaction *(agent reaction to the user's emotional state)*	N/A	recognise
Express-Agent-Opinion	Express Agent Attitude *(agent comments on emotional aspects of an event or influence)*	N/A	inform
Query-Response-to-General-Situation	Comment on Situation *(agent comments on the appropriateness of the user's emotional reaction to the situation)*	Warn *(inappropriate)*	question
Commend-Response-to-General-Situation		Reassure *(appropriate)*	approve
Advise-on-Anticipation-of-Outcome	Comment on Anticipation *(agent comments on whether the user's anticipation of the main event's outcome is consistent with the agent's anticipation)*	Warn *(inconsistent)*	advice
State-Disagreement-with-Anticipation		Deny *(inconsistent)*	disagree
State-Agreement-with-Anticipation		Confirm *(consistent)*	agree
Promote-User-Ability	Comment on User Ability *(agent comments on the user's ability to alter the outcome)*	Promote	praise
Demote-User-Ability		Demote	criticise
Warn-Threat	Comment on Influences *(agent comments on additional events or persons that may have a positive or negative effect on the main event)*	Threat *(negative event)*	warn
Play-Down-Antagonist		Antagonist *(negative person)*	inform
Reassure-Enabler		Enabler *(positive event)*	approve
Commend-Helper		Helper *(positive person)*	propose

Typical events reported by the user can imply a deterioration of her situation (office-move, redundancy, increased-workload), transient difficulties at work (missed deadline, arguments with colleagues) or potential for improvement (promotion, pay-rise). The ASM, upon instantiation of corresponding event templates by the dialogue manager, not only categorises the event in terms of its likely impact on the user's situation, but also analyses the default set of influences for the events at hand: positive influences such as enablers or helpers, negative influences such as threats or antagonists. These are used to implement the influencing strategy of the agent, giving a precise content to reassuring or warning statements: reassurance may play down the reality of a threat to the successful completion of a positive event whilst warnings may identify potential antagonists or emphasise the severity of a negative outcome which the user may appear to have overlooked.

The result of the appraisal phase is used to determine the overall strategy generated by the ECA, and in particular if the agent should encourage, comfort or warn the user. The role of the ASM module is to generate a short narrative whose backbone is constituted by a set of argumentative statements based on emotional operators (Empathise) or specific communicative (influence) operators. In common with both narrative generation [16] and textual generation [17], the ASM is based on planning technologies, more specifically a Hierarchical Task Network (HTN) planner [18], which works through recursive decomposition of a high level task into sub-tasks until a plan of sub-tasks is reached that can be directly executed. Here the tasks correspond to the various strategies for influencing the user (reassuring, cautionary, congratulatory... each of which can be decomposed into multiple tactics). The HTN planning process uses the information from the event templates along with results from the appraisal step as heuristics to guide its decomposition process. When combined with the fact that this heuristic selection process occurs at multiple levels of the HTN, it allows for considerably more complexity and variance than is achievable with a scripted approach.

The operators constituting the plan generated by the HTN implement Bremond's theory of influence by basing their advice on the structure and roles of the reported events. For instance, various operators can emphasise or play down the event consequences (Express-Likelihood-of-Result, Play-Down-Worry-About-Result, Express-Happiness-About-Result) or comment on additional factors that may affect the course of events (Commend-Enabler, Reassure-Helper). The planner uses a set of 40 operators, each of which can be in addition instantiated (parameterised) to incorporate specific elements of the event. Overall this supports the seamless generation of hundreds of significantly different influencing strategies from the base set of influence operators. A typical strategy corresponds to a sequence of operators, each of which will be translated into an utterance, the Natural Language Generation module mapping each operator to a communicative act (see Table 1).

It is worth observing at this point that the appraisal, and thus the strategy selection, can also be influenced to some degree by the 'personality' defined for the Companion. Currently there are three different parameters modelled to represent changes in personality between a Companion; whether the Companion is supportive towards the user or not, whether the Companion is self-focussed or user-focussed and whether the Companion's outlook is optimistic or pessimistic. The last of these can come into play with strategy selection as, for borderline cases, whether the Companion is optimistic or pessimistic will determine both the agent's anticipation of events and thus also the appropriateness of the user's anticipation.

```
<Op1> ((EMPATHISE POSITIVE LOW))
<Op2> ((QUERY-RESPONSE-TO-GENERAL-SITUATION       DETERIORATION
POSITIVE))
<Op3> ((STATE-AGREEMENT-WITH-ANTICIPATION          MERGER
DETERIORATION COMPLETE COMPLETE))
<Op4> ((WARN-THREAT  REDUNDANCY_OTHER  DETERIORATION  COMPLETE
MERGER))
<Op5> ((EXPRESS-WORRY-ABOUT-RESULT  INCREASE-WORKSTRESS   NIL
NIL MERGER))
<Op6> ((PROVIDE-MORAL WARNING MERGER DETERIORATION COMPLETE))
```

Fig. 4. Example of an influencing strategy generated by the HTN Planner for the Affective Strategy Module (ASM). The sequence of operators will be translated into a set of communicative acts constitutive of a short narrative influencing the user's emotional state.

5 Persuasive Dialogue for Attitude Change

In this section, we present more extensive excerpts of dialogue between the user and the system which illustrate the ECA's influencing strategy in the context of real dialogue sessions. The following dialogue corresponds to a warning strategy triggered by the finding that the user's emotional state, as detected through emotional speech recognition, is at odds with the situation s/he describes. This dialogue also corresponds to the screen capture of Figure 6.

```
<System12>: Hello, John. How did your day go?
(EmoVoice: Positive-Passive)
<User13>: hello Sam Weller my day has been a bit dramatic
<System14>: Indeed! Please, tell me more.
(EmoVoice: Positive-Passive)
<User15>: we've  just  lent  her  department  is  going  to  be
merged  with  the  Barcelona  one  I've  always  liked  working  in
the final department
<System16>: What do you think will happen next?
(EmoVoice: Positive-Passive)
<User17>: I  heard  some  people  will  be  moved  to  the  other
office  in  the  next  couple  of  months  hopefully  I  won't  get
laid  off  or  forced  on  with  their<System18>: You seem to be in
a good mood.
<System19>: But  are  you  sure  this  is  appropriate  for  the
situation?
<System20>: I also think the merger will go ahead.
<System21>: What  is  more  the  merger  is  likely  to  create
redundancies.
<System22>: I'm  worried  that  this  may  mean  more  stress  for
you.
<System23>: Remember  that  the  consequences  of  the  merger  are
likely to be bad.
```

Fig. 5. An example dialogue corresponding to a warning strategy: the Companion has detected a discrepancy between the emotional state of the user and the nature of the events under discussion (see also Figure 4 for the operators' sequence).

The last six system utterances of Figure 5 correspond to an influencing strategy (whose operators are represented on Figure 4), which aims at countering the user's casual attitude towards the announcement of a departmental merger. After acknowledging the user's mood the ECA immediately questions the user reaction (<Op2> Query-Response-to-General-Situation). This example illustrates how the generic operators are instantiated with event parameters specific to the situation at hand. If we consider the operator <Op4> Warn-Threat, it is instantiated with both the event (merger) and the specific type of threat (redundancy_other) to give the utterance <System21>. In a similar fashion, the operator <Op5> Express-Worry-About-Result is instantiated by default knowledge associated with the event category (work_stress) to give the utterance <System22>.

This typical example illustrates the many determinants contributing to the variability of the ECA's conversation: i) variations in strategies from the planner, ii) instantiation with the event's data, iii) use of default knowledge associated with event categories and iv) variability of surface expression from the natural language generation system.

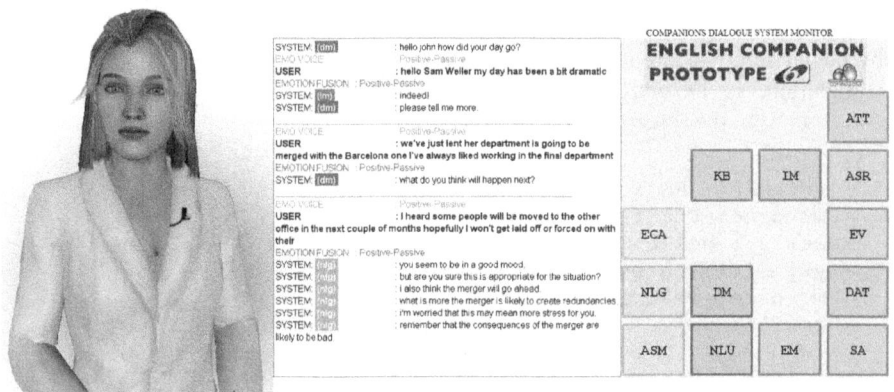

Fig. 6. The ECA in operation during the dialogue of Figure 5. The long utterances (tirades) corresponding to the influencing strategy are visible at the lower centre of the interface screen.

6   System Validation: Sentiment Analysis of the ECA's Affective Output

The evaluation of persuasive systems is a notoriously difficult task, even more so for attitude-changing persuasive systems, as the realistic evaluation of affective dialogue systems is faced with considerable difficulties related to the need to collect or induce actual affective situations. In our case, this would also involve prolonged use of the system by users in their everyday environment, without this being part of a structured behaviour-changing programme [8], as our scenario deals with a generic everyday aspect. In lieu of such user evaluation, which we hope to complete in the future, we present a validation of the affective output of the system.

We have devised a preliminary validation method which evaluates the appropriateness [19] of the ECA's utterances with respect to the appraisal of the user's attitude. This method is based on the independent analysis of the ECA's utterances by a Sentiment Analysis (SA) module, which has been independently tested and validated on large corpora.

The SA parser, described in [20], uses part-of-speech tagging, dependency parsing, large manually compiled sentiment lexica, a hand-written sentiment grammar, and compositional sentiment logic to assign positive/neutral/negative sentiment scores to individual words, syntactic phrases, entities, sentences, and documents.

The parser, tested on the SemEval-2007 Task #14 data set[2] of 1000 news headlines [21], reached an accuracy of 65.6~77.36% (86.06~91.33% on strong cases). At the level of noun phrases, it reached an accuracy of 73.39~85.87% (80.33~89.51% on strong cases) against 1541 explicit NPs from the FBS[3] product feature dataset [22].

The underlying hypothesis of the validation method is that the ECA's influencing strategy can be mapped onto the three categories of SA (positive, neutral and negative). A global mapping from the agent's narrative text to an SA category would probably be too crude to be helpful; this is why we are considering mapping at the utterance level. Influencing strategies correspond to a sequence of influence operators, such as Figure 4, to which an SA pattern can be associated, through the mapping of influence operators to their default emotional text appearance (e.g. comforting statements will map onto POS sentiment, whilst warnings will map onto NEG). For instance, an overall warning strategy such as depicted in Figures 4 and 5 would be compatible with an SA pattern such as [POS NEG POS NEG NEG NEG].

We carried out testing of the effectiveness of the influencing strategies by generating a total of 60 plans with 5 datasets (relating to 5 prototypical dialogue strategies utilising a range of different events and requiring separate affective strategies for each example). For each plan we then generated 5 tirades to account for the range of surface variation introduced by the natural language generation. This led to a total of 1395 utterances being generated (an average of 4.65 utterances per tirade).

We then calculated two sets of metrics for comparing the sentiment of the generated utterances against the target sentiment of the original influence operator. The first metric consisted of a scoring attributing 1 for a perfect match, 0 for a substitution of POS/NEG to NTR (Neutral) and -1 for all other cases. The second metric consisted of a scoring attributing 1 for a perfect match, -1 for a substitution of POS/NEG to NTR and -2 for all other cases.

Using the first metric, we received a total score of 1130 for the 1395 total utterances (an average score of 3.77 per tirade). This is a 'correctness' score of 81%[4]. Using the second metric, we received a total score of 994 for the 1395 total utterances (an average score of 3.31 per tirade). This is a 'correctness' score of 71%. The conclusion is that even for the more demanding metric, the overall sentiment of a tirade will almost always be in line with the ECA's goal in terms of positive or negative influence.

---

[2] http://www.cs.unt.edu/~rada/affectivetext
[3] http://www.cs.uic.edu/~liub/FBS/FBS.html
[4] Note that this is not a true percentage of correct answers due to negative marking.

Table 2. Details of the ECA's output used in the automatic sentiment analysis of the influencing utterances

Total Plans	Total Tirades	Total Utterances	Average Utterances (Per Tirade)
60	300	1395	4.65

Table 3. Evaluation of the ECA's output using automatic sentiment analysis of the influencing utterances (see text for comments)

Metric	Total Score	Correctness (%)	Average Score (Per Tirade)
Metric 1	1130	81	3.77
Metric 2	994	71	3.31

7 Conclusions

A Companion ECA may include various forms of persuasive dialogue: whilst some may correspond to traditional coaching features similar to those of previously described systems [2] [8], we have discussed in this paper a different form of persuasion, related to the most basic role of a Companion, that of a sympathetic listener. The main target of our ECA is the immediate user attitude, and it aims at influencing the user's affective state almost in real-time, at the end of his/her working day. We have shown that such influence can be embedded within the natural flow of dialogue, supporting the kind of light conversation a Companion should be able to support. The affective content of the ECA utterances, as measured independently by a SA module, is an accurate reflection of the intended influencing strategy determined from an appraisal of the user reaction. This now opens the way to a more traditional form of experimental evaluation.

Acknowledgments. This work was funded by the Companions project (http://www.companions-project.org) sponsored by the European Commission as part of the Information Society Technologies (IST) programme under EC grant number IST-FP6-034434. The EmoVoice system has been used courtesy of the Multimedia Concepts and Applications Group of the University of Augsburg.

References

1. André, E., Dybkjær, L., Minker, W., Heisterkamp, P. (eds.): ADS 2004. LNCS (LNAI), vol. 3068. Springer, Heidelberg (2004)
2. Cavalluzzi, A., Carofiglio, V., de Rosis, F.: Affective Advice Giving Dialogs. In: André, E., Dybkjær, L., Minker, W., Heisterkamp, P. (eds.) ADS 2004. LNCS (LNAI), vol. 3068, pp. 77–88. Springer, Heidelberg (2004)
3. Hernández, A., López, B., Pardo, D., Santos, R., Hernández, L., Relaño Gil, J., Rodríguez, M.C.: Modular definition of multimodal ECA communication acts to improve dialogue robustness and depth of intention. In: Heylen, D., Kopp, S., Marsella, S., Pelachaud, C., Vilhjálmsson, H. (eds.) AAMAS 2008 Workshop on Functional Markup Language (2008)

4. Heylen, D., Kopp, S., Marsella, S., Pelachaud, C., Vilhjálmsson, H.H.: The Next Step towards a Function Markup Language. In: Prendinger, H., Lester, J.C., Ishizuka, M. (eds.) IVA 2008. LNCS (LNAI), vol. 5208, pp. 270–280. Springer, Heidelberg (2008)
5. Tørning, K., Oinas-Kukkonen, H.: Persuasive system design: state of the art and future directions. In: Proceedings of the fourth International Conference on Persuasive Technology, Persuasive 2009, New York, NY, USA, vol. 350 (2009)
6. Cavazza, M., Santos de la Camara, R., Turunen, M., and the Companions consortium: How was your day? A Companion ECA. In: Proceedings of AAMAS 2010, accepted for publication (demonstration paper), Toronto (2010)
7. Smith, C., Cavazza, M., Charlton, D., Zhang, L., Turunen, M., Hakulinen, J.: Integrating Planning and Dialogue in a Lifestyle Agent. In: Prendinger, H., Lester, J.C., Ishizuka, M. (eds.) IVA 2008. LNCS (LNAI), vol. 5208, pp. 146–153. Springer, Heidelberg (2008)
8. Bickmore, T., Sidner, C.L.: Towards Plan-based Health Behavior Change Counseling Systems. In: Proceedings of AAAI Spring Symposium on Argumentation for Consumers of Healthcare, Stanford, CA (2006)
9. Prochaska, J., Di Clemente, C., Norcross, H.: In search of how people change: applications to addictive behavior. Americal Psychologist 47, 1102–1114 (1992)
10. Grasso, F., Cawsey, A., Jones, R.: Dialectical argumentation to solve conflicts in advice giving: a case study in the promotion of healthy nutrition. Int. J. Human-Computer Studies 53, 1077–1115 (2000)
11. Tørning, K.: Persuasive Technology Design – A Rhetorical Approach. In: Oinas-Kukkonen, H., Hasle, P., Harjumaa, M., Segerståhl, K., Øhrstrøm, P. (eds.) PERSUASIVE 2008. LNCS, vol. 5033, pp. 83–93. Springer, Heidelberg (2008)
12. Bremond, C.: Logique du Recit. Editions du Seuil, Paris (1973) (in French)
13. Roland, B.: Rhétorique de l'image. Communications 4, 40–51 (1964) (in French)
14. Nakasone, A., Ishizuka, M.: SRST: A Storytelling Model Using Rhetorical Relations. In: Göbel, S., Malkewitz, R., Iurgel, I. (eds.) TIDSE 2006. LNCS, vol. 4326, pp. 127–138. Springer, Heidelberg (2006)
15. Marsella, G., Gratch, J.: Modeling Coping Behavior in Virtual Humans: Don't Worry, Be Happy. In: Proceedings of AAMAS 2003, Melbourne, Australia, pp. 313–320 (2003)
16. Pizzi, D., Charles, F., Lugrin, J.-L., Cavazza, M.: Interactive Storytelling with Literary Feelings. In: Paiva, A.C.R., Prada, R., Picard, R.W. (eds.) ACII 2007. LNCS, vol. 4738, pp. 630–641. Springer, Heidelberg (2007)
17. Appelt, D.E.: Planning English Sentences. Cambridge University Press, Cambridge (1985)
18. Nau, D., Ghallab, M., Traverso, P.: Automated Planning: Theory & Practice. Morgan Kaufmann Publishers Inc., San Francisco (2004)
19. Traum, D.R., Robinson, S., Stephan, J.: Evaluation of multi-party virtual reality dialogue interaction. In: Proceedings of Fourth International Conference on Language Resources and Evaluation (LREC), pp. 1699–1702 (2004)
20. Moilanen, K., Pulman, S.: Sentiment Composition. In: Proceedings of the Recent Advances in Natural Language Processing International Conference (RANLP 2007), Borovets, pp. 378–382 (2007)
21. Strapparava, C., Mihalcea, R.: SemEval-2007 Task 14: Affective Text. In: The Proceedings of the fourth International Workshop on Semantic Evaluations (SemEval 2007), Association for Computational Linguistics, Prague, pp. 70–74 (2007)
22. Hu, M., Liu, B.: Mining and Summarizing Customer Reviews. In: The Proceedings of the Tenth ACM SIGKDD International Conference on Knowledge Discovery and Data Mining (KDD 2004), Association for Computing Machinery, Seattle, pp. 168–177 (2004)

Generating Directions for Persuasive Technology Design with the Inspiration Card Workshop

Janet Davis

Dept. of Computer Science
Grinnell College
Grinnell, IA 50112, USA
davisjan@cs.grinnell.edu

Abstract. Participatory design methods may help account for the ethical implications of persuasive technology. But how can participatory design methods both address ethical issues and lead to effective persuasive technologies? This paper presents the early stages of participatory design with a college EcoHouse. I discuss concepts resulting from an Inspiration Card Workshop [1], finally considering further development of participatory methods for designing persuasive technology.

Keywords: Persuasive technology, participatory design, Inspiration Card Workshop, conceptual design, design materials.

1   Introduction

The discourses of persuasive technology [2,3] and human-computer interaction more broadly [4] have engendered many technological interventions intended to promote more environmentally sustainable behavior. Although most would agree that helping people to reduce their environmental impacts is a good end, even design to a good end brings moral responsibility. The designer must be concerned not only with the ethical implications of persuasive strategies—for example, privacy in systems that monitor activity—but also issues of autonomy and consent raised by the act of persuasion itself [5].

While some have developed ethical principles for persuasive technology [2,6], Davis argues that designers need methods to help them account for their ethical responsibilities [5]. Participatory design, with its commitment to engaging future users as full partners in the design process [7], has some promise. Moreover, Goodman argues that participatory design can help account for stakeholders' differing beliefs about the human relationship to nature [4]. In reference to the work of DiSalvo, et al. [8], Goodman explains that participatory design "can help empower potential users to surface, reflect upon, and creatively respond to their own unmet needs" [4]. But with the exception of recent work by DiSalvo [8] and Miller, Rich, and Davis [9], there has been little exploration of participatory approaches to persuasive technology design or to sustainable interaction design.

I aim to further such exploration through work with a student project house, EcoHouse. The design goal is to implement persuasive technology to support

T. Ploug, P. Hasle, H. Oinas-Kukkonen (Eds.): PERSUASIVE 2010, LNCS 6137, pp. 262–273, 2010.
© Springer-Verlag Berlin Heidelberg 2010

EcoHouse's mission of enacting and promoting environmentally sustainable campus life. The research goal is to consider two questions. First, how can participatory design methods lead to effective persuasive technologies? Second, what are the ethical outcomes? How do participants and non-participants relate to the resulting persuasive technology—both the intentions behind it and the strategies it employs? Prior work in this space does not fully address these questions. DiSalvo, et al. focused on participation as empowerment and technology as rhetoric [8]; there is no evident intent to deploy any technologies. Although Miller, Rich, and Davis had this intent and used a participatory approach, the final concept was developed mainly by the designers [9]. This paper begins to address these questions by relating the early stages of participatory design with EcoHouse.

Thus far, there are few published methods for designing persuasive technology to draw upon. Fogg's 8-step process [10] is appealing in a participatory context because it provides a flexible framework for the early stages of design and is intended for new persuasive technology designers. Though deviating in significant ways, this work is informed by Fogg's recommendations.

In this paper, I will briefly present the design context, report on exploring the space through field study and generative tools [11], explain how the Inspiration Card Workshop [1] generated design concepts, and finally discuss this participatory approach and future directions in light of the questions above.

2   Design Context

This work is set at a small, residential liberal arts college in the midwestern United States. The college has three *project houses*, student residences allocated through an annual competitive process. EcoHouse's proposal for the 2009-2010 academic year sets forth not only a broad goal for residents to live sustainably, but also three more specific goals, each supported by a committee: first, to conduct educational outreach through events and workshops; second, to raise a garden in EcoHouse's backyard and use its produce; and third, to collaborate with the college's Facilities Management (FM) unit in testing new technologies and practices for possible use elsewhere on campus. I chose to approach EcoHouse as an opportunity space, "where many new things are possible but there is no clear requirement" [12], and therefore scoped the early stages of the design process to consider all aspects of EcoHouse's mission.

All ten of EcoHouse's residents for the fall 2009 semester (4 men, 6 women) initially agreed to participate in this design project. However, one resident left the house mid-term and withdrew from the project. The remaining nine residents participated to varying degrees over the course of the semester.

3   Exploring the Space

This project began with ethnographically-inspired field methods, which have a longstanding role in participatory design [13]. I briefly interviewed participants about their goals, hopes, and concerns for living in EcoHouse, their relation to EcoHouse's mission, and their comfort with potential technology channels. I also obtained documents such as the aforementioned proposal. Finally, I acted as a participant-observer in EcoHouse's weekly dinner meetings. Although field study informed my work in other ways, here I will focus on persuasive technology channels and on one persuasive technology already in use at EcoHouse.

Fogg points out that designers should choose a persuasive technology channel based not only on the target behavior, but also on the habits of the target audience [10]. Somewhat surprisingly, not all of the college student participants reported being active Facebook or mobile phone users. Several participants have Facebook accounts but rarely use them; one has no account. Although all participants have mobile phones, some keep them turned off, due to cost, poor reception, or personal preference. Participants did report using email and the Web on a daily basis, making these potentially appropriate technology channels. Moreover, the common space of EcoHouse itself could support ambient displays.

Field study revealed a few simple, ad hoc persuasive systems already in place at EcoHouse. Most relevant here is a metering system installed last year to help residents monitor their energy and water consumption. This system has been a mixed success. On one hand, the system is inaccessible and hard to use. Some residents described the system as a mysterious thing lurking in the basement. On the other hand, members of the FM committee produced monthly and daily trend graphs, from which they have identified high-consumption activities (heating, cooking, and showering) as targets for behavior change.

Beyond my own analysis of the site, I wanted participants to be active partners in reflecting on their own behaviors and intentions. However, participatory methods for understanding workplace tasks seemed problematic in EcoHouse's home setting. Instead, I designed a package of materials for participants to complete and reflect upon on their own time, that would feed into later stages of the design process. While these generative tools are similar in form to those in a cultural probes package [14], in a participatory context they are intended to serve as "primes" to begin engaging the participants' creativity [11], as well as a source of information and inspiration for design.

I delivered the materials at the house's second weekly meeting, stressing the opportunity for fun and reflection. I told participants that the materials could be completed in groups or individually, and that there was no need for consensus, nor to complete them all. In keeping with the environmental focus, I constructed a display and many of the individual items from reused materials. The generative tools remained for four weeks in EcoHouse's living room. The package included

- Cards with questions and images to evoke stories, reflection, and analysis;
- Three cards offering "three wishes" for new things for EcoHouse [15], to get participants imagining changes to the house;
- A disposable camera with prompts to take photos of scenes such as "something to use more" and "a guilty pleasure", to promote playful reflection;
- Floorplans of the house with instructions to annotate them with activities and resources consumed in different locations;

– A Sustainability Diary asking participants to complete the sentence "Today I'm proud of myself because I..." on a "green day" and "Today I wanted to...but I didn't because..." on a "not so green day".

These last three items were intended in part as a kind of "investigative participation" [16] to help participants identify desirable behaviors and barriers that prevent those behaviors, both early steps of Fogg's 8-step process [10].

Participants responded well to the generative tools, completing more than half the materials. Several participants contributed, sometimes even to a single item. Their enjoyment was apparent in some elaborate responses. Though not systematic, the responses revealed desires for behavior change—for example, to reduce food waste, take fewer or shorter showers, do chores more reliably, and avoid buying "cheap, industrial" food. Although some participants clearly desired these changes for themselves, some comments seemed more directed at others. One item, a blank pie chart, unexpectedly inspired a participant to classify ways in which EcoHousers act or fail to act sustainably. He divided sustainable actions into individual decisions such as turning off lights and group decisions such as buying a farm share. But he also considered *barriers* to sustainable action: "unconscious actions" or habits, "accidental unsustainability" due to a "lack of knowledge," "devil's bargains" where there is no good choice; and finally "laziness/apathy." Even in this group organized around environmental sustainability, the most apparent barrier was a lack of motivation to prioritize sustainability over other conflicting desires—for example, participants wrote in the Sustainability Diary about giving in to the desire to buy a favorite flavor of ice cream or overcoming the aversion to working outdoors on a muddy morning. Beyond the desire for comfort, three different participants cited a lack of time as a barrier to achieving house goals. The participants have some freedom in managing their time commitments, but may prioritize other highly valued activities, such as their academic work, over work for EcoHouse. Thus, although a lack of motivation may simply be "apathy," it may arise from competing values.

4   Inspiration Card Workshop

To move from analysis and reflection to design, I used Halskov and Dalsgård's Inspiration Card Workshop [1]. As suggested by the name, the key materials are the Inspiration Cards, which provide simple, tangible representations of domain concepts and inspirational technologies. During the workshop, participants and designers select and combine cards to create new design concepts. Below, I discuss the the Domain and Technology Cards, the workshop, and its results.

4.1   Domain Cards

Domain Cards represent concepts from the design domain: in this case, Eco-House. The front of each Domain Card comprises a title and an image; the back

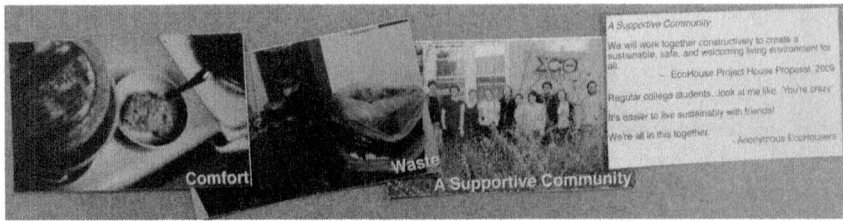

Fig. 1. *Comfort, Waste,* and *A Supportive Community* (shown front and back) are three examples from the 27 Domain Cards used to represent concepts from EcoHouse

uses words to further evoke or explicate the concept (figure 1). The Domain Cards are intended to support participants in making design moves such as juxtaposing concepts or shifting from the concrete to the abstract [1].

Halskov and Dalsgård suggest that Domain Cards can be created either by the designers or by participants [1]. In the interest of both fostering participation and respecting participants' time, I first identified 55 possible Domain Cards by reviewing EcoHouse documents, interview transcripts, my notes from participant-observation, and the generative tools and then I met with three participants to validate and prioritize the concepts. Groups of "unimportant," "vague," and "redundant" cards emerged. Of the final 27 Domain Cards, participants helped to distill, augment, clarify, or rename ten concepts, more than a third of the total; participants also proposed two entirely new cards. Finally, I chose pictures and words to illustrate each concept. When possible, I selected a photo from the results of the generative tools, thus reflecting participants' own work back to them in this intermediate product [17]. For the remainder, I enlisted a participant's help in taking additional photos at EcoHouse, or chose stock photos. For the backs of the cards, in most cases I used participants' own words. For concepts that were clearly important but less explicitly discussed, such as *Water*, I used quotations from published sources.

4.2   Technology Cards

Technology Cards depict inspirational technologies. Like the Domain Cards, these serve as tokens to support design moves, but also to educate participants about technological options. The front of each card shows a photograph or screen shot, while the back gives a description and a citation (Figure 2).

Halskov and Dalsgård recommend that the designers determine the set of technology cards based on their expertise [1]. In selecting the Technology Cards, I followed Fogg's recommendation to work from example persuasive technologies that share an audience, technology channel, or target behavior with the design problem at hand [10]. However, because of the broad scope, the 18 Technology Cards cover a range of behaviors related to environmental sustainability: conserving energy (4 cards), water (2), and paper (1), making sustainable choices while shopping (1), and increasing recycling (1). I also included two persuasive

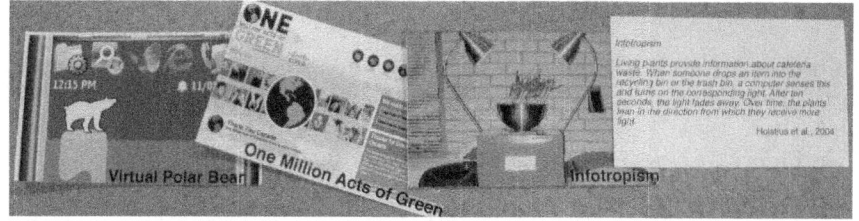

Fig. 2. The *Virtual Polar Bear* [18], *One Million Acts of Green* [19], and *Infotropism* [20] (shown front and back) are examples of the 18 Technology Cards

web sites concerned with "sharing goals" for environmental sustainability, as classified by Zapico, Turpeinen, and Brandt [3]. Based on the interviews, I included both ambient displays (8 cards) and web sites (5) as preferred technology channels. Finally, I considered not only the college student audience (5 cards), but also the context of home (5). Some Technology Cards fall into multiple categories: for example, Oberlin's dorm energy competition [21] overlaps the current project in audience, technology channel, *and* target behavior.

I included as provocation two cards that arguably fall on the borderline of persuasive technology. First, the Shower Manager [22], marketed to parents of teenagers, reduces the water pressure after a pre-set time has elapsed as negative feedback to discourage long showers. Second, "These Come from Trees" stickers [23] are not a computational technology at all, but are an excellent example of the *kairos* strategy [2] when placed on a paper towel dispenser.

4.3   Workshop Agenda

The Inspiration Cards served as the basis for two, two-hour workshops on consecutive Saturdays, one with four participants and the other with three. These workshops were audio recorded, and took place in my research lab in order to gain distance from the context of use and shift into a design mind-set.

First, I introduced the agenda and goal for the workshop: to generate ideas for new technologies in support of EcoHouse's mission of promoting sustainable living. The Domain Cards were presented by one of the participants who had helped to review them, while I presented the Technology Cards. Where the domain concepts were familiar to participants, the technologies were mostly new and prompted questions and discussion. The main part of the workshop is the Combination and Co-Creation phase. I explained that participants could select any cards to create a new idea; illustrate the idea as a poster using the cards, tape, and markers; and use blank cards to introduce other inspirational technologies or domain concepts. As Halskov and Dalsgård recommend [1], the workshop had no rules for taking turns or combining cards, so participants could use the cards in a variety of ways. At the end of the workshop, participants explained their ideas to each other; I photographed each poster to capture its final state. At the participants' request, this became a discussion of next steps.

4.4 Workshop Results

The primary results of the workshops are the posters depicting design concepts. Participants generated a total of 26 concepts, 14 in the first workshop and 12 in the second. Table 1 gives participants' spoken descriptions of selected posters, while Figure 3 shows examples of the posters themselves.

Design concepts combined as many as eight cards and as few as one, with a median of one Technology Card and three Domain Cards. One pattern was to combine a single Technology Card with a few Domain Cards showing how the technology could support EcoHouse's mission. For example, a participant explains how the *Weather Beacon* [24] could help them to proactively manage the house's heating system, in relation to *Energy* and *Changing with the Seasons* (Table 1, B8). However, other ideas were more innovative in their combinations: for example, combining the domain concepts of *Energy* and *Cooking and Eating* with the *Breakaway* [25] technology to produce an ambient display that suggests taking advantage of the oven's residual heat after it is turned off (Table 1, B10).

All the design concepts reflect an intent to change behavior. By my analysis of the posters and participants' spoken descriptions, each concept employs at least one persuasive strategy. Moreover, as shown in Figure 4a, the strategies used by participants are similar to those represented in the Technology Cards. While most strategies are drawn from the taxonomy of Oinas-Kukkonen and Harjumaa [26], I decided to include negative feedback because it is the strategy used by the provocative *Shower Manager* [22]. I also included setting goals [27] and connection with nature [18] as strategies evident in the Technology Cards.

Furthermore, nearly all the design concepts target behaviors related to Eco-House's mission. Conserving energy was the single behavior most frequently targeted by participants (8 of 26 concepts). However, 9 of the 26 concepts, including that described in Table 1, A14, aimed to generally promote sustainable behaviors and sustainability projects, falling into Zapico, Turpeinen, and Brandt's "sharing goals" category of climate persuasive services [3].

Participants considered themselves an audience for most (20/26) of the design concepts. However, in keeping with the domain concepts of *Educational Outreach* and EcoHouse as *A Testing Ground* and *An Example for Others*, eleven of the design concepts explicitly consider other students; in four cases, other students are the sole or primary audience. Moreover, participants in each workshop proposed engaging with students with similar goals at other colleges or universities.

The technology channels used in participants' concepts reflect the Technology Cards, but with some differences (Figure 4b). Participants based more than a third (10/26) of their design concepts on the Web, perhaps because of its familiarity. Participants also envisioned two email-based persuasive technologies, even though email was not represented in the Technology Cards. Two types of design concepts were questionably persuasive *technology*. First, one poster proposed a policy concerning technology distribution: "Every Student Gets a Power Strip" to help reduce standby power consumption on campus. Second, six of the design concepts are uses of non-computational devices that nonetheless embody persuasive strategies. For example, one participant proposed a salad spinner to store

Table 1. Participants' descriptions of selected design concepts

ID	Participant's Description
A1	"A way to provide feedback on how much water we're using and...not to exceed our stated goal.... When you use water, it drains water out of the fish tank, and if you you too much water, you risk killing the fish."
A5	"Some sort of visual display of how much energy you're using.... Option one is like the mug where when you put hot water into it the glaciers melt and the water floods the land. And then option two is that the globe would glow red if you're using a lot of energy and glow blue if you're not."
A12	"Send a picture in an email of the delicious food that you are cooking, and that can be an extra incentive for hungry people [to come share it]."
A14	"Using online tools...so that we can share what kinds of projects we're doing, what ideas we have...talking to other eco-houses about what they're doing and ideas that they have, how they overcame their conflicts with sustainability.... That would offer us motivation, kind of like the competitive urge to do more...."
B5	"The journal in the Cultural Probes was good for making us think of what we were actually doing in EcoHouse and what we were succeeding at, and also, the ones that said, today I am not so proud of myself because I ... those were also a good way to keep us on track. And we don't have anything like that right now."
B8	"If we had something that had a very visual forecast of the weather, then we could anticipate changes in the weather, and adjust the heating system accordingly.... If it's going to get warmer, we could turn the heat off in advance. If it's going to get colder, we could close the windows."
B10	"Every time people use the oven, maybe the thing would perk up, and then gradually settle down as the oven cooled. So that if people were walking by, they could see someone had used the oven recently...and say, I was planning to bake later, but I'll bake now...go ahead and use that energy."
B11	"Especially with greens, a lot of the time they didn't get eaten...and part of it for me was just that I didn't want to have to worry about taking them out and washing them. But with the salad spinner we could prepare everything when the CSA comes so that it's ready and available to eat."

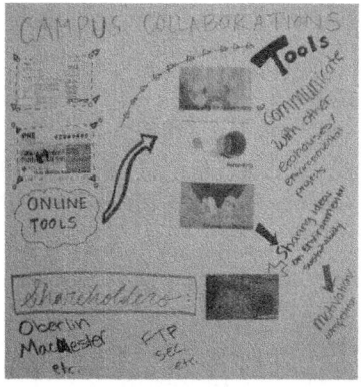
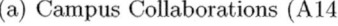

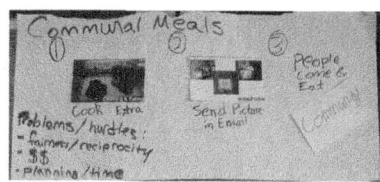

(b) Communal meals (A12)

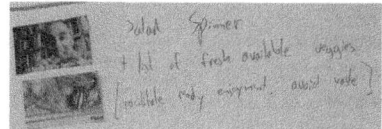

(a) Campus Collaborations (A14)   (c) Using a salad spinner (B11)

Fig. 3. Sample design concept posters from the Inspiration Card Workshops

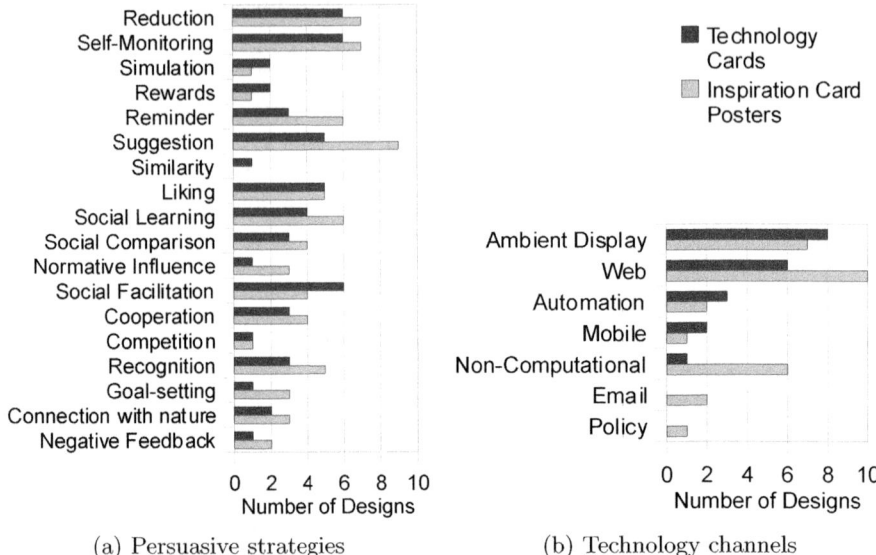

Fig. 4. Persuasive strategies and technology channels in the participants' design concepts versus the input Technology Cards

clean salad greens; he intended a reduction strategy [2], simplifying preparation of the greens when they are used (Table 1, B11).

Finally, the design concepts are all feasible, though some require more fleshing out. Indeed, we are working towards implementation of several. At the end of each workshop, participants identified a non-computational design to implement immediately: A "Props Board" to promote positive recognition of each others' contributions, and a return of the Sustainability Diary, described in Table 1, B5. In plenary discussions, we decided on four other directions:

- The oven tell-tale described in Table 1, B10, a fairly simple intervention;
- Evolving the "Every Student Gets a Power Strip" policy, to consider "smart" power strips and targeted distribution;
- Systems to make feedback on resource consumption more visible and frequent, perhaps through an ambient display such as those of Table 1, A5;
- A social networking site to connect college eco-houses, promoting sustainable behaviors through recognition, social learning, and so on.

I began this exploration with concern about the ethical implications of persuasive technology. Although participants were not prompted to discuss ethical issues, some such discussions arose. Indeed, the very first concept, involving a live goldfish (Table 1, A1), understandably raised concerns about the welfare of the fish and the users: "You'd have to set [the target consumption] high enough that you'd have to try pretty hard to kill the fish. But then if you did, how traumatic is that?" Arguably, the stakes are high enough that this is coercion rather than persuasion. One participant seemed to recognize the potentially co-ercive nature of the Shower Manager [22], saying, "I just resent the fact that we might need technology to enforce that." In considering its use in college locker rooms, one participant said, "the danger is that there would be a backlash.... We're infringing on their right to have a long shower, so [we must] inform peo-ple as to why it is important." Although "informing" might not be enough, the participant seems aware that the Shower Manager might change behaviors but is unlikely to positively affect attitudes. Furthermore, in one case participants questioned not only the means of behavior change, but the change itself. They proposed a system to facilitate impromptu communal meals (Figure 3b and Table 1, A12), to promote community and save energy. But they soon realized this could cause not only practical problems with planning meals, but also prob-lems with "reciprocity and fairness in terms of who's cooking all the time."

5   Conclusions and Future Work

The EcoHouse Inspiration Card Workshop succeeded in several ways. Partici-pants generated a range of feasible design concepts. The Technology Cards seem to have guided participants to use persuasive strategies in their designs. And the workshop created a space for participants to reflect upon desired behavior changes in EcoHouse and on campus, and consider means for achieving those changes. One participant said, "I wish everyone could have been here."

However, the method as applied also had shortcomings. In the space of persua-sive technologies, the concepts generated by participants are not wildly innova-tive: social networking sites are already being used for persuasion, and there are off-the-shelf systems for monitoring resource consumption and reducing phan-tom load. Furthermore, participants' non-computational approaches to persua-sion were a surprise. But, the research problem here is not to develop novel persuasive media or strategies, rather to explore participatory design methods. A successful participatory design project could adapt *existing* technology to par-ticipants' needs. Moreover, Fogg's 8-step process suggests that novice persuasive technology designers learn and build confidence by closely imitating existing per-suasive technologies [10]. At the same time, the broad scope of this Inspiration Card Workshop means that concepts differ in behavior, audience, and technology channel, and cannot be directly compared as Fogg recommends [10].

My process thus far has made use of established design methods, filling in the blanks with topics and examples related to persuasive technology. In future work, I plan to explore further development of participatory design methods to directly address persuasion and its attendant ethical issues. With more specific couplings of target behavior, audience, and technology channel now identified, one approach is to conduct further Inspiration Card Workshops. Technology Cards could be more tightly focused; Domain Cards could more directly repre-sent contexts for the desired behavior and the barriers that prevent the behavior. Where a number of possibilities have already been identified—notably, in consid-ering the many commercial devices that help reduce phantom load—we can move directly into a participatory process of gaining concrete experience [28] with the technologies, testing them more or less as Fogg suggests [10]. But, when should ethical issues be an explicit focus? How could design activities or materials help foreground these issues in a participatory process?

Returning to the earlier steps of Fogg's process [10], it seems that an audience and target behavior must be identified to bring participants together. Selecting a single technology channel may create opportunities for more structured participatory design activities. For example, DiSalvo, et al. [8] and Miller, et al. [9] both selected sensor-actuator systems, and developed games in which participants explored a physical space to identify possible target behaviors. Could a similar approach be effective for mobile persuasion? How might games or other activities get at behaviors that are better suited to other technology channels? And how might participatory methods go beyond the generative tools used here to facilitate reflection on value conflicts and other barriers to desired behaviors?

Finally, EcoHouse is interesting as an extreme group: not only are participants already committed to sustainable living, but many have some expertise. .expertise. What, then, might be the role of experts in a participatory design process where users desire behavior change but are not experts themselves?

Acknowledgments. Thanks to the fall 2009 EcoHouse residents for their investment in this work, to Kim Halskov for answering my questions, and to the reviewers of an earlier version of this paper for their helpful advice.

References

1. Halskov, K., Dalsgård, P.: Inspiration card workshops. In: 6th Conference on Designing Interactive systems, pp. 2–11. ACM, New York (2006)
2. Fogg, B.: Persuasive Technology: Using Computers to Change What We Think and Do. Morgan Kaufmann, San Francisco (2003)
3. Zapico, J.L., Turpeinen, M., Brandt, N.: Climate persuasive services: changing behavior towards low-carbon lifestyles. In: 4th International Conference on Persuasive Technology. ACM, New York (2009)
4. Goodman, E.: Three environmental discourses in human-computer interaction. In: CHI 2009 Extended Abstracts on Human Factors in Computing Systems, pp. 2535–2544. ACM, New York (2009)
5. Davis, J.: Design methods for ethical persuasive computing. In: 4th International Conference on Persuasive Technology. ACM, New York (2009)
6. Berdichevsky, D., Neuenschwander, E.: Toward an ethics of persuasive technology. Communications of the ACM 43(5), 51–58 (1999)
7. Bødker, S., Grønbæk, K., Kyng, M.: Cooperative design: Techniques and experiences from the Scandanavian scene. In: Schuler, D., Namioka, A. (eds.) Participatory Design: Principles and Practices, pp. 157–175. Lawrence Erlbaum, Mahwah (1993)
8. DiSalvo, C., Nourbakhsh, I., Holstius, D., Akin, A., Louw, M.: The neighborhood networks project: A case study of critical engagement and creative expression through participatory design. In: Tenth Anniversary Conference on Participatory Design, Indiana University Conferences, Bloomington, IN, USA, pp. 41–50 (2008)

9. Miller, T.M., Rich, P., Davis, J.: ADAPT: Audience design of ambient persuasive technology. In: CHI 2009 Extended Abstracts on Human Factors in Computing Systems, pp. 4165–4170. ACM, New York (2009)
10. Fogg, B.: Creating persuasive technologies: An eight-step design process. In: 4th International Conference on Persuasive Technology. ACM, New York (2009)
11. Sanders, E.B.N.: Design research in 2006. Design Research Quarterly 1(1), 4–8 (2006)
12. Hornecker, E., Halloran, J., Fitzpatrick, G., Weal, M., Millard, D., Michaelides, D., Cruickshank, D., De Roure, D.: Ubicomp in opportunity spaces: Challenges for participatory design. In: 9th Conference on Participatory Design, pp. 47–56. ACM, New York (2006)
13. Blomberg, J., Giocomi, J., Mosher, A., Swenton-Wall, P.: Ethnographic field methods and the relation to design. In: Schuler, D., Namioka, A. (eds.) Participatory Design: Principles and Practices, Lawrence Erlbaum Associates, Mahwah (1993)
14. Gaver, B., Dunne, T., Pacenti, E.: Cultural probes. Interactions 6(1), 21–29 (1999)
15. Blythe, M., Monk, A., Park, J.: Technology biographies: Field study techniques for home use product development. In: CHI 2002 Extended Abstracts on Human Factors in Computing Systems, pp. 658–659. ACM, New York (2002)
16. Graham, C., Rouncefield, M.: Probes and participation. In: Tenth Anniversary Conference on Participatory Design, Indiana University Conferences, Bloomington, IN, USA, pp. 194–197 (2008)
17. van Rijn, H., Stappers, P.J.: Expressions of ownership: Motivating users in a co-design process. In: Tenth Anniversary Conference on Participatory Design, Indiana University Conferences, Bloomington, IN, USA, pp. 178–181 (2008)
18. Froehlich, J., Dillahunt, T., Klasnja, P., Mankoff, J., Consolvo, S., Harrison, B., Landay, J.A.: UbiGreen: Investigating a mobile tool for tracking and supporting green transportation habits. In: CHI 2009 Conference on Human Factors in Computing Systems, pp. 1043–1052. ACM, New York (2009)
19. One million acts of green, http://www.cbc.ca/green/
20. Holstius, D., Kembel, J., Hurst, A., Wan, P.H., Forlizzi, J.: Infotropism: Living and robotic plants as interactive displays. In: 5th Conference on Designing Interactive Systems, pp. 215–221. ACM, New York (2004)
21. Petersen, J.E., Shunturov, V., Janda, K., Platt, G., Weinberger, K.: Dormitory residents reduce electricity consumption when exposed to real-time visual feedback and incentives. Int. Journal of Sustainability in Higher Ed. 8, 16–33 (2007)
22. Shower Manager, http://www.showermanager.com/
23. These come from trees, http://thesecomefromtrees.blogspot.com/
24. Weather beacon, http://www.ambientdevices.com/cat/beacon/
25. Jafarinaimi, N., Forlizzi, J., Hurst, A., Zimmerman, J.: Breakaway: An ambient display designed to change human behavior. In: CHI 2005 Extended Abstracts on Human Factors in Computing Systems, pp. 1945–1948. ACM, New York (2005)
26. Oinas-Kukkonen, H., Harjumaa, M.: A systematic framework for designing and evaluating persuasive systems. In: Oinas-Kukkonen, H., Hasle, P., Harjumaa, M., Segerståhl, K., Øhrstrøm, P. (eds.) PERSUASIVE 2008. LNCS, vol. 5033, pp. 164–176. Springer, Heidelberg (2008)
27. Consolvo, S., Klasnja, P., McDonald, D.W., Landay, J.A.: Goal-setting considerations for persuasive technologies that encourage physical activity. In: 4th International Conference on Persuasive Technology. ACM, New York (2009)
28. Kensing, F., Munk-Madsen, A.: PD: Structure in the toolbox. Communications of the ACM 36, 78–85 (1993)

Designing Effective Persuasive Systems Utilizing the Power of Entanglement: Communication Channel, Strategy and Affect

Haiqing Li and Samir Chatterjee

School of Information Systems and Technology, Claremont Graduate University,
130 E. 9th Street, Claremont, CA, 91711, USA
{Haiqing.Li,Samir.Chatterjee}@cgu.edu

Abstract. With rapid advances in information and communication technology, computer-mediated communication (CMC) technologies are utilizing multiple IT platforms such as email, websites, cell-phones/PDAs, social networking sites, and gaming environments. However, no studies have compared the effectiveness of a persuasive system using such alternative channels and various persuasive techniques. Moreover, how affective computing impacts the effectiveness of persuasive systems is not clear. This study proposes (1) persuasive technology channels in combination with persuasive strategies will have different persuasive effectiveness; (2) Adding positive emotion to a message that leads to a better overall user experience could increase persuasive effectiveness. The affective computing or emotion information was added to the experiment using emoticons. The initial results of a pilot study show that computer-mediated communication channels along with various persuasive strategies can affect the persuasive effectiveness to varying degrees. These results also shows that adding a positive emoticon to a message leads to a better user experience which increases the overall persuasive effectiveness of a system.

Keywords: persuasive effectiveness, affective computing, emotions, design, user experience, experiment design, simulation mock-ups.

1 Introduction

A persuasive system is a system to communicate with a persuadee using communication messages with different strategies to influence and change her/his behavior and/or attitude [1]. With advances in computers and communication technologies, several domains such as healthcare, marketing and politics are rapidly developing IT-enabled persuasive systems. Using persuasive technology to promote healthy behavior has become one of the most important domains [2]. Research studies in persuasive technologies and the associated usage of IT systems show a high potential for improving healthy living, reducing the cost of the healthcare system, and allowing people to maintain a more independent lifestyle [2, 3].

New communication technologies give researchers and developers more communication channel options to deliver messages and, at the same time, raise the

T. Ploug, P. Hasle, H. Oinas-Kukkonen (Eds.): PERSUASIVE 2010, LNCS 6137, pp. 274–285, 2010.
© Springer-Verlag Berlin Heidelberg 2010

challenge of selecting the right communication channels for the system in order to maximize persuasive impact. With advances in communication technology, the CMC channel becomes an umbrella for multiple technologies, such as email, mobile devices with short message service (SMS), social networking sites (SNS), multimedia websites, and gaming environments or virtual worlds. Does the persuasive effectiveness vary by the CMC channel used in the persuasive system? If there are differences, which kind of CMC channel is the most effective for a specific persuasive strategy? These questions motivate our study. Until now, there has been no comprehensive comparison study to evaluate the persuasive effectiveness of different CMC channels.

Affective computing is a new technology that can add emotional appeal to digital interfaces. It proposes to integrate the exchange of emotional information into the communication and interaction between the user and the computer in a natural and comfortable way [4]. Recent studies show that adding affect via affective computing interaction can impact the performance of a persuasive system [5-7]. This study posits that affective computing does not directly impact the effectiveness of persuasion. Instead, affective computing impacts the overall user experience (UX)[8], which acts as an intermediate factor between affective computing and persuasive effectiveness. Therefore, this study explores how the delivery of affective computing information using different communication channels impacts the overall persuasive effectiveness on the user.

The study uses both design science research (DSR) [9] and quantitative research methodology [10]. A simulation system, which represents communication channel and persuasive strategy combinations, was designed and developed using mock-up technology. This study will adapt the DSR methodology to guide the development of the mock-up, which will then be used to conduct an experiment to evaluate the effectiveness of the persuasive system. A pilot study with a small population size was initially conducted. The preliminary results of the pilot study showed the positive impact of the affective computing on UX and persuasive effectiveness.

In section 2, we provide an overview of related works on persuasive technology, affective computing and user experience. We describe the research questions and propose a deterministic model of persuasive system effectiveness in Section 3. Then, we describe the methodology and the experimental design in Section 4. We present the initial results of the pilot study in section 5, discuss our findings in section 6, and conclude with some future research directions in section 7.

2   Literature Review

2.1   Persuasive Technology Revolution and Strategy

Persuasion is "a symbolic process in which communicators try to convince other people to change their attitudes or behavior regarding an issue through the transmission of a message, in an atmosphere of free of choice" [11]. Fogg [12] defined the term persuasive technology as "a computing system, device, or application intentionally designed to change a person's attitude or behavior in a predetermined way", and coined the term "Captology," which refers to the study of computers as persuasive technology. Chatterjee and Price [2] provided an overview of the evolution of the persuasive-based computing technology in healthcare (see Fig. 1), which categorizes the available persuasive technologies into four generations. The results of this study will benefit the third and future generation persuasive system designers.

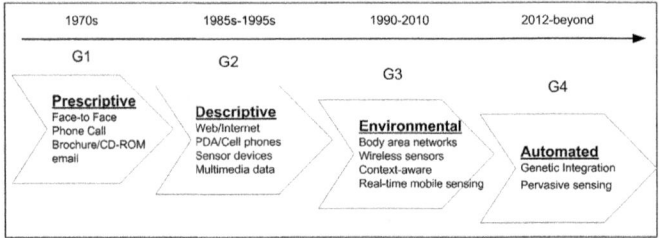

Fig. 1. A roadmap showing the evolution of Persuasive Technology (adopted from [2])

We design a persuasive system using a simple model as shown in Fig. 2. In this model, the persuader sets up a goal of the persuasion (such as to promote more physical exercise or encourage a healthy diet). The communication messages are developed using different strategies. Those messages will be delivered to the persuadee using different communication channels with the intent of achieving behavior change.

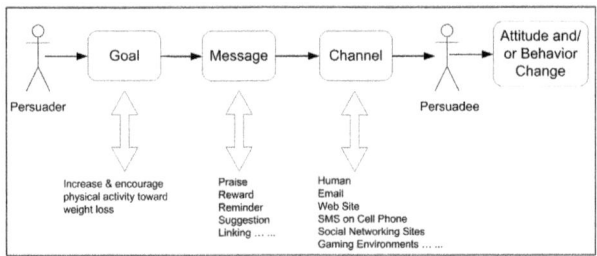

Fig. 2. General Persuasion System

There are many different typologies that categorize the persuasive message strategies, such as rewarding compliance versus punishing non-compliance [3], rational arguments versus non-rational arguments, or positive message versus negative message. This study focuses on computer-human interaction implemented through dialogue support [1] and selects four main message strategies: praise, reward, reminder, and suggestion.

2.2 Persuasion and Communication Channel

The communication channel is one of the key factors of persuasive systems [13, 14]. Selecting the right channel to deliver a persuasive message is also one of the critical steps toward designing an IT-Persuasive System [15].

There are multiple communication theories for scientific research on persuasive communication. Information Processing Theory (IPT) dominates persuasive communication research because it considers the different communication capability between face-to-face and computer-mediated-communication. Information Processing Theory assumes that receivers of the persuasive communication can be engaging in an active process of analyzing and elaborating on the information presented. Petty and Cacioppo's Elaboration Likelihood Model (ELM) hypothesized that the persuasion result is a function of the way in which the information is elaborated [16]. Depending on the motivation and ability of the persuadee to process the message, persuasion communication can use either a central route or a peripheral route.

In the early stage of persuasive communication research, the studies focused on the face-to-face communication channel and traditional publication channels, such as newspapers and magazines. The Digital revolution has changed the usual modes of communicating [16]. Recent studies consider CMC as one channel, generally using email as its representation; and compare the persuasive effect with the human based face-to-face communication channel [3, 16-19]. However, the effectiveness of persuasion over different CMC channels is not well understood [17, 20].

2.3 Affective Computing, Emotion, and Persuasion

Affective computing is a new research area which proposes that emotional information be communicated between the user and the computer in a natural and comfortable way [4]. This communication can improve computer interaction with users by recognizing users' emotional status and/or influencing users' mood with emotional information such as color, font style and size, image, voice, face expression, and multimedia. The key to establishing affective computing is the ability to recognize peoples' feelings and to express appropriate empathic feedback through both language and non-verbal gestures [4, 21].

Picard proposed a 2x2 framework that guides affective computing research (Fig. 3) in two dimensions [4]: one dimension is for computers that can or cannot express affect, and the other is for computers that can or cannot perceive affect. Because building a system that meets case III of the affective computing research model requirements takes considerable resources, this study focuses on case II, which addresses to the computer systems that can express affect.

Computer	Cannot express affect	Can express affect
Cannot perceive affect	I	II
Can perceive affect	III	IV

Fig. 3. Four categories of affective computing, focusing on expression and recognition [4]

Most research suggests that the persuasive effects of emotion are generated through the impacts of information processing, and either minimize the information processing (heuristics), stimulate careful information processing, or promote selective information processing [22]. Unlike previous research, this study investigates the impact of emotion on the effectiveness of persuasion systems from different points of view. This study proposes that emotion may vary persuasive effectiveness through user experiences, which will be described in next section. To simplify the analysis, this study uses the bipolar valence model and focuses on positive emotion.

Emoticons (such as :-) or ;-)) are widely known and commonly recognized by users of CMC and are used as emotion substitutes [23]. This study uses emoticons "smiley" and "wink" to deliver positive emotion in CMC. They allow individuals to express some of their emotions and help to communicate more clearly the current mood or mental state of the author [24]. Huang et al [25] analyzed the effects of emoticons and concluded that a user of emoticons felt a positive effect on enjoyment, personal interaction, perceived information richness, and perceived usefulness of the system. The authors also suggested that emoticons are a valuable addition to communication methods.

2.4 User Experience

User Experience (UX) is a term that describes the overall experience and satisfaction a user has when using a product or system [26]. This concept has been widely disseminated and readily accepted in the Human-Computer Interaction (HCI) community [27]. Compared with usability, which is widely used in technology acceptance research, UX is a broader concept. Besides the pragmatic experiential aspects, UX also covers the hedonic experiential aspects, such as affection and emotion, from a user perspective [26].

The ways in which a user experiences different persuasive systems may vary with the task context and with time, but an understanding of the overall user experience may contribute to better design and generate a positive impact on the overall effectiveness of the persuasive system[28].

3 Research Questions and Model

This study proposes a deterministic model of persuasive system effectiveness (Fig. 4), which consists of persuasive system and user experience. In the original persuasive system, the communication channel and the persuasive strategy are the two primary determining factors of the persuasive system. The interaction between the communication channel and the persuasive strategy mainly impacts the usability and utility of the persuasive system, which are two direct factors of the pragmatic aspect of the overall user experience. When the persuasive system adds affect and emotion support using affective computing design technology (such as emoticons), it generates an effect on the hedonic aspect of the overall user experience. The user experience of the persuasive system then influences the degree of persuasive effectiveness. This framework investigates several direct and indirect relationships that impact the effectiveness of the persuasive system. Regarding the measurement of effectiveness, this study focuses on perceived persuasive effectiveness [3], which measures the users' perceptions. Although we anticipate the results of this study will cross domains, for the purpose of this study, the application domain for the persuasive system is healthy lifestyle persuasion.

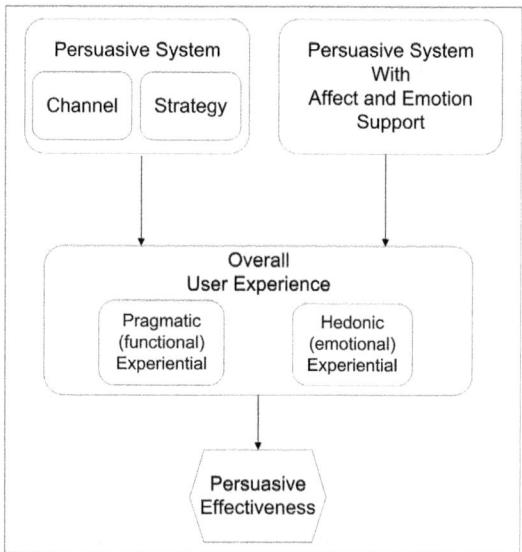

Fig. 4. Theoretical framework of the persuasive system effectiveness

Two research questions are proposed to explore these effects and their relationships. The first research question of this study explores the persuasive effectiveness of computer-mediated communication channels using different message strategies.

RQ 1: *Can computer-mediated communication channels, along with various persuasive strategies, affect the persuasive effectiveness to varying degrees?*

No research shows consistent direct correlation between the elements of affective computing and the persuasive effectiveness of the system. User experience (UX) is an important factor in the success of an information system. As described by Walther and D'Addario [23], affective computing has a direct effect on the user experience. In this study, we propose that the user experience is the mediating factor between the persuasive system and persuasive effectiveness. The second research question of this study is to explore how affective computing could impact persuasive effectiveness over different computer-mediated communication channels.

RQ 2: *Can adding a positive emoticon to a message leading to a better user experience which increase the overall persuasive effectiveness of a system?*

4   Methodology and Research Design

A new simulation system was designed and created to conduct experiments in this study. The simulation system is a set of mock-ups of persuasive systems. Fig. 5 shows examples of the mockups. This simulation system is used to establish an experiment that is designed to measure the effectiveness of persuasion, which uses different combinations of persuasive strategies, communication channels, and affect add-ons. In this study, the mock-up represents the user interface of a persuasive system with different communication channels.

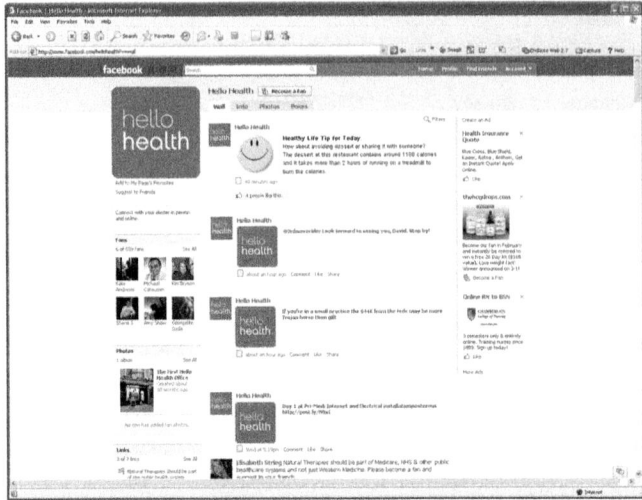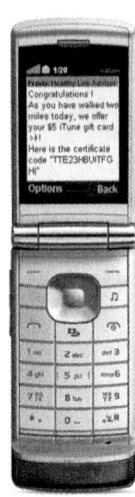

Fig. 5. Examples of the mock-ups: On the left is the mock-up for the suggestion message with smiley emoticon on one facebook social site; and on the right is the mock-up of a reward message using a text message over a cell phone

We investigated four different communication channels (email, web, facebook social site, and cell-phones with SMS) and four different persuasive message strategies (suggestion, reward, reminder, and praise). A total of 16 mock-ups were created for those channel/strategy combinations. Then, emoticons were added to create a second set of mock-ups that represented an affective computing integrated persuasive system. The content/text of these communication messages were chosen from a prior study [29] and from the US Department of Health & Human Services and CDC's(Centers for Disease Control and Prevention) healthy life campaigns. The templates of the mock-up are collected from instances of real healthy life interventions online. This study uses a well established healthcare social networking site "HelloHealth" [30] from facebook.com as the template of the SNS mock-up, and uses "www.smallstep.gov" as the template of the persuasive web site mockup. For text messages on cell phones, this study uses a general model of a cell phone with a common screen size (2.2 inch) as the template. The size of all mock-ups are same as the real system.

In order to observe the effects of affective computing, the participants were divided into two groups using a randomized controlled trial. The first group reviewed the persuasive messages without any specific affect add-on. The second group reviewed the persuasive messages with an affect add-on that is implemented using an emoticon. There is no difference in the persuasive message context and communication channel features besides the emoticon added according to the mode of the message. The subjects were asked to review all 16 mock-ups of the persuasive system. In order to control the source effect of the persuasive system, participants were told that these persuasive systems were created by healthcare professional organizations. For each mock-up, participants were asked to view the persuasive message presented in it. Then, participants filled out an evaluation survey that followed each mock-up interface before they moved to the next mock-up. The sequence of the 16 mock-ups was random for each subject in order to control the experiment system bias.

This study measures the receivers' perceptions of persuasive effectiveness. For user experience measurement, two sets of questionnaires were used in this study to cover the pragmatic experience and the hedonic experience of the simulated persuasive system.

One challenge to measuring persuasive effectiveness is "contamination" that occurs in a research design [31]. When a study tries to use behavioral intention as the measure of the attribute changes, the pre-measure can introduce a direct and contaminating effect on the subject of this experiment. This study uses a perceived persuasion effectiveness measure without a pre-measure to attempt to reduce this type of contamination.

5 Results

A pilot study with 13 participants was conducted in a controlled lab setting. Participants were randomly assigned to two groups. The first group reviewed the mock-ups without emoticons and the second group reviewed the mock-ups with emoticons.

Table 1. The persuasive effectiveness of various channel and strategy combinations: a) without emoticon; b) with emoticon; c) the influence of affective computing

a)

	praise	reminder	reward	suggestion
email	3.43	3.21	3.79	3.71
facebook	3.36	2.64	3.50	3.57
Cell phone with SMS	3.36	3.36	3.71	3.43
Web Site	3.21	2.93	3.79	2.93

b)

	praise	reminder	reward	suggestion
email	3.92	3.92	4.08	3.83
facebook	3.58	3.33	3.67	3.50
Cell phone with SMS	3.67	3.67	3.83	3.42
Web Site	3.33	3.50	4.08	3.33

c)

	praise	reminder	reward	suggestion
email	14%	22%	8%	3%
facebook	7%	26%	5%	-2%
Cell phone with SMS	9%	9%	3%	0%
Web Site	4%	20%	8%	14%

The first set of results (Table 1a) shows persuasive effectiveness in terms of various channel and strategy combination without emoticons. The next set of results (Table 1b) shows the same for emoticons. As seen in the results, certain combinations of channel and persuasive strategy have greater impact on the user than others. For example, Table 1a shows that praise message works best via email, and reminder message works best via cell phone with SMS. Table 1b shows the strong impacts of the affective computing on persuasive effectiveness. Table 1c shows that 14 of 16 channel/strategy combinations increase persuasive effectiveness with emoticons.

6 Discussion

We expect it should have a positive impact on a user's hedonic experience when we add affect and emotion support to the persuasive system. Table 2 shows the changes in the hedonic UX of these 16 combinations, and 11 of them have positive emotional influence that is more than 5%.

The messages on facebook show negative impact with added emotional influence. The reason could be that most pilot study participants have a privacy concern regarding communicating personal health information on a social networking site. The reminder message on facebook does show positive emotional influence because we use a general healthy lifestyle content in this message ("drink more water"), and it does not raise the privacy concerns of the participants.

Both reward and praise messages show negative emotional influence compared with reminder and suggestions messages on all channels. The reason for this observation is that praise and reward messages already use positive emotional appeals in the message content. The emoticon cannot generate much positive gain based on that level. For reminder and suggestion messages, which could be considered as neutral emotion messages, the affect add-on (such as emoticons) could generate much higher positive emotional influence.

Table 2. Impact of emotions on hedonic UX

	praise	reminder	reward	suggestion
email	7%	34%	0%	11%
facebook	-2%	24%	-1%	-6%
Cell phone with SMS	9%	9%	5%	11%
Web Site	6%	15%	2%	12%

Table 3 shows the changes in usability and utility of the interface after we added emoticons to the messages. There were no changes on the mock-ups other than the emoticon we added to the message. We expected that this would not impact the users' pragmatic experience. The results show that 11 of 16 combinations have a delta change of only 5% or less on UX. However, the results show the emoticons impact the functional user experience of several channel/strategy combinations, such as praise message over email, reminder message over email and facebook, and reward message on facebook. Huang et al [25] reports that emoticons could increase the users' enjoyment level of the system, then increase the perceived information richness and perceived usefulness of the system. The relationship found in [25] could be the reason for this observation in this pilot study. Moreover, the results of this study shows that perceived usefulness impacts the these channel/strategy combinations differently.

Table 3. Impact of emoticons on usability and utility

	praise	reminder	reward	suggestion
email	17%	22%	3%	5%
facebook	0%	27%	10%	3%
Cell phone with SMS	-4%	-3%	5%	-3%
Web Site	5%	0%	5%	7%

7 Conclusion

In this study, we proposed a new research framework for persuasive effectiveness that brings user experience into play as a mediating factor. To measure persuasive effectiveness and user experience, we designed and created an experiment using mock-ups. The pilot study results show that computer-mediated communication channels along with various persuasive strategies could affect persuasive effectiveness to varying degrees. Meanwhile, the results also show that adding positive emoticons to a message leading to a better user experience increases the overall persuasive effectiveness of a system. The study provides a guideline for the designers of persuasive systems, who can optimize the effectiveness of their systems based on this study.

The pilot study validated the experiment and tested the surveys. The size of the population is a limitation of this pilot study. In our continuing research, we will optimize the mock-ups and surveys to conduct a full subjective controlled study. With a larger sample size, we hope to conduct t-tests, ANOVA and significance results. We will also investigate the potential correlations between the media richness of the channel and the amount of information in the message (information entropy) to determine the impact on persuasive effectiveness.

References

1. Oinas-Kukkonen, H., Harjumaa, M.: Persuasive Systems Design: Key Issues, Process Model, and System Features. Communications of the Association for Information Systems 24 (2009)
2. Chatterjee, S., Price, A.: Healthy Living with Persuasive Technologies: Framework, Issues, and Challenges. Journal of the American Medical Information Association 16, 171–178 (2009)
3. Wilson, E.V.: Perceived effectiveness of interpersonal persuasion strategies in computer-mediated communication. Computers in Human Behavior 19, 537–552 (2003)
4. Picard, R.W.: Affective computing (1995)
5. Nguyen, H., Masthoff, J.: Designing empathic computers: the effect of multimodal empathic feedback using animated agent. In: Proceedings of the 4th International Conference on Persuasive Technology, pp. 1–9. ACM, Claremont (2009)
6. Reitberger, W., Meschtscherjakov, A., Mirlacher, T., Scherndl, T., Huber, H., Tscheligi, M.: A persuasive interactive mannequin for shop windows. In: Proceedings of the 4th International Conference on Persuasive Technology, pp. 1–8. ACM, Claremont (2009)

7. Torning, K., Oinas-Kukkonen, H.: Persuasive system design: state of the art and future directions. In: Proceedings of the 4th International Conference on Persuasive Technology, pp. 1–8. ACM, Claremont (2009)
8. Roto, V., Rautava, M.: User Experience Elements and Brand Promise. In: International Engagability & Design Conference, in conjunction with NordiCHI 2008, Lund, Sweden (2008)
9. Hevner, A., Chatterjee, S.: Design Science Research in Infomration Systems. In: Hevner, A., Chatterjee, S. (eds.) Design Research in Information Systems: Theory and Practice, ch. 2. Springer, Heidelberg (2010)
10. Creswell, J.W.: Research Design: Qualitative & Quantitative Approaches. SAGE Publications, Inc., Thousand Oaks (1994)
11. Perloff, R.M.: The dynamics of persuasion: communication and attitudes in the 21st century. Lawrence Erlbaum, Mahwah (2007)
12. Fogg, B.J.: Overview of captology. Persuasive Technology, pp. 15–22. Morgan Kaufmann, San Francisco (2003)
13. Ajzen, I.: Persuasive Communication Theory in Social Psychology: A Historical Psychology. In: Manfredo, M.J. (ed.) Influencing Human Behavior Theory and Applications in Recreation and Tourism Natural Resources. Sagamore Publishing (1992)
14. Holbert, R.L.: Embodied meaning of media form. In: Dillard, J.P., Pfau, M. (eds.) The persuasion handbook: developments in theory and practice. Sage Publications, Inc., Thousand Oaks (2002)
15. Fogg, B.: Creating persuasive technologies: An eight-step design process. In: Proceedings of the 4th International Conference on Persuasive Technology, pp. 1–6. ACM, Claremont (2009)
16. Paola, D.B., Luca, M.: Computer-mediated communication and persuasion: Peripheral vs. Central route to opinion shift. Computers in Human Behavior 24(3), 798–815 (2007)
17. Cugelman, B., Thelwall, M., Dawes, P.: Communication-based influence components model. In: Proceedings of the 4th International Conference on Persuasive Technology, pp. 1–9. ACM, Claremont (2009)
18. Ramachandran, D., Canny, J.: The Persuasive Power of Human-Machine Dialogue. In: Oinas-Kukkonen, H., Hasle, P., Harjumaa, M., Segerståhl, K., Øhrstrøm, P. (eds.) PERSUASIVE 2008. LNCS, vol. 5033, pp. 189–200. Springer, Heidelberg (2008)
19. Guadagno, R.E., Cialdini, R.B.: Online persuasion: An examination of gender differences in computer-mediated interpersonal influence. Group Dynamics: Theory, Research, and Practice 6, 38–51 (2002)
20. Zhu, W.: Promoting Physical Activity Through Internet: A Persuasive Technology View. In: de Kort, Y.A.W., IJsselsteijn, W.A., Midden, C., Eggen, B., Fogg, B.J. (eds.) PERSUASIVE 2007. LNCS, vol. 4744, pp. 12–17. Springer, Heidelberg (2007)
21. Reynolds, C., Picard, R.W.: Designing for Affective Interactions. In: Processding of 9th International Conf. on HumanComputer Interaction, New Orleans, p. 499 (2001)
22. Nabi, R.L.: Discrete Emotions and Persuasion. In: Dillard, J.P., Pfau, M. (eds.) The persuasion handbook: developments in theory and practice. Sage Publications, Inc., Thousand Oaks (2002)
23. Walther, J.B., D'Addario, K.P.: The impact of Emotions on Message Intrepretation in Computer Mediated Communication. Social Science Computer Review 19(3), 324–347 (2001)
24. Derks, D., Fischerb, A.H., Bosc, A.E.R.: The role of emotion in computer-mediated communication: A review. Computers in Human Behavior 24, 766–785 (2008)

25. Huang, A.H., Yen, D.C., Zhang, X.: Exploring the potential effects of emoticons. Information & Management 45, 466–473 (2008)
26. Bevan, N.: UX, Usability and ISO Standards. In: CHI 2008. ACM, Florence (2008)
27. Law, E.L.-C., Roto, V., Hassenzahl, M., Vermeeren, A.P.O.S., Kort, J.: Understanding, scoping and defining user experience: a survey approach. In: Proceedings of the 27th international conference on Human factors in computing systems, pp. 719–728. ACM, Boston (2009)
28. Segerstahl, K., Oinas-Kukkonen, H.: Distributed User Experience in Persuasive Technology Environments. In: de Kort, Y.A.W., IJsselsteijn, W.A., Midden, C., Eggen, B., Fogg, B.J. (eds.) PERSUASIVE 2007. LNCS, vol. 4744, pp. 80–91. Springer, Heidelberg (2007)
29. Megha, M., Samir, C., David, D.: Exploring the Persuasiveness of "Just-in-time" Motivational Messages for Obesity Management. In: Oinas-Kukkonen, H., Hasle, P., Harjumaa, M., Segerståhl, K., Øhrstrøm, P. (eds.) PERSUASIVE 2008. LNCS, vol. 5033, pp. 258–261. Springer, Heidelberg (2008)
30. Hawn, C.: Take two aspirin and tweet me in the morning: How Twitter, Facebook, and other social media are reshaping health care. Health Aff. (Millwood) 28, 361–368
31. Bettinghaus, E.P.: Health promotion and the knowledge-attitude-behavior continuum. Preventive Medicine 15, 475–491 (1986)

Embodied Agents, E-SQ and Stickiness: Improving Existing Cognitive and Affective Models

Pablo Brice de Diesbach

Ecole Hôtelière de Lausanne-LHR, 1000 Lausanne 25, CH
pablo.diesbach@ehl.ch

Abstract. This paper synthesizes results from two previous studies of embodied virtual agents on commercial websites. We analyze and criticize the proposed models and discuss the limits of the experimental findings. Results from other important research in the literature are integrated. We also integrate concepts from profound, more business-related, analysis that deepens on the mechanisms of rhetoric in marketing and communication, and the possible role of E-SQ in man-agent interaction. We finally suggest a refined model for the impacts of these agents on web site users, and limits of the improved model are commented.

Keywords: Modelling, Experimentation, EVA, attitude, affect, E-SQ.

1 Introduction

The role of a website has been seen as mainly informational in most research publications in the first ten years of the Internet era, within a dominant cognitive paradigm. A branding website was therefore used as a mostly informative tool, being even mostly called an "online catalog". Then, researchers started integrating the possible effects of affective cues, often in a pure ergonomic approach and then in a theoretically and conceptually more open approach integrating affective cues [e.g. 1,2]. Interestingly, this evolution parallels another, more ancient, similar evolution in marketing and in communication in general, to a theoretical framework which tries to integrate the role of affect: in Marketing in [3, 4, 5; 6, 7, 8], or in Communication sciences as the seminal works of Burgoon [9, 10] and Ekman [11, 12] show. That leads to rethinking theoretical frameworks, and to sharp oppositions among academics, as the acknowledgement of the place of Affect is actually in play [13, 13; 15, 16, 17]. This is the general context in which research on virtual agents takes place.

2 Conceptual Framework

Marketing or E-Marketing is not *Selling* or *Communicating*. It rather consists of building a relationship, creating more value for customer and corporation [18, 19; 20]. Research on the role of human counterparts in marketing show that the way they are perceived may deeply impact users' behavior [21, 22; 23]. Affect actually impacts cognition, and affective reactions to the message sender impacts our attitude to the

T. Ploug, P. Hasle, H. Oinas-Kukkonen (Eds.): PERSUASIVE 2010, LNCS 6137, pp. 286–298, 2010.
© Springer-Verlag Berlin Heidelberg 2010

object of the message. If human counterparts do play such a role in a marketing context, virtual counterparts or EVAs, should do so. This might first be related to the fact that machines such as robots or computers are treated as social counterparts, as Picard and Nass [24; 25, 26, 27] or other scholars [28, 29, 30], show; second, to the fact that Virtual agents are even more logically treated as social counterparts as a number of works by Cassel and Bickmore [31; 32, 33, 34; 35] show.

3 Contributions and Limits of Previous Research

The need for modeling agents effects
As Nass posits (opening speech, Persuasive Technology, Stanford University, May 2007), many research show that EVAs do impact behaviors; but: *"the key issue is the Why of the observed effects"*. We need models integrating mediating – and maybe moderating – variables, through which "something" happens. That means, we need modeling.

Relevance of Website/Interface Stickiness in a user-centered approach
A managerial literature exists on the concept of online or website stickiness, which generally expresses the capacity of a website to retain a user [36, 37]. Unquestioned that was until the internet bubble burst [16, 20]. Mere behavioral retention may be the center of early thinking about internet strategy [39] but it narrows a view. Recent contributions on such issue [40, 41] posit that a more useful construct of stickiness should be composed of both behavioral and attitudinal or intentional measurement, capturing a will to maintain a relationship with the interface. Our Stickiness construct is therefore defined as a "power of retention", i.e. of creating a durable relationship of a website or any interface, with a user. It is operationalised in a single, bi-dimensional construct with a Behavioral dimension (Navigation duration and Number of pages visited), and an Intentional dimension (Intention to recommend and Intention to revisit).Last, it perfectly fits with two important streams of research (and managerial practice) in marketing, as we see hereafter. The first research stream, called Environmental psychology and then Environmental marketing, posits that ambience or design factors may exert effects on affective reactions, conceptualized as a 3-dimensional affective space called the PAD (*Pleasure;Arousal*; and *Dominance* or *feeling of Control*). Those may [46, 61] in turn, impact behaviors or intentions. Such behaviors are called *Approach-Avoidance Behaviors* and can be expressed as Staying-Exploring-Affiliating-Having the intention to come back. Those perfectly match *Website stickiness* in our context, with four variables: *Navigation duration* (Staying) and *Number of clicks* (Exploring) for the *Behavioral stickiness* (1st dimension, composed of 2 variables), and *Intention to recommend* (Affiliating) and *Intention to return* (Intention to return) for the *Intentional* stickiness (2nd dimension, composed of 2 variables). Second, such construct of stickiness perfectly matches the modern conceptualization of marketing in general [19] and E Marketing [20], as a value creation process, build-up through a Relationship construction. Stickiness is a non perfect, but quite elaborated, construct, measuring how much any electronic interface, generates a will to know more, more in depth, to be more loyal and affiliate, . It does not capture the intention to buy online. The fact she spends more time and cognitive resource informing his/herself about a specific product or brand, and affiliating and

willing to come back to it, means she does not dedicate such resources and intentions to another competitive product-brand. Likeliness to buy sooner or later, online or offline, is then quite strongly captured.

Last, for the final dependent variable of Website Stickiness, it was important to go beyond simple behavioral measures of visit duration and pages visited. The two resulting dimensions of *behavioral* and *intentional* stickiness are related, though distinct in nature. Theory makes us assume they are part of a single construct, and statistical analysis will confirm it.

Contributions and limits of the previously tested models

In two recent studies, we attempt to address what we believe to be an important gap in the literature relating to embodied virtual agents and their effects on the users of commercial websites. That is, the lack of model explaining agent effects.

First, we study the effects of a virtual agent through a direct route with no mediating variable, that is, that the Presence of an agent impacts Website stickinessin a direct or black-box approach. Then we identify two additional routes. We keep the idea of a Central vs a Peripheral route or persuasion, inherited from the literature in psychology and advertising relative to the ELM (*Elaboration Likelihood Model*) approach of Petty and Cacioppo [43, 44]: we posit a central, more cognitive, attitudinal route composed of three attitudes [41, 42]. In that first, *Central or Attitudinal persuasion route,* the user's Attitude toward the agent impacts Attitude toward the web . In turn, these attitudes influence the Attitude towards the brand. Measures of the attitudes towards agent, site and brand, were developed building on the literature on attitudes toward messages and sales people [21, 22] and toward web sites [45]. All multi-item measures show high construct reliabilities. Then in the *Peripheral or Affective* route, emotions that agent and site invoke influence Stickiness. Measures of affect were developed from the literature on pleasure, dominance and arousal [46, 47, 48, 61]. Again reliable measures are obtained. We tested our hypotheses using data from a laboratory experiment with 344 randomly selected users [see 40, 41, 42], and 2 web sites, Primolea (French luxury olive oil) and Träser (Swiss diving watches), with the presenceXabsence of an embodied virtual agent (EVA) and, where present, whether this agent's appearance was congruent or non-congruent with the nature of the web site – but this role of congruency is not addressed here. Our purpose is to synthesize what was learned about the three routes - direct, attitudinal and affective; and to suggest ways to expand our knowledge of how embodied agents impact behaviors. We now analyze and criticize the results.

4   Results of the Experiment and Discussion

We are now going to discuss the observed effects across the three possible routes.

Simple effects of the agent on stickiness

We first test a "blck-box" route with no mediating, explanatory variables. The presence of an agent has a very significant effect on navigation duration (H1a***) and a significant effect on the number of pages (H1b*), and no significant effect on either Intention to revisit (H2a NS) and Intention to recommend (H2b NS). Effects are presented in figure 1 hereafter:

Effects into and through the attitudinal hierarchy or Central route

Effects of presence of the agent on the three attitudes (H5, H9 to H12) are examined in the attitudinal hierarchy of effects. For the two attitudes A_{ws} (towards the site) and A_b (towards the brand), the effects are positive and highly significant (effect of presence on A_{ws}: H9**, effect on A_b: H11***). Looking more closely into the hierarchy, *among the attitudes* and then *from each attitude towards Stickiness*, the effects of each attitude on the next one, and on Intentional stickiness, are validated:

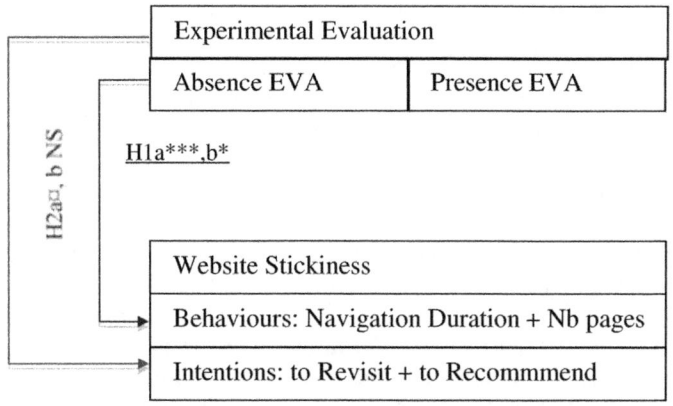

Fig. 1. Results, Hypotheses testing: simple effects

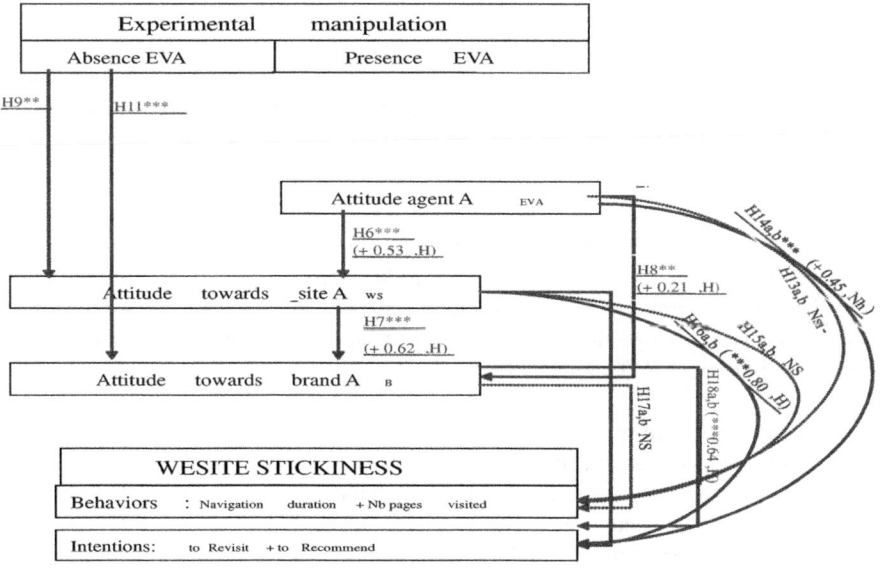

Fig. 2. Research model, effects through the hierarchy of attitudinal effects

But effects of each attitude on the *behavioral stickiness* are *not* validated.

We measure high to very high correlations between Attitudes and Intentional stickiness components ranging from 0.40 to 0.80. All constructs have adequate discriminant validities and such high correlations are not problematic. Effects are *quite homogeneous,* across the two sites (Chow tests on each step of the hierarchy).

Effects observed into and through the affective route

We use the Affective scale inherited from Environmental Psychology and adapted Online by Novak & al.. The exploratory and confirmatory factorial analysis let only 2 affective dimensions emerge (*Pleasure,* and *Dominance*). The first step of the affective model is not confirmed: agent presence has no significant effects on affective reactions (H19 NS). The second step is partly validated, that is, on intentional stickiness only. Pleasure has a very significant effect on intentional stickiness (H21$_{c,d}$***) and Dominance has a significant effect on one component of intentional stickiness (H22c NS on the intention to revisit, H22d* on the intention to recommend). But both affective reactions have no significant effects on behavioral stickiness (H21$_{a,b}$ NS, H22$_{a,b}$ NS) – see figure 3 hereafter:

We also note that the Central (Attitudinal) and Peripheral (Affective) routes are not independent from each other: correlations between attitudes (A$_{EVA}$, A$_{ws}$, A$_{brand}$) and Pleasure and Dominance are highly significant (from +0.13 to +0.55) even though we checked their discriminant validity. This is a very important point for the future model improvements. We have tried to follow Batra and Bagozzi in the idea of assessing attitudes in a multi-item (though mono-dimensional) measurement of attitude, without discarding the possibility that they encapsulate affective dimensions. We nevertheless assess high correlations but *cannot* posit a directional effect: such issue having been *per se* a controversial, non resolved, issue for decades [8, 14, 15, 16 and 17, 52, 59].

Supported hypothesis. The direct route receives support: presence of an agent impacts significantly on behavioral stickiness (Navigation duration and Number of pages visited). The hierarchy of attitudes impacts Intentional stickiness: positive attitudes to the agent enhance attitudes towards the site and to the brand, and increase Intentional stickiness (intentions to revisit or recommend to others). Feelings of pleasure and dominance also increase Intentional stickiness.

Non-supported hypothesis. While feelings of pleasure and dominance increase intentional stickiness, the presence of an agent has no impact on these feelings. We cannot confirm the full peripheral route. Additionally, Affect and Attitudes impact significantly on intentional stickiness, but not on behavioral stickiness: we have so far not found a satisfying model answering the crucial question raised by Nass: "what do we know about the WHY of such effects?".

Critique of these studies

The model is not adequately specified as yet. Affect and attitude play a role but we do not understand their drivers fully, nor do we understand the reasons for the separation of impacts on intentional and behavioral stickiness. We speculate that this model misses important moderators, e.g. the topic addressed by the agent or the design of the agent itself, including its gender, size, appearance or personality expressed by the way the agent talks, moves, and was designed in shape. For instance we tested agents that

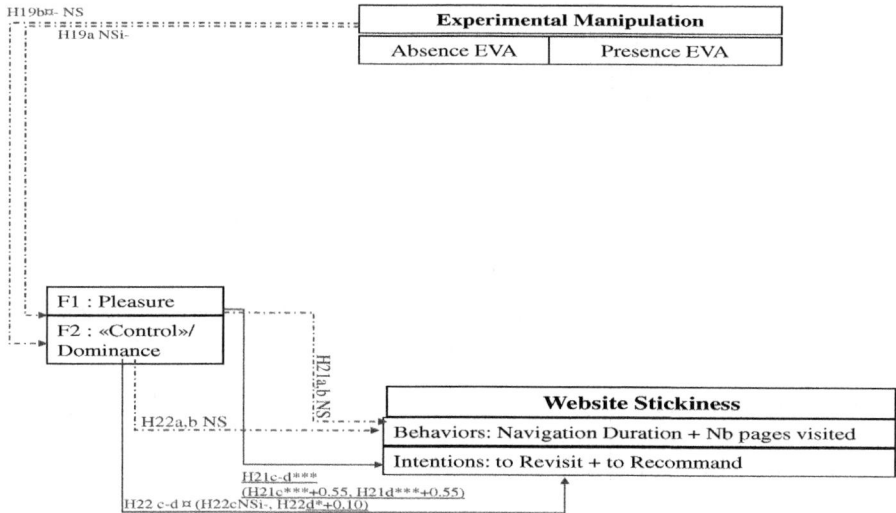

Fig. 3. Research model, effects through the Affective route

were perceived as either Congruent, or Non Congruent, with the website and the brand: that is we varied how much the physical design (body shape, face, body language, etc.) was perceived as congruent in an holistic, global manner, with the site and brand. For the Swiss diving watches, the congruent agent was a sexy girl (vs a teen ager girl with roller skates: refer to images of the agents in annex at the end of the article). We also have not included individual moderators such as personality traits, innovativeness or aesthetic tastes. Both website topic and agent design AND tasks (here the agents were only tour-guides) together with individual characteristics, may impact user's emotions, attitudes, behavior. We now work refining the tested model.

5 Improving the Previous Models

Some effects occur in the direct route and are NOT explainable so far.

A need for concept simplification and a better model specification arises
We have demonstrated that the observed effects are not explained by the attitudinal route as it is. We hence need to enrich or specify our model: first with the concept of E-SQ (E-Service Quality). Effects on stickiness could therefore actually occur through E-SQ, either in a direct route from the agent/agent congruency stimulus, or via the mediation of attitude(s). Second, we modify the constructs use inside the affective and attitudinal route.

Reducing the number of attitudes used in our model
Concerning the attitudinal persuasion route, we have an already complex route with three attitudes, between the stimuli (agent presence+agent congruence or any other

agent design cue) and the criterion variable of stickiness. If we add the E-SQ variable, we again have a two complex model. A broad concept of *Attitude towards the interface* could be sufficient as a possible mediator. It could include components of the attitude towards the Agent and towards the website and brand per se. We hence reduce from 3 to only 1 attitude, and then adding E-SQ does not give a too long or heavy model. Keeping only one super-construct of Attitude towards the interface simplifies our approach without inconvenients as we only want to see from a macro perspective where the routes of influence go. Measuring broad attitudinal reactions, affective (improved) reactions and E-SQ related-reactions is more than enough.

The insufficient dimensionality when conceptualizing the Affective reactions

Affective measure conceptualization and operationalization is difficult and controversial – see e.g. Zajonc, Markus, Bagozzi, Holbrook etc. in extensive literatures on that issue.

We try to improve our conceptualization of affective reactions and among them, of *Pleasure*. Duncker [63] already distinguished in 1941 among 3 types of pleasure: *Sensory* pleasures, *Aesthetic* pleasure and *Accomplishment* pleasure. After an extensive review in the Emotional conditioning, the Environmental Psychology, and the Experiential literatures in the last 30 years, we believe the more profound reflections on Pleasure can be found in the research of Csikszentmihalyi and the Experiential literature. The more usable conceptualization of pleasure is to be found in particular in the conceptualization by Dubé & Le Bel [66]. They conduct 5 studies and propose 4 categories of Pleasures, *Intellectual and Emotional* on the one hand, *Social and Sensorial* on the other hand, forming the 4 dimensions of a mega-construct.

The relevance of such conceptualization to an online interaction context is real. In the case of an interaction with a virtual agent, this approach would hold relevant: a website-an agent can provide knowledge, learning, understanding (Intellectual pleasure); fun, relaxation or excitement (Emotional); reassurance, tranquility, friendliness, importance (Social pleasure). We therefore will focus on the 4 possible facets of Pleasure in our Affective reaction stage online. The other affective dimensions of the PAD (Arousal, Dominance) should be unchanged. We don't address the issue of paradoxical, emotions, though relevant – Mick & Fournier [67].

The mediating role of E-Service Quality

We first comment the relevance of the concept, and dimensionality, of E-Service Quality. A navigation on a website may be approached as a service experience in most cases, e.g. for narration experience, for socializing, enjoying a virtual trip, preparing a purchase (for a future offline or online purchase) etc. Service Quality or SQ might therefore be a mediator of the effects of an EVA on stickiness.

In a wide literature, the team of authors commonly nicknamed as PBZM (Parasuraman, Berry, Zeithaml and Malhotra) because of the so wide literature published on the subject, study the drivers and conceptualization, then operationalization, of the key concept of Service Quality (SQ) [51], and later, E-Service Quality (E-SQ). Parasuraman & al. define Service Quality as: "*the quality on non-internet based customer interactions and experiences with companies*" [51, p.214]. Extensive research conducted on dozens of websites, lead first to the distinction of 11 dimensions of E-SQ [50], and later 4 dimensions [51]. With both mentioned scales, an embodied agent could very logically contribute on SQ or E-SQ, therefore impacting the will to stay on the site, complete the task, make it last more and to return or affiliate other users – that is, on Stickiness. E-SQ then might be a relevant mediator, as a conversation with A. Parasuraman confirmed. We hence propose to insert E-SQ as a mediator in our original. This proposition is examined.

An issue is How E-SQ could be located in our model. Actually the rationale of Parasuraman, Zeithaml and Malhotra starts from the observation that a website is NOT only an information-search tool but a service encounter. A first major result is evidenced by Szymanski & Hise who show that Convenience and Site design are more important drivers of E-Satisfaction than Perceived Financial security and Merchandising (i.e. Product offering and Product information). Second, as occurs in a real outlet, the feeling and attitudinal reactions toward sales agent or the outlet (real or virtual) can strongly impact user/consumer reactions and behaviors, for instance purchase intention [21, 22; 64]. Parasuraman & al. offer the most comprehensive approach on the issue. The final E-SQ scale after exploratory and confirmatory factor analysis, consists of 22 items, grouped in 4 dimensions, labeled as follows:

- *"Efficiency: The ease and speed of assessing and using the site.*
- *Fulfillment: The extent to which the site's promises about delivery and item availability are fulfilled.*
- *System availability: The correct technical functioning of the site.*
- *Privacy: The degree to which the site is safe and protects customer information".*

It is suggested here that E-SQ could be positioned as output, at the end of both attitudinal or affective persuasion routes as a partial or complete mediator.

Conclusion of the modeling process

Concerning the right (attitudinal) of the model, we decide then to collapse together the three attitudes towards the IVA, the Website and the Brand, into a single *Attitude towards the interface*, which will consist of the 15 more relevant items selected from the existing literature + from a new factorial analysis on the already collected data.

Concerning the left part of the model we enrich the existing measures of Affective reactions with a 3-dimensional concept of Pleasure, drawn from the mentioned articles, not specifically related to online interaction but to the very concept of Pleasure. As a conclusion, as an element of design able to generate positive affective reactions, an EVA may impact affect, through affect, E-Service Quality, and through it, Stickiness. As an interactive element, such and a social counterpart that provides information to help and ease the navigation, and requires concentration and skills, an EVA is also likely to positively impact attitude toward the interface and through it, E-Service Quality and finally, Stickiness. Last, part of the effects on Stickiness may occur directly, with no mediation of either Attitudes, Affective reaction, and/or E-SQ.

We propose to test the following, improved research model:

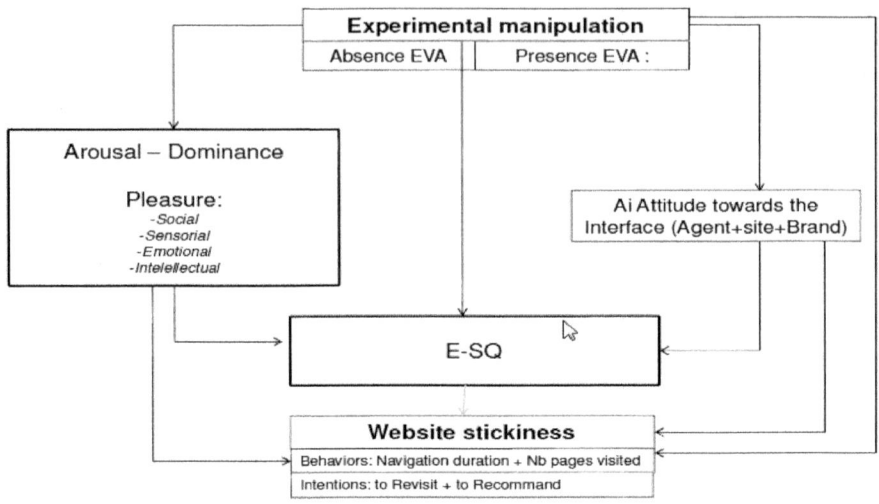

6 Contributions and Limits of the Research

Contributions of the research
As a conclusion we propose a summary and critical analysis of two previous research on the effects of an EVA on website stickiness. We point out the fact that the direct, simple-effects route shows effects of an EVA on Behavioral stickiness, whereas the attitudinal route and the Affective route on the other hand, only evidence effects on Intentional stickiness. Possible moderating variables related to the agent design or the user's characteristics, or experience, were commented [40, 41, 42]: we propose to introduce the role of E-SQ. Many other important variables related to the agent design and the very user's characteristics, are not taken into consideration, which is a strong limitation of our model. Future research should take such concepts into consideration. We conclude on research avenues, related to limits of the present research.

Limits and Research avenues
Basically, the limits of the present research are related to the fact we do not integrate in our improved model, a number of concepts which are nevertheless key in understanding man-machine-being interaction.

The moderating role of the Navigation goal and the feeling of Control: due to the very complex interactions between cognitive and affective reactions, we highlight, without refining more on this point in this article, that the Navigation goal (more goal-oriented or functional, vs more experiential or entertainment-oriented) might be an important moderator of the relative weight of both attitudinal vs affective persuasion route towards stickiness. Other complex issue: the goal of the navigation seems to matter in how design elements impact the user reactions to the same design cues [45, 49]. Issues of privacy level and how much the user controls the situation [42] might play an important role too. Navigation goal and Control could hence moderate how much the Cognitive vs Affective route would dominate in the persuasion process.

The concept of Online Trust, studied e.g. in the banking sector [65], is absent of the model. Neither have we integrated the role of *Flow*, a major concept in online interactions, although Holbrook and Hirschman earlier, and Csikszentmihalyi later, point out the experiential dimension as an important driver of consumption behaviours and satisfaction [52, 52; 54. In a large research production Csikszentmihalyi analyses activities qualified of *autolelic,* that is, that provide *per se,* without the need for some external output, their own benefits to the individual, subject – or better said actor – of such activity. In some cases in such activities, a feeling of Flow, defined as an *"optimal experience"* that is *"intrinsically enjoyable"* [56], may emerge.

As posited in [59]: *"Flow occurs when a person perceives that a situation contains high opportunities for action or challenges that are matched with the person's own capacities to act, or skills".* It characterizes situations when people forget themselves, for being highly involved in the task at hand, doing their best work and enjoying themselves in the process, skill, challenge and concentration being necessary [58]. An integrative model by Hoffman & Novak [59] suggests to integrate Flow online; it makes as its components seem logical drivers of 3 out of 4 components of stickiness.

A survey on internet users shows that Attitudes may mediate effects on Flow: namely Attitude toward the site mediates a large part of the effects of interactivity, level of challenge and focused attention, on flow [60]. Attitude towards the EVA, the website and the brand, might, at different levels and/or altogether, positively impact Flow. Once our improved model with E-SQ will be tested, we then will want to try to study how Flow relates with the Attitudes. Last, Flow should logically interact with the Affective route [62, 63]. The topics addressed here leaves avenues to many improvements: we are in our infancy in attempting to understand the WHY of Nass.

References

[1] Drèze, X., Zufryden, F.: Testing Web site design and promotional Content. Journal of Ad Research, 77–91 (1997)

[2] Diesbach-Lambert, P.: Ambience factors, emotions and web-user behavior: A model integrating an affective and symbolical approach. In: Gallopel, K., Maille, V., Rieunier, S. (eds.) 1st Colloquium on Sensorial Marketing, CERAM, 19 p. (2002)

[3] Rajeev, B.: The Role of Affect in Consumer Behavior. In: Peterson, R., Hoyer, W., William, W. (eds.), pp. 17–52 (1986)

[4] George, B., Michael, B.: Advertising and promotion: An integrated marketing communications perspective. McGraw Hill, New York (1998)

[5] Morris, H., Elisabeth, H.: The experiential aspects of consumption. Journal of Consumer Research 9, 132–140 (1982)

[6] Mihaly, C.: The costs and benefits of consuming. Journal of consumer Research 27, 267–272 (2000)

[7] Christian, D.: The impact of affective reactions on attitudes toward the advertisement and the brand. Journal of Marketing Research 32(4), 470–479 (1995)

[8] Bagozzi, R., Gopinath, M.: The role of emotions in marketing. Journal of the Academy of Marketing Science 27, 184–206 (1999)

[9] Judith, B., Thomas, B., Michel, P.: Nonverbal behaviors, persuasion, and credibility. Human Communication Research 17(1), 140–169 (1990)

[10] Judith, B., Bonito, J.A., Bengtsson, B., Cederberg, C., Lundeberg, M., Allspach, L.: Interactivity in human-computer interaction, a study of credibility, understanding, influence. Computers in Human Behavior 16, 553–574 (2000)

[11] Ekman, P.: What we have learned by measuring facial behavior? In: Ekman, P., Rosenberg, E.L. (eds.) What the face reveals: Basic and applied studies of spontaneous expressions using the FACS, pp. 469–485, 495. Oxford University Press, Oxford (1997)

[12] Ekman, P., Friesen, W., O'Sullivan, M.: Smiles when lying. In: Ekman, P., Rosenberg, E.L. (eds.) ch. 9, pp. 201–215 (1997)

[13] Christian, D., Michel, P.: Affective reactions to consumption situations: A pilot investigation. Journal of Economic Psychology 12(2), 325–365 (1991)

[14] Bagozzi, R.: The role of psychophysiology in consumer research. In: Robertson, R., Kassarjian, H. (eds.) Handbook of Consumer Behavior, pp. 124–161. P. Hall, Englewood Cliffs(1991)

[15] Robert, Z.: Feeling and thinking: Preferences need no inferences. American Psychologist 35, 151–175 (1978)

[16] Robert, Z., Hazel, M.: Affective and cognitive factors in preferences. Journal of Consumer Research 9, 123–131 (1982)

[17] Robert, Z., Hazel, M.: Must all affect be mediated by cognition. Journal of Consumer Research 12, 363–364 (1985)

[18] David, A.: Managing brand equity, 299 p. Free Press, New York (1991)

[19] Armstrong, G., Kotler, P.: Marketing: An Introduction, 522 p. Prentice Hall, Englewood Cliffs (2007)

[20] Yoram, W., Vijay, M., Robert, G.: Convergence Marketing, Strategies for reaching the new hybrid consumer, 336 p. P. Hall, Englewood Cliffs (2002)

[21] Barry, B., James, B., William, D.: Salesperson stereotypes, consumer emotions, and their impact on information processing. Journal of the Academy of Marketing Science 23(2), 94–105 (1995)

[22] Babin, L., Babin, B., Boles, J.: The effects of consumer perceptions of the salesperson, product, and dealer on intentions. Journal of Retailing 6, 91–97 (1999)

[23] Burke, M.C., Edell, J.: The impact of feelings on ad-based affect and cognition. Journal of Marketing Research 27, 69–83 (1989)

[24] Rosalind, P.: Affective computing, 292 p. MIT Press, Cambridge (1998)

[25] Clifford, N., Reeves, B.: The Media Equation, SLI. Cambridge U. Press, Cambridge (1996)

[26] Nass, C., Yongme, M.: Machines and mindlessness: Social responses. Journal of Social Issues 56(1), 81–103 (2000)

[27] Nass, C., Lombard, M., Henriksen, L., Steuer, J.: Anthropocentrism and computers. Behaviour and Information Technology 14(4), 229–238 (1995)

[28] Bruce, B.: Old tricks, new dogs: Ethology and interactive creatures, PhD dissertation, MIT-MEDIALAB, 146 p. (1996)

[29] Cynthia, B.: Designing social robots, 263 p. MIT Press, Cambridge (2002)

[30] Klein, J., Moon, Y., Picard, R.: This computer responds to user frustration: Theory, design and results. Interacting with Computers 14, 119–140 (2002)

[31] Judith, D.: Being real: Questions of Tele-Identity. In: Goldberg, K. (ed.) The Robot in the Garden: Telerobotics & Telepistemology, pp. 296–311. MIT Press, Cambridge (2001)

[32] Cassell, J.: Embodied Conversational Agents: representation and intelligence. AI 22(3), 67–83 (Winter 2001)

[33] Cassell, J., Bickmore, T.: External Manifestations of Trustworthiness in the Interface. ACM 43(12), 50–56 (2000)

[34] Cassell, J., Bickmore, T., Campbell, L., Vilhjálmsson, H., Yan, H.: Human conversation as a system framework: designing embodied conversational agents. In: Embodied Conversational Agents, pp. 29–63. MIT Press, Cambridge (2000a)

[35] Bickmore, T.: Relational agents, Effective change through H-Computer relationships, PhD Dissertation, MIT (2003)

[36] Jaffe, J.: Stickiness: A Ludicrous Metric (2002), http://www.mediapost.com/Admire/AdClickThru.cfm?AutoNumID=4247

[37] Martin, O., Jeff, M.: Ensuring website stickiness. In: ADMAP, pp. 21–24 (2000)

[38] Tim, C., Timothy, D., Alopi, L., David, M.: E-Business: Revolution, Evolution or Hype? California Management Review 44(1), 57–86

[39] Bucklin, R.E., Sismeiro, C.: A model of web site browsing behavior estimated on clickstream data. Journal of Marketing Research 40(3), 249–267 (2003) (working paper 2002, et)

[40] Midgley, D., Diesbach, P.: Embodied agents on a website: Modeling an attitudinal route of influence. In: de Kort, Y.A.W., IJsselsteijn, W.A., Midden, C., Eggen, B., Fogg, B.J. (eds.) PERSUASIVE 2007. LNCS, vol. 4744, 10 p. Springer, Heidelberg (2007)

[41] Diesbach, P., Midgley, D.: Embodied virtual agents: an affective and attitudinal approach. In: HCI, Beijing, 10 p. (2007)

[42] Diesbach, P., Midgley, D.: Embodied Agents: an Affective Persuasion Route. In: Oinas-Kukkonen, H., Hasle, P., Harjumaa, M., Segerståhl, K., Øhrstrøm, P. (eds.) PERSUASIVE 2008. LNCS, vol. 5033, 10 p. Springer, Heidelberg (2008)

[43] Petty, R., Cacioppo, J.: Attitudes and persuasion: Classic and contemporary approaches. Dubuque (1981)

[44] Petty, R., Cacioppo, J., Schumann, D.: Central and peripheral routes to advertising effectiveness. Journal of Consumer Research 10, 135–146 (1983)

[45] Bruner, G.C., Kumar, A.: Web commercials and advertising hierarchy-of-effects. Journal of Advertising Research 40(1/2), 35–42 (2000)

[46] Mehrabian, A., Russell, J.: Environmental Psychology, 221 p. MIT Press, Cambridge (1974)

[47] Robert, D., John, R.: Store atmosphere: An Environmental Psychology approach. Journal of Retailing 58, 34–57 (1982)

[48] Robert, D., John, R., Gilian, M., Andrew, N.: Store atmosphere and purchasing behavior. Journal of Retailing 70(3), 283–294 (1994)

[49] Argyriou, E., Arnott, D.: Website evaluation in goal-directed search behavior: The case for visual processing of website design. In: EMAC, 8 p. (2008)

[50] Zeithaml, V., Parasuraman, A., Malhotra, A.: A conceptual framework for understanding s-Service quality, Marketing Science Institute, Cambridge, MA (2000)

[51] Parasuraman, A., Zeithaml, V., Malhotra, A.: E-S-Qual, A multiple-item scale for assessing electronic service quality. Journal of Service Research 7(3) (February 2005)

[52] Morris, H.: Emotion in the consumption experience. In: Peterson, R., Hoyer, W., Wilson, W. (eds.) The Role of Affect in Consumer Behavior, pp. 17–52 (1986)

[53] Morris, H.: Nostalgia and consumption preferences: some emerging patterns of consumer tastes. Journal of Consumer Research, 245–255 (1993)

[54] Mihaly, C.: The costs and benefits of consuming. Journal of Consumer Research 27, 267–272 (2000)

[55] Mihaly, C.: Conversation with the author, Boston (November 2002)

[56] Mihaly, C.: Finding Flow. Basic Books, NY (1997)

[57] Mihaly, C.: Flow and the Psychology of Discovery and Invention. Harper & Collins, New York (1996)

[58] Donner, E., Mihaly, C.: Transforming stress to flow. Executive Excellence, Provo 9(2), 16–20 (1992)

[59] Hoffman, D., Novak, T.: Marketing in hyper-media computer environments. Journal of Marketing 60, 50–68 (1996)

[60] Luna, D., Perracchio, L., de Juan, M.: Flow in individual websites: Model estimation and cross-cultural validation. ACR 30, 280–281 (2003)

[61] Novak, T., Hoffman, D., Yung, Y.F.: Measuring the customer experience online. Marketing Science 19(1), 22–42 (2000)

[62] Sandra, D.: Virtual stores on the internet: design of emotional online shopping offers on the internet from a behavioral point of view. European Advances in Consumer Research 5, 115–118 (2001)

[63] Duncker, K.: On pleasure, emotion, and striving. Philosophy and Phenomenological Research 1, 391–430 (1941)

[64] David, S., Richard, H.: E-satisfaction: An initial examination. Journal of Retailing 76(3), 309–322 (2000)

[65] Munyoz, P., Pereira, P.: Flow in E-Bank satisfaction measures. In: EMAC, 7 p. (2004)

[66] Dubé, L., Le Bel, J.: Content and structure of laypeople's concept of pleasure. Cognition and Emotion 17(2), 263–295 (2003)

[67] Mick, D., Fournier, S.: Paradoxes of technology: Consumer cognizance, emotions, and coping strategies. Journal of Consumer Research, 123–143 (September 1998)

Annex: Non Congruent and Congruent Agents Tested

Agents tested on the Swiss diving and military-oriented watches website:
Non congruent: little girl with rollers. Congruent: sexy girl, "macho", sex-oriented, imaginaire.

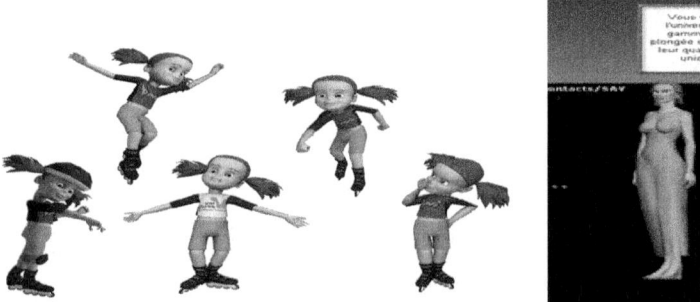

Agents tested on the Olive Oil website: non congruent: a PDA-like agent (form of a personal digital assistant like a I-Phone). Congruent agent: a male *Maître d'Hôtel* dressed with a suit.

Author Index